"A great book that goes into detail about what vegan is and what it is not. Even old vegans might learn something new from this book."
— GoodVeg

"As usual, John puts together another very informative and useful book. It's a great read full of amazing statistics. One of the nice things about this book is that you can pick it up and start reading on any page for a few minutes here and there and get great information that stands on its own. I would recommend this to anyone looking to improve their health, and most certainly to vegans that are forever having to explain or defend their diet."
— Hugh Cruickshank, Raw-Foods-Diet-Center.com

• • •

"The further a society drifts from the truth, the more it will hate those that speak it."
— George Orwell

"If you are right, and you know it, speak your mind. Speak your mind, even if you are a minority of one, the truth is still the truth."
— Mohandas Gandhi

"There are two ways to be fooled. One is to believe what isn't true; the other is to refuse to believe what is true."
— Soren Kierkegaard

"He who cures a disease may be the skillfullest, but he that prevents it is the safest physician."
— Thomas Fuller

"My pigs wait on my back porch begging for a doggie biscuit. Their noses are warm and gentle, and they love a good scratching behind their ears, even though they weigh almost six hundred pounds each.

My pig Scooter ran to see if he could help when one of my calves cried for its momma.

A pig is intelligent with a sense of family. When I sit down next to a tree, my pigs lay down with me.

I could no more kill one of these than I could kill a dog.

I've grown to find the taste of meat distasteful, and knowing from whence it came, despicable. Do not joke about 'tasty animals,' as it is about putting death into your mouth, no more than you would joke about eating a corpse out of a casket."
– David Lay

"I believe all of us secretly know in our hearts that it is wrong. What makes it all that much more disturbing to me is that this 'humane myth' is being perpetuated not only by the industry, but by some animal advocates and organizations as well. Humane farming is a myth. From the moment those animals are taken from those trucks and forced through the slaughtering process, it is the most inhumane treatment that I've ever witnessed."
– Cayce Mell

"Animals who are destined for an abbreviated life that ends in a violent death now called to my conscience and required me to show up, and where I could, show what little bit of mercy I can. Since I have made this conscious decision to show mercy, my life has been blessed a million, million times over and I have found a deep peace. So no, in my experience, there is no such thing as humane animal products, humane farming practices, humane transport, or humane slaughter."
– Harold Brown, former cattle farmer

"I will not kill or hurt any living creature needlessly, nor destroy any beautiful thing, but will strive to save and comfort all gentle life, and guard and perfect all natural beauty upon the Earth."
– John Ruskin

"I used to eat meat when I was a little kid. But I didn't know where it came from. And one day, I cut this piece of meat open, and blood came out of it, and I asked me mother, 'Where did this come from?' She said, 'From animals.' And that was it."
– Geezer Butler, bassist, lyricist for Black Sabbath

VEGAN MYTH
VEGAN TRUTH

OBLITERATING RUMORS AND LIES
ABOUT THE EARTH-SAVING DIET
THAT CAN SAVE YOUR LIFE

A COLLECTION OF WRITINGS BY
JOHN MCCABE

Carmania Books
FOOD • BODY • MIND • SPIRIT • WILDLIFE • AIR • WATER • SOIL • WORLD

Vegan Truth Vegan Myth, by John McCabe $14.95 US

ISBN: 978-1-884702-02-0
Library of Congress Control Number: 2013934041
Dewey CIP: 641.563.   **OCLC:** 213839254
Edition: First edition: February 2013
Editing: Brenda Koplin
Cover: Photo of 12318 Addison tree by Rich Marchewka of Marchewka.com

Carmania Books POB 1272, Santa Monica, CA 90406-1272, USA
Wholesale: Nelson's Books, NelsonsBooks.com, 800-877-1267; and Ingram
Retail: Amazon.com, BarnesAndNoble.com, natural food stores, bookstores, raw restaurants.

Books by John McCabe
Sunfood Diet Infusion: Transforming Health Through Raw Veganism
Igniting Your Life: Pathways to the Zenith of Health and Success
Sunfood Traveler: Guide to Raw Food Culture
Marijuana & Hemp: History, Uses, Laws, and Controversy
Sunfood Living: Resource Guide for Global Health
Extinction: The Death of Waterlife on Planet Earth
Surgery Electives: What to Know Before the Doctor Operates

TABLE OF CONTENTS

"Who's the real extremist? The person who tries to stop unnecessary suffering by cutting out animal products, or the person who says, 'I like the way that tastes, so a sentient being needs to suffer and die'?"
– Ari Solomon

"But for the sake of some little mouthful of flesh, we deprive a soul of the sun, and light, and of that proportion of life and time it had been born into the world to enjoy."
– Plutarch

"The idea that humans belong atop the 'food chain' is a long promoted fallacy used to justify the senseless and cruel exploiting, abusing, confining, killing, and eating of animals."
– Andrew Kirschner

"All beings tremble before violence. All fear death, all love life. See yourself in others. Then whom can you hurt? What harm can you do?"
– Buddha

"Basically, it boils down to cold logic. If we are going to care about the suffering of other humans then logically we should care about the suffering of nonhumans, too."
– Richard Ryder

"Too many people only consider cats and dogs when they think about loving animals. They don't realize how every animal out there has feelings, has a heart and soul, has emotions. It only takes meeting them once to really feel that."
– Shannon Elizabeth

"Animals are the innocent casualties of the world view that asserts that some lives are more valuable than others, that the powerful are entitled to exploit the powerless, and that the weak must be sacrificed for the greater good."
– Steven Simmons

"Animals do feel like us, also joy, love, fear, and pain, but they cannot grasp the spoken word. It is our obligation to take their part and continue to resist the people who profit by them, who slaughter them, and who torture them."
– Denis De Roughement

THE HUMAN BODY

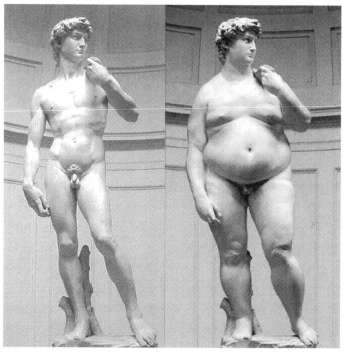

The human body is an amazing mechanism that responds to what the person thinks, eats, says, and does. The physical appearance of the body reflects what is going on with the person. This is often most evident in the shape of the body. Because of this, it can be very easy to tell certain things about how people live simply by observing body shape.

Because of low-quality dietary choices and lack of movement, more and more people are suffering from obesity, heart disease, diabetes, arthritis, kidney disease, cancers, back strains, knee injuries, hernias, learning disorders, and a slew of other problems.

You are making a choice with the quality of foods you consume and the physical activities you do or don't engage in.

A person who remains physically active while following a diet consisting chiefly of raw fruits and vegetables is more likely to resemble the person on the left. A person lacking physical activity while following the modern junk diet is more likely to resemble the body on the right.

Which diet would you rather follow?

"Animals do have a voice. If you ignore their suffering, I will remind you of it. If you don't understand them, I will translate. If you don't hear them, I will be their voice. You may silence them, but you cannot silence me as long as I live."
– Anita Mahdessian

"If people are vegetarian for ethical reasons – because they believe that killing and eating animals is wrong – they really ought to be vegan, too. The average human eats more than 11,000 animals in his or her lifetime, but millions of calves and chicks are also killed every year as 'waste products' of milk and egg production."
– Kerry McCarthy

"I am sometimes asked, 'Why do you spend so much of your time and money talking about kindness to animals when there is so much cruelty done to men?' I answer, 'I am working at the roots.'"
– George T. Angell

"If only we can overcome cruelty, to human and animal, with love and compassion we shall stand at the threshold of a new era in human moral and spiritual evolution – and realize, at last, our most unique quality: humanity.'"
– Jane Goodall

"Animals have done us no harm and they have no power of resistance. Cruelty to animals is as if man did not love God. There is something so very dreadful, so Satanic, in tormenting those who have never harmed us, who cannot defend themselves, who are utterly in our power."
– Cardinal John Henry Newman

"There can be no doubt as to which side is right and which side is wrong, for compassionate defense of life is a force of good and sadistic mass destruction of life is a force for evil."
– Captain Paul Watson, SeaShepherd.org

"There are many noteworthy examples of ordinary evil in every culture and country around the globe, but in terms of preventable evil, I am hard pressed to find any examples that approach those systematically perpetrated by humans against the members of other species."
– Lawrence Pope

Search: **269Life**

INTRODUCTION

Probably the most common question asked of vegans is, "Where do you get your protein?" Those asking that question are displaying their lack of knowledge about protein. As I explain later in the book, fruits, vegetables, nuts, and seeds are rich in the amino acids our bodies need to produce protein. When you eat enough calories from plants, which is easy to do, you get more than enough protein. The human nutritional requirement for animal protein is absolutely zero. The amino acids in fruits, vegetables, nuts, and seeds are more than adequate for our nutrition needs.

Another misconception common among those who don't understand nutrition is that vegans must eat a lot of tofu to make up for the lack of animal protein in their diet. Tofu is bean curd that has been so processed that it no longer contains some of the nutrients of the raw soybean – which are best eaten raw, if at all. Tofu also includes a chemical that forms in starches heated above 247 degrees. The heat-generated chemicals formed when starches are cooked are acrylamides, which can trigger a response from the immune system, cause inflammation, are identified as carcinogenic, and can damage the nerves.

There are plenty of misconceptions swirling around vegan nutrition, often fueled by the misunderstanding and mistruths surrounding what the body needs for maintaining health.

Because I've written a number of books relating to veganism, I've been asked and told just about everything imaginable about the vegan diet.

There are a lot of fearmongering rumors about veganism. I've been told rather sincerely that you can't be a vegan for more than a couple of years, or your system will collapse. Oh? I've been vegan for more than 20 years.

I've heard people say they were extremely unhealthy as a vegan, which is entirely possible. Simply eat a lot of fried, baked, and processed, sugary, salty, and oily things, and skip out on eating a variety of raw fruits and vegetables. Use a microwave. Eat a lot of gluten grains and stuff that has been cooked to the point of being brown. If you want, you can eat vegan cookies and potato chips all day while slurping beer, and you can call yourself a vegan. Yes, you can be unhealthy as a vegan.

I know of a person who sells nutritional supplements and is continually telling vegans that their diets are deficient, and they need to eat meat. But he is a nutritional supplement salesperson, and is continually telling people which nutritional supplements they need to take – especially the products he sells. He claims that he was once a vegan, and his health suffered. However, he was a person who ate a junk vegan diet – fried stuff, lots of tofu, packaged things with labels stating that the product was "vegan," and other low-quality "vegan" foods. During the time that he was a vegan, he was also a drug addict – which is also something he says, but not in the same storyline – maybe because it might interfere with his sales pitch of selling nutritional supplements to vegans he says are not getting the nutrition they need. So, he was a drug addict and a junk food junkie vegan, and now he eats meat, because he says you can't get the nutrients you need by eating a vegan diet, and he also sells supplements, that he also says he takes. His actions reveal his belief that the meat eating diet isn't supplying him with the nutrients he needs, so he is taking nutritional supplements, and selling them.

Humans get an abundance of all of the nutrients they need by following a low-fat vegan diet rich in raw fruits and vegetables. Humans have no nutritional need for meat, dairy, or eggs. In fact, meat, dairy, and eggs introduce a variety of substances that damage health, including free radicals, saturated fat, and excess cholesterol, arachidonic acid, and carnitine, and also farm chemical residues. Eggs contain lecithin that converts to trimethylamine, raising risk of cancer and cardiovascular disease. Milk and mammal meat contain the sialic acid sugar protein molecule called Neu5Gc (N-glycolylneuraminic acid), which is found on human cancer cells – and only gets into the body by way of eating milk, milk products, and mammal meat.

Fruits, vegetables, sprouts, germinated seeds, nuts, and seaweeds contain all of the components the body needs for experiencing vibrant health, including vitamins, minerals, essential fatty acids, amino acids, antioxidants, fiber, biophotons, and other nutrients. Meat, dairy, and eggs are lacking in some of those components, including fiber. In fact, meat, dairy, and eggs do not contain fiber. A low-fiber diet is associated with a number of health risks, including cardiovascular disease, colon cancer, diabetes, Alzheimer's disease, Crohn's disease, arthritis, and MS, and also with an increased risk of heart attacks and strokes.

"A low-fat plant-base diet would not only lower the heart-attack rate about 85 percent, but would lower the cancer rate 60 percent."
– William Castelli, Framingham Cardiovascular Institute

Another criticism leveled at vegans is that they behave as if they are superior, or uppity. If anything, the vegan diet is more compassionate, such as to their fellow animals – by seeing no need to mass breed, confine, and slay them for eating. It also doesn't use the amount of resources needed to maintain a meat eating diet. A diet heavy in meat uses a disproportionate amount of everything from water, soil, space, and fuel. The resources needed to maintain the supply of meat to feed the population of humans that are eating meat every day are far greater than what it would take to supply food for the same number of vegans. As I explain later, the animal protein-heavy diet is impacting the global economy and environment in all sorts of ways. More and more people are eating a variety of meats every day, and what their diet is doing to the planet is what should be considered an arrogant disregard not only for humanity, but for wildlife and the workings of Nature.

"I don't feel superior because I'm vegan. The truth is, I am vegan because I don't feel superior to others."
– Michele McCowan

More than sometimes, if someone who eats an unhealthful diet hears a vegan talking about nutrition and the benefits of following a plant-rich diet, the vegan can be accused of preaching. As if meat eaters never do that through the culture they are tentpoling. Drive through any city or town, look through newspapers and magazines, listen to commercial radio and watch common television commercials, and notice how much meat advertising there is. There is a continual and massive flow of advertising centered on eating hamburgers, steak, fish, barbecued meat, fried chicken, flame-broiled cow bits, "deli cuts," meat sandwiches, and other products of the animal farming industry, which kills billions of animals every year. Consuming that meat increases the risk of a variety of diseases, including cardiovascular disease, diabetes, Alzheimer's, Parkinson's, Crohn's, MS, obesity, macular degeneration, colon cancer, breast cancer, prostate cancer, uterine cancer, ovarian cancer, bladder cancer, liver cancer, kidney cancer, kidney dysfunction, arthritis, and varicose veins, erectile dysfunction, and skin disorders. In fact, the more meat, dairy, and eggs people consume, the more likely they will experience the most common chronic and degenerative diseases. Hundreds of thousands of people undergo heart surgery every year because they followed a diet heavy in animal protein and other unhealthful foods. Many people die every year from heart attacks, strokes, cancer, and other health problems simply because they ate a meat-, egg-, and dairy-heavy diet. And veganism is considered extreme?

"Sometimes people don't want to hear the truth because they don't want their illusions destroyed."
– Friedrich Nietzsche

As I mention later in the book, the environmental damage caused by the animal farming industry, including farmed fish, cows, pigs, chickens, turkeys, lamb, and other animals people mass-breed and slaughter, and all of the food grown to feed all of those animals, and all of the land, fuel, water, and other resources used by the animal farming and meat industry, is tremendous.

Why are we killing billions of animals every year to eat them, when we don't need to, and when following a plant-based diet would be much better for our health, and the environment?

> "The fact that man knows right from wrong proves his intellectual superiority to other creatures; but the fact that he can do wrong proves his moral inferiority to any creature that cannot."
> – Mark Twain

Nonhuman animals are so amazingly innocent. Can they be any other way? As humans go about their greedy ways filled with lies and deception, the nonhuman animals are simply doing what they need do to get by. Nonhuman animals are not hoarding mass quantities of resources, enslaving other beings, destroying the environment, acidifying the oceans, clearcutting forests, removing mountaintops, and sending other species into extinction. Some nonhuman animals may be trained to damage other beings, such as dolphins with bombs strapped to them being used in human warfare, and dogs taught to attack.

> "Animals are reliable, many full of love, true in their affections, predictable in their actions, grateful and loyal. Difficult standards for people to live up to."
> – Alfred A. Montapert

> "Lord, help me to become the person my dog believes me to be."
> – Canon Charles Martin

Nonhuman animals show an unwavering devotion to those in their community, and even to human caretakers. What do most animals get in return? An Earth that is increasingly damaged by human activity, which is putting more and more varieties of life in endangered situations, and sending many animals and plants into extinction.

> "If having a soul means being able to feel love and loyalty and gratitude then animals are better off than a lot of humans."
> – James Herriot

In many ways, animals are better off than humans. But, because of human activity, the state of nonhuman animals is becoming increasingly dire. It doesn't have to be that way! We can turn this ship around.

One thing that humans can stop doing is massively breeding and then using enormous amounts of resources to feed and house a few select varieties of animals with the goal of killing them and cooking their tissues for human consumption. Realizing that the human body needs absolutely zero animal protein to flourish in health can help end what some people call "the animal holocaust."

"I think most people agree that not committing violence against another – human or nonhuman – is an ethically superior position to hurting someone. For me, I reflect this ethic by being vegan. Contrary to what some people think, being vegan is not an end in itself; it's the means to an end. It's the means through which we can – in our daily lives – reflect our value of not causing harm. The truth is I feel humbled being vegan rather than superior to those who aren't. I have no cause to be self-righteous. There was a time when I ate animals and made excuses, and I feel grateful to be armed with knowledge and awareness and to be able to act on my values of compassion and kindness. Rather than feel morally superior to people who eat animals, I feel great sorrow for the animals who suffer and for the humans who inflict that suffering. If we keep this big picture in mind, we can create the compassionate world we all envision."
– Colleen Patrick-Goudreau

There are so many ways in which humans can benefit by not eating animals, not mass breeding them, and not using tremendous amounts of land, water, and fuel to grow food to feed billions of animals, to slaughter billions of animals, and to process and cook the meat from billions of animals, that it is a wonder why it isn't an obvious reality across the continents.

Many humans pose themselves as moral creatures, aiming to do what is right, claiming that they have a goal of living peacefully, yet they engage in violence through their food choices as they choose to eat animals that have been killed to feed a want, and not a need.

Many humans these days are so disconnected from their food that they have only a vague idea about where their food comes from, or how it got to their dinner table. If they knew more about their food, about where it originates, and about what is involved in producing it, and what it contains, they would likely make different dietary choices. Certainly, many people who eat meat, dairy, and eggs would make different food choices if they knew about the animals, the family structure of the animals, the way animals communicate, and what it is the animals feel – as in the suffering and pain experienced by animals raised for food.

> "There is no fundamental difference between man and the higher mammals in their mental faculties. Nevertheless, the difference in mind between man and the higher animals, great as it is, certainly is one of degree and not of kind. We have seen that the senses and intuitions, the various emotions and faculties, such as love, memory, attention, curiosity, imitation, reason, etc., of which man boasts, may be found in an incipient, or even sometimes in a well-developed condition, in the lower animals."
> – Charles Darwin

Is it not odd that people have cats and dogs, and think that killing and eating those animals would be a repulsive and heinous act, yet the very same humans commonly eat other types of animals at every meal? Is there a difference between the pain a cat or dog feels and the pain felt by farm animals? Is there a difference in the blood that spills from the neck of a slaughtered farm animal, and the blood flowing through the veins of a dog or cat? Are the eyes of a farm animal much different from the eyes of a dog or cat? Do the farm animals not see, feel, smell, taste, and have desires similar to the cats and dogs? Are the senses of the farm animals and the domestic pets much different from the senses of humans? No. Farm animals and human animals are very similar in their sensory mechanisms, in the way they feel joy and pain, and in how they will defend themselves and do what they can to escape pain and suffering.

> "It seems rather bizarre to me, and somewhat Jekyll and Hyde, to be sitting at your table devouring a creature while at the same time lovingly stroking another as your pet. But then again, when one's raised that way, I guess the irony (some would say hypocrisy) isn't so easily seen."
> – Lance Landall

So, there on the plate is that piece of meat that was once the part of a body of an animal that had preferences, felt pain, smelled scents, breathed air, tasted food, digested nutrients, saw things, had a family, played, and reproduced in ways similar to the human eating the bit of flesh taken from the body of a slaughtered animal.

> "Why should man expect his prayer for mercy to be heard by what is above him when he shows no mercy to what is under him?"
> – Pierre Troubetzkoy

6

If you are praying for peace, and want a more peaceful world, why not start with your food choices? Why not take the spilling of blood out of your food? Why not choose to follow a plant-based diet that has many proven health benefits, including reducing risk of cancer, cardiovascular disease, stroke, heart attack, diabetes, vision degeneration, Alzheimer's, Parkinson's, muscular sclerosis, Crohn's, kidney disorder, osteoporosis, skin diseases, and obesity? Why, if you want a more peaceful world, would you continue to eat the flesh of slaughtered animals when you would be better off following a low-fat vegan diet rich in raw fruits and vegetables, nuts, and seeds?

> "If you don't want to be beaten, imprisoned, mutilated, killed, or tortured, then you shouldn't condone such behavior towards anyone, be they human or not."
> – Moby

As I write this, there are billions of farm animals living on farms and in pens on the land and off the coasts for the sole purpose of being slaughtered for human food. These mass-bred animals are eating tremendous amounts of food that take enormous resources to produce. Billions of animals are breathing, seeing, smelling, feeling, and experiencing incarcerated lives as they are being fed to fatten them for slaughter so that humans, who would be better off not eating the meat, will be able to munch on the flesh of these creatures.

The living conditions that billions of farm animals are experiencing right now are stressful, unnatural, cramped, loud, filthy, and cause a great amount of pain and suffering. Not only animals raised for food, but dogs, ferrets, bunnies, cats, birds, alligators, snakes, bears, and other animals that are being raised for their fur, feathers, skin, and even bones.

> "We have enslaved the rest of animal creation, and have treated our distant cousins in fur and feathers so badly that beyond doubt, if they were able to formulate a religion, they would depict the Devil in human form."
> – William Ralph Inge

Why are humans being so clueless about these issues? It is cultural? Does culture make them blind to the sensory abilities of animals? Is being hidden from the processes of animal farming, slaughter, and meat processing keeping humans in a state of perpetual ignorance? Are humans largely that cold and uncaring about fellow creatures that have the same senses, the same reproductive urges, and the same need for food, water, air, safety, and relationships?

> "Alas, what wickedness to swallow flesh into our flesh, to fatten

our greedy bodies by cramming in other bodies, to have one living creature fed by the death of another."
– Pythagoras

At no time in the history of humanity have so many people been eating such an assortment of meat, dairy, and eggs. It is gluttony at its worst, and it is not only causing the death of animals, but is also causing the death of many humans who suffer from eating diets so rich in meat, dairy, and eggs. It is also causing the spread of cheap meat production at the cost of the environment and human rights, such as in poorer countries, where people are kicked off their land so cattle grazing can be expanded, or so thousands of acres of grain can be planted to feed the global animal farming industry. In many regions, poorer people are shoved out of coastal areas so that fish farms can be put in, which then employ some of the former villagers at low wages to produce fish sent off to distant, wealthier countries.

Previous to the invention of refrigeration, humans did not consume such quantities of meat, dairy, and eggs. Often, meat was used as an ingredient in stews, soups, and other dishes. People weren't eating several types of meat every day, or consuming mass quantities of eggs or milk products.

In addition to billions of animals being killed every year for meat, many hundreds of thousands, and likely millions, of animals are killed every year to protect farm animals, to protect food being grown for farmed animals, and in the general spread of the livestock industry. Predator animals on every continent have been killed off, some into extinction, for the sole purpose of expanding the livestock industry. The livestock industry is also using more and more seafood as a protein source in feed, which is contributing to the problems of overfishing – which, because of the circle of life and how Nature works, is a threat to all life on the planet.

The only way I can reason that humans are eating the amount of meat, dairy, and eggs they are consuming is because they are ignorant both of the processes involved and of the environmental damage, extinction issues, and human rights violations caused by producing that amount of animal protein.

"A meat eater eats animals because they are presented to him as mere abstract nuggets on a plate. We are not carnivores or even predators. We do not even crave animal flesh unless it is divorced from the animal it once was and transformed into an abstraction: a piece of 'meat.' The image of eating a real animal repulses us."
– Robert Grillo

8

One issue with meat eating is the complete separation of the realities of the meat industry. People see the plastic-wrapped meat products, the pop-in-the-oven boxed meat products, like pizzas and potpies, and the canned foods containing meat. What they don't see is the blood spilling in the slaughterhouses; the animals being decapitated, and having their legs cut off, their skin removed, and the carcasses cut into pieces; the fish and other creatures struggling to avoid dying; and the environmental damage being done by the meat industry.

"One cannot look deeply into the eyes of an animal and not see the same depth, complexity and feeling we humans lay exclusive claim to."
– Nan Sea Love

Have you ever been around a baby bull? They are the sweetest, most kind, gentle beings. People may see the milk, cheese, butter, creamer, ice cream, yogurt, and other milk products in stores, restaurants, and in their kitchens. What people don't see are the baby male calves (bulls) being killed by the millions. That is how the dairy industry exists, by killing baby bulls and taking the milk those bulls would have survived on and selling it as human food.

Yes, animals die so you can have milk. Many people are unaware of this. In the comforts of towns, cities, and suburbia, they are not exposed to the dirty little secret of the dairy industry – the killing of millions of baby bulls every year.

As I explain later in the book, when cows on dairy farms give birth to male babies, those babies are of no worth to the dairy farm. Male calves don't grow up to produce milk.

Most male babies (bulls) from dairy farms are killed within days or weeks after birth. Much of their sliced-up muscles are sold as a product called veal. Their tender skin is sold as leather. Their stomach lining may be used as an ingredient called rennet in cheese. The milk they would have fed on for the first months of their lives is collected and sold as human food in the form of milk, butter, cheese, cream, creamer, ice cream, kefir, yogurt, whey, and casein.

"All dairy operations, whether conventional or organic, exist solely by doing to millions of defenseless females the worst thing anyone can do to a mother."
– Peaceful Prairie Sanctuary

When female calves are born on dairies, they are raised to adulthood. As soon as they can be mechanically impregnated, they are put in what is called the "rape rack." As the pregnancy advances, the female starts to produce milk, and that is what is wanted on the dairy farm so that it can be sold for human food.

When the dairy cow starts to slow in her milk production, she is often sent off to the slaughterhouse, her muscle ending up as hamburger, as processed and canned meats, and as beef jerky.

> "I know in my soul that to eat a creature who is raised to be eaten, and who never has a chance to be a real being, is unhealthy. You're just eating misery."
> – Alice Walker

What happens to male calves on dairy farms is similar to what happens to male baby chickens on egg farms. Just as bulls are of no use to dairy farms, the male chicks are of no use to the egg industry, so they are put to death soon after they hatch. The female chicks are raised so they can produce eggs. But, because they are of no use to egg farms, billions of male chicks are tossed into grinding machines, or are gassed, or thrown in a bag and smothered, then tossed away as garbage.

Billions of fish, birds, and mammals are dying every year so the stores, restaurants, cafes, cafeterias, industrial kitchens, hotels, and even prisons can keep serving meat, milk, and eggs.

Oh, meat eater, milk drinker, and egg consumer, animals are dying because of your ignorance.

> "To get mud off your hands, use soap and water. To get blood off your hands, go vegan."
> – John Sakars

That is what it is about, this veganism. Not participating in the slaughter of the innocents, avoiding doing harm to other beings, and not supporting companies that are ravaging Nature and depleting the wildlife diversity of the planet. It is also about choosing to avoid foods that induce disease. Veganism is also about supporting the growing of the foods that nurture vibrant health: fruits, vegetables, nuts, and seeds.

Some will say the common derogatory things about vegans and veganism, such as "vegans are weak." As I point out in the book, there are a variety of top athletes, including boxers, bikers, wrestlers, runners, and tennis, football, and baseball players that follow a vegan diet.

> "Some people say vegans should 'stop trying to push their beliefs on others.' Guess what? Eating meat is the ultimate form of pushing your beliefs on others. When you eat meat, you're forcing others to die for your beliefs. If that's not forcing your beliefs on others, I don't know what is."
> – John Sakars

Spewing the common derogatory and ridiculous comments about vegans doesn't reveal a high level of intelligence, but does expose ignorance. It may be the extreme ones who say they enjoy hunting, and enjoy the taste of meat. Maybe so, but they can't argue with the nutritional and environmental science revealing that a meat-heavy diet is not good for the planet, and greatly increases the risk of a variety of human diseases, and of erectile dysfunction.

> "Animal rights provokes hostility from the arrogant people who enjoy power over animals, from the insecure who boost themselves by demeaning and exploiting animals, and from the guilty who do not want to confront their ignorance and implication in violence against animals."
> – Dr. Steve Best

Then, there are the brainy ones. Oh, yes, those who climbed out of the dark ages with the enlightenment telling them that humans need to eat meat, milk, and eggs to survive. Of course. Keep opening that mouth and inserting the foot. And, when you experience the health issues formed by that animal-protein-heavy diet, you will likely turn to synthetic drugs, medical procedures, and surgeries to try to survive. But, the best thing you can do for your health is to adapt a plant-based diet, clean out the junk, and avoid animal products.

> "'I didn't climb to the top of the food chain to eat vegetables?' Really? You did that? You, Frank from Staten Island, climbed to the top of the food chain for all of us?
> Or, was it you, Frank from Staten Island, who drove your SUV two blocks to the store, then got out, did your sad waddle to the front, and had to ask where the meat section is because bright lights confuse you? Then you, Frank from Staten Island, grabbed some pre-packaged, dead thing that you didn't even kill yourself, it was killed by illegal immigrants that are getting paid minimum wage with the bonus of 'hopefully not being deported,' then you, Frank from Staten Island, have to give it to your wife to cook 'cause the last time you made dinner you burnt the hot pockets. Then you, Frank from Staten Island, put on Fox News, insert your hand down your pants and think, 'Yeah, it's good to be at the top of the food chain.'
> Darwin would have killed himself if he knew you were what was coming."
> – Jamie Kilstein

Among the accusations flung to vegans is that they are idealists. Oh, and we are going against the will of God, because some debatable words in some book have been misinterpreted to mean that we are supposed to eat animals. Or, that man has always eaten animals. Really? Some cultures have also enslaved other humans, so should we continue that practice? Some cultures killed people suspected of witchcraft. Should we start up that practice? Some cultures have killed and eaten other people. Should we all get into cannibalism? Some people have believed that eating bull balls make them more viral. Should we all have bull balls for dinner? Should we continue doing things because our ancestors did them, even if those things cause harm?

> "We are evolving as a species. What our caveman ancestors ate is of little import to us now. The question is what is the best diet for modern human beings? Medical literature is clearly showing that the less animal fat and animal protein you put in your system, the healthier you are going to be."
> – Dr. Michael Klaper

> "You don't hate vegans. You hate that vegans make you look at your participation in the exploitation of animals."
> – Gary Smith

Humans are animals. Like other animals, we have sex, care for our babies, eat food, drink water, breathe air, feel pain, see, think, avoid harm, and die. Working to protect animals by ending animal farming isn't working against humans. Humans are better off not eating animals, and humans flourish in health following a low-fat vegan diet rich in raw fruits and raw vegetables. If anything, working against animal farming is pro-human, pro-environment, pro-health, and pro-peace.

> "To be 'for animals' is not to be 'against humanity.' To require others to treat animals justly, as their rights require, is not to ask for anything more nor less in their case than in the case of any human to whom just treatment is due. The animal rights movement is a part of, not opposed to, the human rights movement. Attempts to dismiss it as anti-human are mere rhetoric."
> – Tom Regan

If you present a child with a choice of a garden full of edible plants, including tree fruits, berries, vegetables, nuts, and seeds and also present the child with a cow, pig, lamb, goat, turkey, and chicken, the child is going to eat the edible plants, and will not kill the animals. Can the child survive solely on the plant matter? Of course. Fruits, vegetables, nuts, and seeds contain all of the substances we need to obtain from food.

How would an innocent human, unexposed to meat, be able to kill an animal? Clearly, not with the human teeth, which aren't sharp enough to bite through the skin of an animal and kill it. Not with their claws, because humans don't have those. Why would the human kill the animal? With such a variety of fruits, including berries, and of vegetables, nuts, and seeds, the human wouldn't be hungry. When humans got hungry, would they look at the animal and think that it would taste good slaughtered and heated? That would defy logic.

> "If you had to kill your own calf before you ate him, most likely you would not be able to do it. To hear the calf scream, to see the blood spill, to see the baby being taken away from his momma, and to see the look of death in the animal's eyes would turn your stomach. So, you get the man at the packing house to do the killing for you."
> – Dick Gregory

Clearly, meat eating is a learned practice. And, unlike simply eating edible plants, meat eating takes practice and preparation. As I say later in the book, humans don't like the taste of raw meat, and even cooked meat is often treated with a variety of herbs, spices, sauces, and other things to give it flavor.

With all of that said, veganism isn't perfect. Its a goal is not causing harm, of eating foods that do not cause bloodshed, and of leaving wildlife to live their lives. Of course, digging in soil and planting and harvesting foods will result in some sort of manipulation of the natural environment, and sometimes small animals are lost by digging or using mechanical harvesting. But veganism is far more in harmony with nature, and greatly more protective of animals than the direct harm done by the meat, dairy, and egg diet.

As I explain later, millions of animals have been deliberately killed to protect the meat industry. Some wild animals are killed off because they will prey upon farm animals. Other wild animals are killed off because they will eat farm animal feed, or they dig holes for their dens, which may cause cattle to break their legs. These wild animals that are being killed to protect the meat industry include fox, deer, coyote, beaver, groundhog, raccoon, mountain lion, bobcat, bear, snakes, bunnies, mice, cats, and even certain types of birds. So many varieties of wild animals are killed off by the meat industry that it has led to the plunging of their populations, and that has negatively impacted plant life, soil stability, and even the fertilization and formation of forests.

> "People look at me as a vegan and conclude that since I stepped on a snail or because the vegetables I eat resulted in a tractor death for a squirrel somewhere in Paraguay that somehow vegans are hypocrites, which of course they're not since perfection is an unattainable goal and is something to be driven towards, never

actually achieved. The difference between you and the vegan standing next to you is that while you're both going to step on a bug tomorrow, they've decided to dedicate their lives to as little harm as possible, completely independent from what you do. So in a way does the protozoan life form they step on negate your responsibility for the lamb you're paying a stranger to cut tomorrow? And falling 1 percent short of an unattainable goal is really good when you're standing next to someone who won't even try."
    – Shelley Williams

The growing of fruits, vegetables, nuts, and seeds is clearly more healthful for the environment and wildlife than mass breeding billions of farmed animals, and the processes involved in raising food for them, incarcerating them, and slaughtering and cooking them. As I say repeatedly, the consumption of dead animals, dairy products, and eggs is not only **not** needed for human health to flourish, the consumption of meat, dairy, and eggs increases the incidence of human disease.

For the best nutrition, eat a variety of edible plants. And eat them as close to their original form as you can get them.

Stay away from eating anything that had a face, was born, or hatched. Instead, experience the vibrant health that can be gained through following a diet consisting of the best food on the planet, one that is low-fat and rich in raw fruits and vegetables that are naturally abundant in nutrients that infuse health.

I am not a person who endorses packaged foods or nutritional supplements.

Because the books I've written sell around the world and have inspired many people to follow a clean-food, plant-based diet, I've been approached by various food product and nutrition companies offering me money to endorse their products. They have presented the idea of having my signature on their labels and in their advertising, of sending me to food product conventions, and essentially of being their spokesmodel. I have no interest in that.

The closest I come to endorsing a product is telling people that Billy Merritt's Infinity Greens is a good product. I don't get any money from that company, which you can find on the Internet.

There is really no reason to support all of these food companies vying for the attention of vegans. Just because a product label states that the product is "vegan" does not necessarily mean that the product is good for you.

We can get plentiful amounts of nutrients in fresh plant matter, and in preparing easy-to-make unheated or barely heated foods using some combination of fruits, vegetables, sprouts, nuts, seeds, and seaweed as ingredients.

I can understand why some people would use packaged foods, such as when they are traveling, are in dire straits, or are in a region where fresh foods simply aren't available.

The best form of nutrition you can get is from eating fresh foods, and not from anything canned, bottled, processed, heated to high temperatures, or that contains synthetic chemicals. In other words, you can ignore any food products introduced since the start of the industrial revolution, and instead rely on what has been growing out of Earth since humans have existed on this planet: edible plant matter.

I do not present nonsense about eating for your blood type, or that you should eat a diet rich in protein and lacking in carbohydrates. The whole group of books advising you to do such things can be tossed into the recycle bin.

"*Eat Right for Your Type* contains just enough scientific sounding nonsense to actually seem convincing to the uninitiated. (Peter) D'Adamo has pieced together the outrageous hypothesis that blood type determines which foods an individual should or should not eat. Browsing through what at first glance appears to be a fairly impressive list of references, we found none that seem to support a connection between diet and blood type. He could just as easily have chosen to link food with eye color – and have been no further off target."
– Frederick J. Stare, MD, Founder and former Chairman of Nutrition Department at Harvard School of Public Health

If you stay away from junk food, consume a low-fat vegan diet, and get daily exercise, you will get sick less, experience better health, and will be much less likely to spend any time or money on, or have to deal with, the medical industry.

"I lost both of my parents to operations and medications – the third greatest cause of death in the U.S. after heart disease and cancer. It's called iatrogenic disease – induced unintentionally by the medical treatment of a physician."
– Karen Ranzi, M.A., CCC-SLP; author of *Creating Healthy Children: Through Attachment Parenting and Raw Foods*; SuperHealthyChildren.com

One thing about the medical industry is that it is truly corrupted by corporate interests, especially by publicly traded corporations most interested in making profits for shareholders. These include hospital corporations, medical device companies, medical technology companies, pharmaceutical companies, and insurance companies. In medical schools, students are not taught about nutrition, but are instructed on chemistry, pharmaceutical drugs, medical technology, and surgery.

I recently went into the snack store/cafeteria area of a hospital. I noticed cigarettes for sale behind the cash register. I knew I was going to find typical junk foods, including potato chips, cookies, candy, chocolate, and colas, energy drinks, and canned or bottled gourmet coffee drinks. I also knew I was going to see low-quality foods being served in the cafeteria, but I didn't expect them to be selling a variety of brands of cigarettes. When I mentioned to the cashier that they shouldn't be selling cigarettes, she agreed with me. She also told me that the main people purchasing the cigarettes are the doctors and nurses.

Their selling and use of such health-defeating substances as cigarettes, fried foods, colas, candy, and things containing corn syrup, rancid oils, clarified sugars, animal protein, synthetic food chemicals, and other junk reveals how clueless the medical industry remains.

If you rely on the medical industry for health, you are more likely to be presented with medical procedures, drugs, and surgery, and not with what brings real health: a clean, low-fat plant-based diet accompanied by exercise, intellectual stimulation, including the practicing of talents and skills, and a regular sleep pattern.

I was once caught up in the medical industry. I nearly died at their hands as they were mistreating me for kidney disorders. That was over twenty years ago. They said I needed a kidney transplant as soon as possible. I refused their advice and their prognosis of death.

Like a growing number of kidney patients, I found that following a low-fat vegan diet rich in raw fruits and vegetables is most beneficial to preventing harm to my kidneys. Like many people with kidney disorder, through following a low-fat vegan diet, I have seen my health issues nearly vanish. Not bad for being told decades ago that I would soon die.

I also had back problems, and was advised to undergo spine surgery to fuse my backbones and to implant iron rods along my spine. I also rejected those surgical procedures. Instead, I slowly got active and healthy through diet and exercise – and a change in the way I approached life.

Had I listened to doctors, it is highly likely that I would have died a long time ago. I almost did – dozens of times. Then I went vegan.

The doctors seemed to be overlooking something: the incredible ability of the body to heal through diet, exercise, and a change of thinking processes.

"An increasing number of doctors are aware that diet plays a crucial role in health, and that nutritional changes such as those I recommend can have dramatic effects on the development and

16

progression of disease. But for a number of reasons, current medical practice places little emphasis on primary and secondary prevention. For most physicians, nutrition is not of significant interest. It is not an essential pillar of medical education; each generation of medical students learn about a different set of pills and procedures, but receives almost no training in disease prevention. And in practice, doctors are not rewarded for educating patients about the merits of truly healthy lifestyles."

    – Dr. Caldwell B. Esselstyn, author of *Prevent and Reverse Heart Disease*; HeartAttackProof.com. See the documentary *Forks over Knives*.

Defying the prognosis of the doctors, I'm alive – and some of them have died. I largely credit my health transformation to a change in my diet. Specifically, a largely raw, low-fat vegan diet.

    "He who does not know food, how can he understand the diseases of man?"
    – Hippocrates

Had I listened to the doctors, and undergone the kidney transplant and the procedures they advised, including removal of my thyroid and implanting of rods in my back, I would have been permanently attached to the financially and physically draining whirlpool that is the American medical industry. A lifetime of using a variety of prescription drugs and undergoing more surgeries would have been my future. I am glad I did not listen to those doctors, but did listen to my intuition.

When I was 45 years old I was offered a free physical at a heart institute. I was put through the various tests, including a treadmill test done while I had a bunch of wires taped to various parts of my torso. This is a guy who, because of back injuries, was told more than ten years previous that he would never walk without a cane, would never run, and would never ride a bike.

After the treadmill test was completed, the doctor asked if he could speak with me in his office. I had a feeling that it wasn't for something unfortunate. I was correct.

When we got into his office, this doctor told me that I had the heart of a twelve-year-old, I did very well on all of the tests, and he was surprised that I was able to carry on a conversation with his assistant while I was on the treadmill (the young lady was obese and had asked me about what types of foods she could eat to lose weight). The doctor wanted to know what I ate, which restaurants served the types of foods I eat, and what books he could read to learn about this raw vegan diet stuff. He took notes as he questioned me and we spoke for about 40 minutes.

Just recently, I had been to the dentist. He had started asking me about my diet, and I answered any question he asked. He ended up taking a list of books I advised him to read, and a list of documentaries I advised him to watch. He had recently seen a documentary titled *Forks over Knives*, and he wanted to adapt a more vegan-centric diet – if not vegan, at least close to it. Over the past ten years, the dentist had become concerned about his weight gain, and he was determined to rid himself of it. He found that following a more vegan diet was helping him to lose weight and feel more energetic.

I think it would be helpful for people to learn about veganism. Following a low-fat diet consisting totally or largely of raw plant matter will help them avoid most of the degenerative diseases that are becoming increasingly common among people living in an industrialized society.

"One thing is for sure: We are getting sicker and more obese than our health care system can handle, and the conventional methods of dealing with disease often have harmful side effects and are ineffective for some patients.

As it is now, one out of every two of us will get cancer or heart disease and die from it – an ugly and painful death as anyone who has witnessed it can attest. And starting in the year 2000, one out of every three children who are born after that year will develop diabetes – a disease that for most sufferers (those with Type-2 diabetes) is largely preventable with lifestyle changes. This is a rapidly emerging crisis, the seriousness of which I'm not sure we have yet recognized. The good news is, the means to prevent and heal disease seems to be right in front of us; it's in our food. Quite frankly, our food choices can either kill us – which mounting studies say that they are, or they can lift us right out of the disease process and into soaring health."

– Kathy Freston, A Cure for Cancer? Eating a Plant-based Diet, *Huffington Post*, September 24, 2009; Freston is the author of the book, *Veganist;* KathyFreston.com. In the article, she interviewed Dr. T. Colin Campbell, Ph.D., Cornell University, co-author of *The China Study* and *Whole: Rethinking the Science of Nutrition*; TColinCampbell.org.

While heart disease, diabetes, kidney disease, obesity, osteoporosis, Alzheimer's, Parkinson's, arthritis, Crohn's, and MS, and also colorectal cancer, breast cancer, liver cancer, brain cancer, lung cancer, prostate cancer, uterine cancer, ovarian cancer, stomach cancer, leukemia, and other neoplasms continue to debilitate and shorten lives, an abundance of scientific studies continue to conclude that there is one thing that lowers the risk of experiencing them, can slow them, and can help rid the body of them, and that is a low-fat vegan diet rich in raw fruits and vegetables and free of additives. This is pointed out in the book, *The China Study*, by Dr. T. Colin Campbell. Please read it, and his new book, *Whole*. Watch the documentaries *Forks over Knives; Fat, Sick, and Nearly Dead,* and *A Delicate Balance* (access: ADelicateBalance.com.au).

A growing number of doctors agree that a vegan diet can prevent and reverse common health conditions. They include Dean Ornish, Milton Mills, John McDougall, Caldwell Esselstyn, Joel Fuhrman, Neal Barnard, Marion Nestle, Michael Klaper, Terry Mason, William C. Roberts, Bill Castelli, and Baxter Montgomery. A variety of nutritionists are also advising people to follow vegan diets rich in raw fruits and vegetables. Among them are Brenda Davis and Vesanto Melina, who authored the book, *Becoming Raw*. Throughout this book, I include quotations from many of these and other heath professionals, along with information from various studies and reports.

> "Although we think we are, and we act as if we are, human beings are not natural carnivores. When we kill animals to eat them, they end up killing us, because their flesh, which contains cholesterol and saturated fat, was never intended for human beings, who are natural herbivores."
> – Dr. William C. Roberts, editor of the *American Journal of Cardiology*

Obviously, this book is not suggesting that people eat the foods that have become typical in much of the world today. Because of this, the diet suggested in this book will also bring people to experience a level of health that is increasingly uncommon in a society where obesity, diabetes, cardiovascular disease, Alzheimer's disease, Parkinson's disease, Crohn's disease, and certain other chronic, degenerative, and truly debilitating diseases are increasingly common.

If you are a person who has been eating a typical American diet, you are likely experiencing some level of the typical dietary related health issues. Reading this book and following its advice on food choices will radically transform your health.

If you are already vegan, you will also likely find information in this book that you had not previously known or considered, and your diet will also likely become cleaner, benefiting your health.

There are currently an estimated 24 million Americans with diabetes, and one in five healthcare dollars is being spent on diabetic patients. Also, obesity is so common that one of the most popular elective surgeries in the U.S. is for stomach-reduction surgery.

Clearly, food has something to do with the rates of obesity and diabetes. While these health problems are becoming more common, so has the consumption of processed foods containing toxic farming chemical residues, synthetic chemical food additives, clarified sugars, animal protein, and genetically modified organisms.

Artificial sweeteners are offered as one solution to the obesity problem. These toxic chemicals we call "no-calorie sweeteners" are no answer to health problems. Artificial sweeteners are being marketed as if they are a healthy choice. As I point out in the book, artificial sweeteners, which are known as excitotoxins, create health problems, including nerve damage and brain lesions. Some of these are known as Acesulfame K, Aspartame, Saccharin, Sorbitol, and Sucralose.

When you consider the foods that contain artificial sweeteners and other synthetic toxins, you may realize that the first way you heard about them was through advertising. If a food has to be advertised, there is a strong likelihood that it is not good for you.

Many of the same foods containing artificial sweeteners also contain a variety of other ingredients that are horrible for health, such as synthetic chemical dyes; emulsifiers like brominated vegetable oil (BVO), carrageenan, and polysorbate 80; anticaking agents like alumino-calcium silicate, aluminum silicate, and sodium alumino-silicate; antifoaming agents like Dimethylpolysiloxane and TBHQ (tertiary butylhydroquin-one); sodium benzoate, sodium nitrates (nitrosamines), MSG, whey, casein, and problematic oils, such as canola oil, soy oil, corn oil, palm oil, and margarine (hydrogenated vegetable oils). You can do an Internet search for any one of these, and add the words "health problems" after the word, and you will find a variety of sources detailing how these substances are not good for health.

People seem to think that any food that is advertised is safe to eat, has been tested to high standards, and is allowed on store shelves only after some approving body of the government gave its approval for the product to be sold as food. That thinking is not reality.

The so-called gatekeepers that you may be thinking exist to protect our health, such as the U.S. Food and Drug Administration, the U.S. Department of Agriculture, and the U.S. Centers for Disease Control and Prevention, act more as concierge services for corporate America and the executives that run them. When legislation is written to protect consumers, these organizations often give in to corporate lobbying so that the laws act not in the best interest of consumers, but in the best interest of company profits. Some of the people who run the various offices of the government that seem to exist to protect consumers directly and financially benefit by approving or allowing questionable products to be sold.

Many elected officials in Washington, D.C., also own stock or are somehow financially connected to the large corporations that employ parades of lobbyists to guide politicians to vote in favor of legislation favoring the profits of corporate America, which very often means that the legislation doesn't favor the health of the people, or of wildlife and the environment.

> "The answer to the American health crisis is the food that each of us chooses to put in our mouths each day. It's as simple as that."
> – T. Colin Campbell, Ph.D., Cornell University; author of *The China Study* and *Whole: Rethinking the Science of Nutrition*; TColinCampbell.org

As I mention, people who eat what have become the typical American foods also go on to experience the common health problems and conditions common among people following what has become known as the "standard American diet," which is often called "the SAD diet." (Yes, I know, that reads "the standard American diet diet.")

Other health conditions that are more common among people who follow the junk diet that is deficient in omega-3 fatty acids and fiber, rich in fried and rancid fats, nearly or completely void of biophotons, heavy in animal protein, filled with bleached starches, clogged with gluten, abundant in bottled oils, saturated with synthetic chemicals, and lacking in raw fruits and vegetables include high blood pressure, cardiovascular disease, kidney disorders, liver toxicity, visual degeneration, colorectal cancer, and various organ issues, including erectile dysfunction and prostate cancer in males and diseases of the sex and reproductive organs in females.

This book came about because I considered that the message contained in some of my books was being limited to a certain audience. I wanted to make the information available to more people, to clarify some points, and to present some additional information not contained in my previous books. I wanted to make it known that there are specific things being said about the vegan diet that are misinformation, or simply bold lies. The meat, dairy, and egg industries helps spread these lies.

Also, I wanted to turn people away from unhealthful foods that are being marketed as "vegan" and "healthy." The foods might be vegan, but that does not mean the very same foods are healthy to eat. These vegan junk foods row the shelves of typical natural foods store, and are often sold at premium prices – even though they are not premium nutrition. Many of the marketing campaigns used to sell these products can be very convincing, but there is really no major benefit from the products, and the reason they are being sold is largely because someone is out to get money by selling them; there are a lot of charming salespeople, and the vegan industry seems to have no shortage of them.

There are also a number of vegans who are misinformed, and are spreading misinformation about vegan nutrition and issues relating to it. As a way of counteracting this, I encourage people to do their own research. Throughout the book, I include a list of documentaries and Websites people can use to learn more about a variety of issues relating to the food industry and environmental issues. Without a healthy environment, healthful foods cannot be grown.

One excellent source of information about vegan nutrition is Dr. Michael Greger's Website videos, NutritionFacts.org. Greger does his research, and presents information about various studies confirming the health benefits of following a plant-based diet that is rich in raw fruits and raw vegetables.

It is good to get all or a majority of your foods from your region, including from your own garden, from organic local farmers, from local farmers' markets, from local natural foods co-ops, and maybe some wild edible foods. You may be able to locate an organic fruit and vegetable wholesaler that will sell you cases of food at discount rates that are far below the prices you would pay at a store. There also may be a local CSA membership group that you can join to get a regular delivery or pick-up box of locally grown foods.

What you don't need is to purchase all of the high-priced packaged items, supplements, and especially "vegan" foods containing an abundance of oils, sugars, salts, gluten grains, and clarified extracts. Bottled juices and products "sweetened with fruit juice" are also not the best foods to eat. While they aren't going to kill you, it is still better to simply eat raw fruit, and if you want juice, to make fresh juice using a juicer or blender – avoiding pasteurized and reconstituted juices.

Know that the vegan food industry is a multibillion-dollar industry, and it is the focus of companies selling products containing ingredients from unreliable sources and of questionable or unknown origin. Just because a label boasts the product as healthful, it does not necessarily mean that the product or ingredient is that thing. Labels often mislead.

It is a bummer that so many companies are flinging unhealthy products using claims that the products are healthy. It is especially unethical when there are many people switching to a vegan diet to rid themselves of some pretty terrible health problems. What they don't need is to eat more low-quality nutrients. No matter how the products are labeled, many of these products are not exactly great for health.

If you are one who is wishing to clean up your diet, and especially if you are aiming to reverse health problems, and reclaim your health, this book is one that contains information you may want to consider. I also encourage you to read Dr. Esselstyn's book about heart disease.

> "The dietary changes that have helped my patients over the past twenty years can help you, too. They can actually make you immune to heart attacks. And there is considerable evidence that they have

benefits far beyond coronary artery disease. If you eat to save your heart, you eat to save yourself from other diseases of nutritional extravagance: from strokes, hypertension, obesity, osteoporosis, adult-onset diabetes, and possibly senile mental impairment, as well. You gain protection from a host of other ailments that have been linked to dietary factors, including impotence and cancers of the breast, prostate, colon, rectum, uterus, and ovaries. And if you are eating for good health in this way, here's a side benefit you might not have expected: For the rest of your life, you will never again have to count calories or worry about your weight."

    – Dr. Caldwell B. Esselstyn, author of *Prevent and Reverse Heart Disease*; HeartAttackProof.com

If you eat healthfully, you are likely to be more healthy, to have a better mood, to enjoy physical and sexual activities. This is especially true if you get daily exercise. Following a clean food low-fat vegan diet rich in raw fruits and raw vegetables will strongly increase the chances that you will have a longer, healthier life. And it will decrease the chances that you will be susceptible to bad medicine, to taking toxic prescription drugs, and to being injured by neglect, infection, or injury in a medical facility.

Decades of scientific studies have concluded that consuming a diet rich in raw fruits and vegetables and other edible plant matter is beneficial to human health. We know that a plant-based diet completely free of animal protein is most beneficial to the environment, to wildlife, and to global health – especially when that diet is based on organically grown and local fruits and vegetables.

I hope you find this book to be useful, helpful, inspiring, and worthy of your time and energy, and that you share it with others.

During the time it took you to read this opening, hundreds of thousands of animals were killed for human consumption, including pigs, horses, deer, cows, turkeys, chickens, ducks, rabbits, lobster, clams, shrimp, tuna, salmon, trout, sharks, lambs, goats, snakes, frogs, dogs, cats, whales, and other beings that were born or hatched, and had families, felt pain, experienced joy or sadness, and had eyes.

    "It is not only for what we do that we are held responsible, but also for what we do not do."
    – Moliere

    "Your inability to communicate with animals does not render them 'stupid,' nor does it justify eating them."
    – Holly Goheavy

WHAT IS A VEGETARIAN?

"I don't eat meat because meat brings out negative qualities
such as fear, anger, anxiety, aggressiveness, etc. Vegetables
peacefully offer themselves to the earth when ripe, thus allowing a
sublime and peaceful thought consciousness."
– Carlos Santana

THE simple answer is: A vegetarian is someone who doesn't consume
meat (including the flesh of cows, deer, bear, snakes, hogs, chickens,
turkeys, ducks, fish, shellfish, and other "born" or "hatched" beings).
Pure vegetarians do not eat any kind of animal product derived from
killed animals, including oils (such as lard or fish liver oil), bouillon
(from the meat of chicken or cows), gelatin (which is made from bone
and or cartilage), or rennet (stomach lining often used in cheeses).

There are a variety of people who consider themselves vegetarians.
(Access the Website for The Vegetarian Resource Group: VRG.org)

• PESCOTARIAN OR PESCO-VEGETARIAN:

These people consume fish. They might also consume dairy and eggs.
They may also consume honey and other bee products, such as royal
jelly, propolis, and bee pollen.

I don't consider these people to be vegetarian, because the flesh of
fish isn't a vegetable, it is the flesh of a living creature that had a family,
and had been killed and sliced into pieces. The consumption of fish is
not necessary for humans to experience health.

The oceans are in serious trouble as they have been so depleted of
populations of fish to the point of being on the edge of collapse. Sea life,
including in the most distant parts of the oceans, from the Arctic to
Antarctica, are being found with varieties of pollutants in their tissues.
People consuming fish are also consuming the heavy metals and other
industrial and commercial society pollutants in the tissues of those fish.
Additionally, ocean acidification and changing temperatures are
threatening all life in the oceans. For more information on the issues
facing the sea creatures and how they are risking all life on the planet,
please read my book, *Extinction: The Death of Waterlife on Planet Earth*.

Additionally, pescotarians may want to consider the origins of the
dairy and eggs they may also be consuming. The support of the milk and

egg industries is supporting industries that kill billions of animals in the form of baby bulls and baby male chicks as they are not needed because they do not produce milk or eggs. The dairy and eggs may also be saturated with farming chemical residues, synthetic drugs, and health-depleting chemicals formed by heating animal protein.

• LACTO-OVO VEGETARIAN:

These people include eggs and dairy (milk, butter, cream, ice cream, cheese, yogurt, kefir, casein, and whey) in their diet.

Those who think they are vegetarian but are eating cheese containing rennet may be interested to know that rennet is the stomach lining of a slaughtered calf.

Also, because of the way milk is obtained from cows, there remains the question of how vegetarian people are if they are consuming milk products. To get milk from a cow, she needs to produce milk. To get her to produce milk, she needs to get pregnant. The way most dairy cows get pregnant are by way of putting her in a "rape rack" and then mechanically impregnating her. When the cow has a baby, the calf is taken away (usually within hours or days after its birth). The female calves are kept for future milk production. Very few of the male calves are raised to adulthood, and often only for their stud service. The vast majority of male calves are sold off, and they are often killed for their tender meat, which is sold as veal (the flesh of baby bulls), and their skin is sold and made into soft leather products. Other male calves are raised to adulthood, and then killed for their meat. When the milk of the dairy cow slows, she is impregnated again. The female cows that get too old to produce enough milk to earn their keep are also sold off and slaughtered for their meat, and much of that meat ends up as hamburger, as processed meats, and as meat for canned chili and stew. (Access: NoVeal.org, FarmUSA.org, PETA.com, VeganOutreach.org, and MercyForAnimals.org. See the documentaries *Earthlings* and *Meet Your Meat*).

While following a lacto-ovo vegetarian diet is more healthful than following a diet that contains meat, one is still participating in the animal slaughter industry. Raising billions of farm animals on the planet so that people can eat milk and eggs uses up tremendous resources, including vast quantities of land, water, fuel, and food, and is not sustainable.

Milk and dairy are not necessary for humans to experience vibrant health.

The nutritional requirement for cow milk in the human diet is absolute zero. The chemistry in the milk is best for turning a small calf into a huge animal within months. (Access: MilkSucks.com, VegSource.com,

NotMilk.com, MilkIsCruel.com, and HeartAttackProof.com.)

• OVO-VEGETARIAN:

These people include eggs in their diet. They might also consume honey and other bee products, such as royal jelly, propolis, and bee pollen.

"The use of eggs as food is just another good example of man's wholesale exploitation of the subhuman creation. We should indeed be ashamed at making the poor hen into an egg-laying machine, especially in that solitary confinement method known as the battery system. Eggs were meant to produce chickens and not omelets! Like cows, hens do not receive old-age pensions, and disobedience to the laws of nature always involves disease or suffering."
– Dugald Semple in his 1956 book, *The Sunfood Way to Health*

By 2007 estimates, there were over two billion chickens being raised in the U.S. alone. Most are raised in factory farms in which they are never allowed outside, eat an unnatural diet, are treated with numerous drugs and chemicals, and spend their entire lives in small cages.

"The attitude we have toward our personal pets as opposed to the animals that suffer under the factory farm is hypocritical and delusional."
– James Cromwell

"If you caught your kid raising cats in tiny boxes, forcing them to live in their own feces without clean air or sunlight, pulling their teeth and claws out with pliers to keep them from hurting each other, then skinning them alive to make collars to sell to their friends, you'd rush him to a psychiatrist. But you support that very behavior every time you buy meat, eggs, dairy, or fur."
– Dan Piraro

"Promoting the consumption of 'free-range' or 'happy' animal products as an 'ethical' way to eat is like promoting not beating a victim too hard as an 'ethical' way to engage in battery."
– Gary L. Francione

"Not having known anything better does not alleviate the suffering of the animal. Its fundamental desires remain and it is the frustration of those desires that is a great part of its suffering. There are so many examples: the dairy cow who is never allowed to raise her young, the battery hen who can never walk or stretch her wings, the sow who can never build a nest or root for food in the forest litter, etc. Eventually we frustrate the animal's most fundamental

desire of all – to live."
– David Cowles-Hamar

"We are the lucky ones – we are not standing day after day in a tiny space, breathing the stench of our own waste, waiting only to be slaughtered. We must do everything possible for those suffering lives of pain and terror."
– Matt Ball

"Imagine living your life in a small, filthy cage constantly in pain, unable to stand or lie down comfortably. After months of agony, your torture finally ends, but not at the slaughterhouse. Instead, two gentle hands reach down to lift you out of the darkness, and bring you to a safe, loving place. For the first time in your life you can stretch your wings and legs and feel soft straw and cool grass beneath your feet."
– Dr. Karen Davis, United Poultry Concerns; UPC–Online.org

"Do you think from your perception that the birds have a sense of what is going to happen to them? Yes. They try everything in their power to get away from the killing machine and to get away from you. They have been stunned, so their muscles don't work, but their eyes do, and you can tell by them looking at you, they're scared to death."
– Virgil Butler, former Tyson slaughterhouse worker

"An animal's eyes have the power to speak a great language."
– Martin Buber

"We cannot glimpse the essential life of a caged animal, only the shadow of its former beauty."
– Julia Allen Field

"Factory farms constitute the most intense cruelty that the human race is capable of. They are, in fact, concentration camps in which sentient, sensitive beings live out their all-too-brief lives deprived of fresh air, sunlight, space in which to move about and stretch their legs or wings, and the ability to live in social communities suited to their natures. Their suffering is so intense and unrelieved from birth to death that insanity is a regular consequence of life in an animal factory. The helpless animals' minds are simply crushed by pain and deprivation."
– Norm Phelps

"I don't see why someone should lose their life just so you can have a snack."
– Russell Brand

Billions of male chicks are killed soon after they hatch. They are put to death because they are of no use in the egg industry. Often, they are killed by simply dropping them into a grinding machine, gassing them, or loading them into plastic bags and suffocating them.

"About twenty four hours before chicks are ready to hatch, they start peeping to notify their mother and siblings that they're ready to emerge from their shells. This activity, which biologists call 'clicking,' helps to synchronize the hatching of the baby chicks. The peeping, sawing and breaking of eggs can go on for as long as two days. As soon as all the eggs are hatched, the mother and her brood go forth eagerly to eat, drink, scratch and explore. When chicks venture away from their mother, they communicate back and forth all the while by peeps and clucks. The hen keeps track of her little ones by counting the peeps of each chick and noting the emotional tones of their voices. In industrial farming chicks and their mums never meet. Eggs are hatched in giant incubators. In the egg laying industry female chicks are destined for a short life of around 18 months and then they will be slaughtered. Male chicks are either ground up alive or gassed at a day old as they are the wrong sex to lay eggs, (around 40 million male chicks a year in the UK). Chickens bred for meat will be slaughtered when they're between 39 and 45 days old. There are videos on this link showing a UK hatchery, the new 'enrichment cages' and so called 'free range' farming systems."
 – VIVA.org.UK

The need for egg protein in the human diet is absolute zero. As is pointed out later in the book, men who consume eggs are much more likely to experience prostate cancer.

Eggs contain cholesterol, which contributes to hardening of the arteries, heart attacks, strokes, and erectile dysfunction.

(Access: UPC-Online.org and MercyForAnimals.org.)

•VEGAN:
These people avoid all animal protein, including meat (mammals, reptiles, amphibians, fish, crustaceans, birds, etc.), eggs, and all dairy products (milk, cream, creamer, ice cream, butter, cheese, yogurt, kefir, casein, whey, etc.).

Vegans also avoid wines that may have been made with the use of casein (a milk protein), egg white, bull blood, or isinglass (dried fish bladder) in the process.

Gelatin is made by boiling connective tissue from slaughtered animals. Vegans avoid gelatin, which is used in desserts, candy, and some other packaged foods, and also in some types of medicine, including dissolvable capsules. If you purchase supplements in capsules, look for those in vegetable gel caps, or vegan gel caps.

L-cysteine that is used in some bread, donut, muffin, scone, cake, bagel, and pastry products is an amino acid that may originate from feathers. It also can be derived from human hair.

Lanolin is in some brands of gum, and is derived from sheep's wool. It is also used in some types of skincare, haircare, sunscreen, baby care products, and cosmetics. It may also be in non-mushroom vitamin D.

Another nonvegan substance used in some foods is red dye made from dried, ground-up cochineal beetles. This dye may be used in some brands of ice cream, yogurt, cake, bagels, pastry, maraschino cherries, some brands of prepared tomato products and foods containing them, and some types of prepared or gourmet coffee drinks.

In addition to casein, lanolin, L-cysteine, isinglass and crushed beetles, there are other reasons why vegans may avoid a wide variety of prepared and packaged foods. Some brands of "natural" raspberry food flavoring and also vanilla may contain urine extract and the anal gland secretions of beavers. Some fried foods may contain lard, which is animal fat. Lard also may be in some breads, cookies, crackers, pastries, icing, chocolates with cream centers, and other foods.

Ingredient concerns include more reasons why vegans go to vegan restaurants and shop at natural foods stores, farmers' markets, and food co-ops, and join CSAs (organic produce delivery or pick-up), rather than go to typical supermarkets and restaurants.

"If a man earnestly seeks a righteous life, his first act of abstinence is from animal food."
– Leo Tolstoy

There are those following a vegan diet, but are not necessarily living a fully vegan lifestyle, for instance, they may still wear leather shoes and belts. People who are fully vegan refuse to wear leather, silk, and fur.

Vegans also avoid products containing derivatives of animals, such as some brands of soaps and cosmetics, and some types of medicine. (Access: Vegan.org.)

Some people consider themselves vegan even though they consume honey and other bee products. Those who are vegan often say that they refuse to eat honey and other bee products, including propolis, bee pollen, and royal jelly. They believe that bees are collecting pollen and nectar for their own families, and that taking the food of the bees is stealing, and relying on bees to make honey and pollen is enslaving the bees. If vegans with this belief think that they aren't participating in the honey industry, but are eating fruits and vegetables, they may like to know that many farms use managed hives to pollinate the crops. Taking the honey and pollen from the hives gets the bees to collect more, thus pollinating more crops.

My diet is vegan, although I may sometimes consume something that contains honey or bee pollen. I'm also aware that many of the foods I eat are from farms where managed beehives are used to pollinate the crops. I grow some of my foods, and get some of my foods from friends who also have gardens. So I am less reliant on store-bought foods than many other people. But I do know that some of the foods I consume originate from farms that use managed beehives. Am I concerned, offended, or appalled by that? No.

Although my diet is basically vegan, my life isn't. I am not some perfect being.

Then there are the issues of plastic "vegan" clothing and leather, which is a two-sided sword. I am aware that leather is grim and plastic production ends up polluting the environment and plastic poses a variety of environmental problems. But I also have leather shoes and belts, including from second-hand stores. Some vegans will wear belts and shoes made of plastic. I see no need to pollute the planet with more plastic that may linger on the planet as pollution, as plastic may last hundreds or thousands of years. Unlike plastic, leather is biodegradable – although many toxic chemicals are now being used to treat leather before it is made into clothing, and that is not good. Most leather is a byproduct of the meat industry, and the animals aren't being killed for their leather, but for their meat. Other than the unsustainable aspects of animal agriculture, the most polluting thing about leather is in the processing. It is still considered more environmentally friendly than plastic, which is and will be causing problems for the environment and wildlife for many years. The creation of plastic also utilizes a lot of resources, and it uses toxic chemicals that end up in the environment.

When you consider the damage that is being done to the environment to produce leather, and the mass quantities of plastic pollution, including in the rivers, lakes, and oceans, where plastic kills wildlife that eat it, it is easy to understand why people who follow a vegan diet also might choose to continue wearing leather – instead of wearing plastic shoes and belts.

Plastic in the form of various clothing products is one of the problems with ocean pollution, and pollution in many other areas of earth. Many birds, ocean mammals, fish, and land animals die every year after eating plastic, including bits of brightly colored plastic clothing. Truly biodegradable plastic isn't common.

"I think vegan is a beautiful word. It is more than just a description for our diet. I see it as a visible template for an ethical, healthy, responsible, and rational life. Because it describes our character, it says we do not take the life of another living being to satisfy our wants."
– Philip Wollen, KindnessTrust.com

• SUNFOODIST, RAW FOOD VEGAN, OR RAW BEEGAN:

The term *sunfoodist* has been around for more than 100 years, being used among some raw foodists in Scotland. A sunfoodist is a vegan who follows a completely raw, or largely raw diet consisting of unheated fruits, vegetables, nuts, seeds, germinated seeds (such as quinoa, chia, and buckwheat), germinated legumes (such as lentils and garbanzos), seaweeds, sprouts, and maybe some edible flowers.

A lot of people say that I coined the term "raw vegan." In his book, *Raw Controversies*, Frederic Patenaude says that I did. I guess it could be true. I joke that I also invented sailing ships and butterflies. I'm very creative. My point in starting to use the term back in the 1990s was to clarify the difference between raw foodists who are vegan and raw foodists who may consume raw milk or raw eggs or raw meat. So, "raw vegan" seemed to be the easiest way to clarify that difference. I started using the term raw vegan, and it caught on – being used in books and magazines, in blog names, in company names, on social media, etc.

Because some "raw foodists" also consume raw dairy, eggs, and meat, the term *sunfoodist* is more accurate when describing a raw vegan (even though many sunfoodists consume honey and other bee products, which some people consider to be nonvegan).

Some people who are otherwise raw vegans might eat some steamed foods or simmered foods (such as soup, beans, quinoa, millet, lentils, and wild rice) in their diet. Some raw vegans may also consume maple syrup, which isn't truly a raw food – because it is low temperature simmered tree sap. Some sunfoodists may also occasionally use organic germinated grain or brown rice tortillas made at low heat, or dehydrated.

Sunfoodists also avoid brewed and distilled drinks. They might consume wine, because wine is fermented. But some wines aren't vegan, because they might contain isinglass, a collagen derived from fish bladders that is used as a refining agent by some wine makers and by beer brewers. Some wine makers use albumen, which is egg white used to clarify wine and some brands of vinegar. Some wines contain casein, which is a milk protein that can also clear wine of impurities. Casein can trigger allergic reactions and mood swings, anxiety, and depression – and autistic-like symptoms. Some wines may also contain gelatin, which is

31

processed from animal bones and/or collagen. Some wines also contain bull's blood, which is illegal to use as a filtering agent in winemaking in the U.S. and Canada, but which is still used in other countries, by winemakers who export their wines to markets in the U.S. and Canada. Many natural foods stores sell vegan wines.

Many raw foodists avoid alcohol altogether, considering it a neurotoxin. Anyone having a history of alcoholism should avoid alcohol. (Access: VeganConnection.com/VeganWine.htm)

• LIVE FOODIST:

This is someone who is a raw vegan, but who consumes seeds and nuts only after they have been soaked in water to turn off their enzyme inhibitors, which then triggers growth of enzymes, essential fatty acids, and other nutrients. Live foodists also eat raw fruits, vegetables, and sprouts, and combinations of them.

Seeds and nuts that are raw are in a dormant state. Live foodists believe that it is best to consume only nuts and seeds that have been brought out of the dormant stage, and which are truly alive with enzymes and other nutrients that form as a seed or nut begins the growth stage.

• LFRV (LOW FAT RAW VEGAN):

Low-fat raw veganism is a dietary approach that is approximately 80 percent of dietary calories from carbohydrates, as in: sweet fruit, including berries, melon, grapes, and also stone, tropical, citrus, and other tree fruits. They also consume nonsweet fruits, such as tomatoes, zucchini, cucumbers, and bell peppers. LFRVs aim to get 10 percent of their dietary calories from fatty foods, such as nuts, seeds, durian, and avocados (durian and avocado are also fruits). The other 10 percent of their calories consists of protein-rich foods, such as greens, including romaine and other lettuces and also celery, chard, kale, spinach, collards, cauliflower leaf, fennel leaf, cilantro, parsley, basil, oregano, broccoli leaf, dandelion, purslane, dill, and other greens.

The LFRV diet is certainly one rich in antioxidants, biophotons, enzymes, amino acids, vitamins, phytochemicals, micronutrients, and soluble and insoluble fiber.

"There are many types of 'extracted' fiber products on the market, including tablets and powders that can be mixed with water and taken as a drink. Most health care professionals would advise a healthy adult to eat a pear or a handful of raisins instead of turning to a supplement. Satisfying your daily fiber needs with food is the

best way to get a healthful balance of soluble and insoluble fiber. It's also a great way to improve the overall quality of your diet, since fiber-rich foods tend to be rich in vitamins, minerals, and disease-fighting phytochemicals."
– Nancy D. Berkoff, RD, EdD, Ask the Nutritionist: How much fiber do I really need?; VegetarianTimes.com

People into the LFRV diet typically avoid salt; refined oils (bottled oils, including olive and flax oils); refined sugars (including white sugar, brown sugar, agave, and corn syrup); stimulant foods (including chocolate, hot peppers, garlic, and onions); and all dairy, eggs, meat (including from fish, birds, mammals, reptiles, and amphibians), and processed foods (including anything containing MSG and any artificial sweeteners, dyes, flavorings, scents, and preservatives). They usually seek organically grown foods. Many LFRVs are into growing food gardens and planting fruit trees and berry bushes.

People may question the "no refined oils" guideline about the LFRV diet. They may ask about olive oil, flax oil, hemp oil, coconut oil, and other refined oils. Hemp oil is a better source of omega-3 fatty acids than any of those oils, and most people in industrial society are deficient in omega-3s. Instead of using bottled hemp seed oil, a better choice would be to add raw hemp seeds to the diet. As mentioned elsewhere in this book, any raw fruit or vegetable also contains omega-3s. The reason people are short on omega-3s is because they don't eat enough raw fruit and raw vegetables, but do eat junk food lacking omega-3s.

I used to add oils to my food, especially hemp, olive, and flax oils. But, years ago, I mostly stopped purchasing those oils. Usually, when I eat foods made by someone else, such as at a raw vegan café, I do consume foods containing added oils. Sometimes at home, there is very little hemp oil or coconut oil used.

"In the United States, where vascular disease is the leading killer, the average citizen eats sixty-five pounds of fat per year – consuming two tons of suet by the age of sixty – and average cholesterol levels hover around 200 mg/dL."
– Dr. Caldwell B. Esselstyn, author of *Prevent and Reverse Heart Disease*; HeartAttackProof.com

Consider the vegan diet suggested by Dr. Caldwell Esselstyn who authored the book *Prevent and Reverse Heart Disease*, which, as mentioned, advises people to stay away from refined oils, including olive oil. Dr. Esselstyn's son, Rip Esselstyn, also wrote a low-fat vegan book, *The Engine 2 Diet: The Texas Firefighter's 28-Day Save-Your-Life Plan That Lowers Cholesterol and Burns Away the Pounds*.

"What about olive oil? It's heart-healthy, right? No, it's not. Extracted oils are the most concentrated source of calories on the planet, at 120 calories per tablespoon, and they have more empty calories than either white sugar or white flour, and it's 15 percent artery-clogging saturated fat, and there's absolutely zero nutrition to speak of. That's olive oil."
– Rip Esselstyn, author of the low-fat vegan book, *The Engine 2 Diet: The Texas Firefighters' 28-Day Save-Your-Life Plan That Lowers Cholesterol and Burns Away the Pounds;* Engine2Diet.com and Farms2Forks.com

People often claim that olive oil is good for the heart, and they mention the "Mediterranean diet" espoused by a variety of people, and especially by olive oil dealers. In his book, *Prevent and Reverse Heart Disease*, Dr. Esselstyn has some interesting things to say about the Mediterranean diet, including that those who follow the diet often experience cardiovascular disease. Monounsaturated oils can raise blood sugar and elevate triglyceride levels. In other words, we shouldn't be considering a diet rich in olive oil to be ideal for experiencing the best of health.

Many athletes follow a LFRV diet, and credit it with improving their performance.

Two of the most active promoters of the low-fat raw vegan lifestyle have been Australians, Harley "Durianrider" Johnstone and Freelee Frugivore. They hold retreats and run the popular social networking site 30BananasADay.com. Harley is a Division One biking athlete and both are runners. They are known for being a bit irreverent, and even harsh, in their approach to educating people about LFRV, and in steering them away from the nonsense of mass-marketed processed foods, fast foods, useless supplements, and meat, dairy, and egg products.

"All of the leading cancer researchers, cardiologists, and health researchers like Doctors Ornish, McDougall, Barnard, Heinrich, Klaper, Fuhrman, etc., recommend a diet that is under 10 percent of total calories from fat over the course of the seasons. Fruit is the best source of vitamins, greens the next best. Greens are the best source of minerals, fruit being the next best. Fresh sweet fruit is the most human, nutrient-dense calorie on the planet."
– Harley "Durianrider" Johnstone, 30BananasADay.com

A popular book promoting low-fat raw veganism is Douglas Graham's *The 80/10/10 Diet: Balancing Your Health, Your Weight, and Your Life One Luscious Bite At a Time*. Graham also wrote the booklet *Grain Damage: Rethinking the High-Starch Diet*, and the book *Nutrition and Athletic Performance*. Graham is a chiropractor who turned his focus to diet and health. His books may be helpful, but it is also good to read others.

Another well-known LFRV is Michael Arnstein. He refers to himself as a *fruitarian*. In July 2011, he won the Vermont 100-mile race. That same year, he placed fourth in a 100-mile race in Colorado. In 2012, he ran the 135-mile Badwater Race, and that same week, he and his wife, Victoria, ran the Vermont 100. He holds the annual event, Woodstock Fruit Festival, in upstate New York. It began in 2011, and is growing in popularity. (Access: TheWoodstockFruitFestival.com).

> "People may *survive* in the short term on diets outside their intended species-specific diet, but they do not *thrive*. There is evidence of it everywhere. We are surrounded by people trying different diets all the time, and we are sicker than ever as a species. The problem is people don't trust nature's guidelines, and instead they trust diets created by the human ego – like metabolic typing, zones, Atkins, blood type, and others."
> – Freelee Frugivore, 30BananasADay.com

Within the LFRV community there are discussions about which percentage of certain foods are the best to maintain high-grade athletic performance. Consuming a variety of edible plant substances gives a broader spectrum of nutrients. It is a high-carbohydrate diet, but there is a difference between what some people think of as carbohydrates and what qualifies as a carbohydrate, what foods contain those carbohydrates, and how the carbohydrates are digested and used within the body. There are also different types of carbohydrates, including disaccharides, monosaccharides, oligosaccharides, and polysaccharides.

While reading Graham's book, *The 80/10/10 Diet*, might be helpful, reading more than one book about raw vegan nutrition can give a broader understanding of nutrients provided on the diet. While it isn't a LFRV book, *Becoming Raw: The Essential Guide to Raw Vegan Diets*, by Davis, Melina, and Berry, is a helpful book. Another book that isn't raw, but provides information on a low-fat vegan diet is Dr. Caldwell Esselstyn's *Prevent and Reverse Heart Disease*. An excellent little low-fat raw vegan recipe booklet is skate boarder Chris Kendall's *101 Fricken' Rawsome Recipes* (Access: TheRawAdvantage.com); there are also books by Megan Elizabeth (Access: MeganElizabeth.com).

Whether or not one follows LFRV, including a variety of raw, unheated, organically grown sweet and nonsweet fruits in the diet is an excellent way of obtaining top quality nutrients, such as antioxidants, biophotons, enzymes, amino acids, minerals, vitamins, certain minerals, soluble fiber, and other beneficial substances.

It is best to limit fats to those obtained by consuming raw plant substances, such as raw fruits and vegetables, and some raw soaked nuts and soaked, germinated, or sprouted seeds, as they contain the omega-3 fatty acids we especially need for health. Raw flax, walnuts, and hemp seeds, and germinated chia seeds and germinated buckwheat are rich in Omega-3 fatty acids. All raw fruits, leafy greens, and other vegetables contain omega-3 fatty acids. There are also omega-3s in sea vegetables, which some LFRVs avoid.

There is no reason to consume raw dairy, eggs, fish oil, or other animal products to obtain omega-3 fatty acids. The animals obtain the raw fatty acids by consuming plants. Eggs that are sold as "rich in omega-3 fatty acids" are from chickens fed raw flax seeds and/or fishmeal (the fish get the omega-3s by eating algae). Grass-fed beef is often sold as being "rich in omega-3 fatty acids," and this is because the cattle are consuming raw greens in the field. To obtain high-quality omega-3 fatty acids, we can skip consuming the flesh of slaughtered animals and other animal products, and simply eat raw fruits, vegetables, nuts, and seeds.

Most people consume an abundance of omega-6 fatty acids, and the majority of people living in the industrialized world consume low-quality fats, such as fried fats, transfats, and animal fat. There are a variety of fats that people obtain from food. Fats that especially should be avoided are transfatty acids and fried and sautéed oils. Many people have learned about and avoid transfats. Foods are often labeled as free of transfats, but transfats and fried fats are very common in processed and restaurant foods.

To obtain fruit, get involved in growing food, in connecting with local organic orchards, and in learning which stores and farmers' markets sell organically grown fruits, including berries and melons. You can likely find a fruit wholesaler in your region selling directly to the public. Purchasing from them will save you money.

Save the seeds and pits from the best-tasting fruits you eat, and plant them someplace, or give them to someone who can.

Many people are involved in planting "fruit forests" either on their own land, on the land of others, or on government or wild land. This involves seeking out fruiting trees and bushes that grow well in the region, and planting a variety of them.

Some people question the energy used to import the tropical fruits often eaten by LFRVs, and say that this is unsustainable. However, it is more sustainable than the typical meat eating diet, which uses up enormous supplies of water, land, fuel, and food to raise and feed the farmed animals, then to transfer them, slaughter them, and then to package the meat, which then has to be transferred to markets, bought, and cooked. The amount of water, fuel, and other resources used to clean up after all of the slaughtering and meat eating is tremendous. Also not to be overlooked is that the methane emitted from cows is more damaging to the environment than the burning of fossil fuels – which are also used to cook the meat, and to heat the water used in cleaning the slaughter-houses, the ovens and stoves, and the grills, pots, pans, and utensils. In other words, if anyone who is following the common standard American diet of meat, dairy, eggs, GMO grains, and processed and junk foods containing fried oils, processed salts and sugars, and synthetic food chemicals is critical of the environmental implications of importing fruit, they are certainly not dealing with the reality of their own diet.

Key to maintaining a LFRV diet is having access to plentiful fruit and other fresh produce, nuts, and seeds. It is even better if the foods are free of pesticides and other toxic farming chemicals.

Some people into a high-fruit diet are constructing greenhouses and growing fruiting trees, berry bushes, and fruiting vines inside these. Some people travel and work as volunteers on organic fruit farms, such as through WWOOF.org (see below). Some people follow lifestyles in which they can travel with the seasons, going to the tropical regions during colder months, and moving north or south into the summer seasons of the hemispheres.

You may be interested in what Kristina Carrillo-Bucaram has been doing in Texas. Kristina, a long-term LFRV, connected with local organic farmers and founded the Rawfully Organic Co-op, which quickly grew into what is now a successful member co-op through which a growing variety of people are getting mostly locally grown organic fruits and vegetables on a weekly basis. (Access: RawfullyOrganic.com, and also Kristina's site, FullyRaw.com.)

The majority of my meals tend to be aligned with the LFRV style of eating, but I don't consider myself to be a LFRV.

The people who closely follow a LFRV style of eating mostly or totally avoid what they call "gourmet raw," which is the food served in many of the raw restaurants, such as raw vegan cheesecake (made largely of creamed nuts), dehydrated seed breads (containing salt and oil), and salads with nut, avocado, or oil-based dressings. Many LFRVs consider the occasional binge on gourmet raw to be fine.

Some people follow a mostly LFRV diet, but don't stick to it so strictly. They may eat some raw gourmet and heated vegan foods.

• NATURAL HYGIENE:

This is a way of eating that some raw foodists are into. Natural hygiene is more than a diet, it involves avoiding polluting the body and avoiding exterior pollution. One guideline of the natural hygiene diet is: Can you make a meal of it? Another is: Would you feed it to a baby? (Well, ideally, babies should be fed nothing but their mother's breast milk for the first months of their life.) Another guideline is: Does it grow naturally in your environment? That can be limiting, especially in a cold climate.

People that have been involved in teaching about natural hygiene include TC Fry, Weston A. Price, Keki Sidhwa, David Klein, Debbie Took, Herbert Shelton, and Marilyn and Harvey Diamond.

As with any dietary plan, anyone who expects those who advocate it to be following the diet to perfection are not dealing with reality.

Natural hygiene dietary guidelines encourage few fatty foods (such as seeds, nuts, and avocados); no sea vegetables; no added oils; no fermented foods; no sprouts; no stimulating foods (ginger, onions, garlic, peppers, coffee, cocoa, etc.); no salt, spices, or condiments; no wheat grass juice; but lots of greens and fruit. Natural hygienists advocate fasting (not for pregnant women, or those who are breast feeding). They advocate paying attention to food combining: not mixing proteins with starches; fruit should be eaten by itself, and not with other food.

My diet is not in alignment with the natural hygiene philosophy.

• RAW VEGAN FUSION (RVF):

This is a diet that is vegan and largely raw, but also includes some heated foods. Probably most raw vegans are RVF. More and more vegan restaurants are becoming RVF, serving some cooked vegan food such as soups, rice tortillas, rice, beans, cooked or raw vegan nonsoy burgers, and some raw platters, while also offering both raw and cooked vegan desserts.

Rather than high-temperature cooked foods such as fried, sautéed, grilled, or baked foods, these heated foods that people who are otherwise raw foodists may consume are likely to be along the lines of simmered vegan soups that don't have any oil or salt added until the soup is in the serving bowl, and steamed vegetables, quinoa, millet, and lentils.

One goal is to avoid cooking starchy foods to above 247 degrees Fahrenheit, which is when acrylamides form. Also, avoid cooking that would make foods brown, which is when glycotoxins form (such as toast). Acrylamides and glycotoxins are chemicals that trigger the immune system and have been shown to increase the risk of cancer, kidney disease, and other health issues.

Water boils at about 212 degrees Fahrenheit at sea level, and at lower temperatures at higher elevations, such as in the mountains. So steaming and simmering foods are ways of avoiding heating foods to the point where harsh, heat-generated chemicals will form.

While heating food does damage or destroy some nutrients, including biophotons, some vitamins, some antioxidants, some amino acids, and also essential fatty acids, a few foods contain beneficial substances that may become more bioavailable when the foods are lightly heated. These include carrots, onions, garlic, broccoli, and tomatoes. And there are also some foods that become more digestible when low-temperature steamed or simmered. These include beans, bamboo shoots, and yams.

For more information on heated foods in an otherwise raw vegan diet, read the book *Becoming Raw: The Essential Guide to Raw Vegan Diets*, by Brenda Davis, Vesanto Melina, and Rynn Berry.

The heated foods that otherwise raw foodists might eat also include truly fermented, organic, whole grain sourdough bread – which is to say, not your typical, low-quality sourdough bread sold at the grocery store. Those avoiding gluten may wish to avoid any bread containing wheat, rye, or barley.

There are some well-known otherwise raw vegan restaurants that have some heated foods on the menu. These include the California restaurant chain Cafe Gratitude, and Rod Rotundi's Leaf Organics in Culver City, California. Also, Cherie Soria of the Living Light Culinary Institute, which is the main raw vegan chef school, knows about preparing some foods at low temperatures, and avoiding putting oil or salt in the foods until after they are ready to serve, as a way of avoiding damaging the essential fatty acids and salts.

Here is what Rod Rotundi says about raw vegan fusion:

"Since I have been a raw foods chef and restaurateur for nearly 10 years, some of you are probably surprised to see that I am offering some cooked vegan foods in addition to my extensive array of raw dishes. Allow me to explain…

While I do believe that raw foods are optimally healthfull food for most people in most situations, I also realize that we don't always eat only for "optimizing health." In fact, there are many other reasons to eat! One of the most obvious ones is pleasure – and it's not a sin! Taking pleasure from our culinary experiences is in my opinion a natural and normal way to eat. In fact, if the food we eat isn't delicious and pleasant tasting then we probably won't continue eating it for very long.

Now I know that some in the raw foods community think that every bite we take should be done with optimal health in mind. And indeed, there is certainly much merit in this approach. However, I believe that the ultimate objective is not optimal health but optimal happiness.

And let me tell you, I love food. I take great pleasure in tasting and eating different foods. Food offers us culture, community and comfort in addition to sustenance. When I was restricting myself to solely raw foods, I was doing it because I wanted to, because it felt right to me and I was enjoying it. After many years eating this way, I found myself wanting to broaden my culinary boundaries to include some cooked vegan foods – especially foods from around the world. And so I have. And I feel good with it.

So while I still eat a predominantly raw foods diet, I also enjoy some cooked foods. And I find that including probiotic foods together with cooked vegan foods helps with the digestion. I have included some of my favorite world cuisines in my new menu: Ethiopian, Indian and Mexican, and combined them with our raw creations and pro-biotic sauerkrauts to create my Vegan Fusion dishes."

– Rod Rotundi, Leaf Organics restaurant, Culver City California; leaforganics.com; author of *Raw Food for Real People*.

• FLEXITARIAN:
This is a person who goes back and forth from being a vegan to a vegetarian, to a meat eater, or a raw foodist, or fast junk foodist.

• OPPORTUNARIAN:
This is a person who eats anything, as long as they like the taste of it.

"For I tell you truly, he who kills, kills himself, and whoso eats the flesh of slain beasts, eats to the body of death."
– Jesus, the Gospel of Peace

"The question is not, Can they reason? Nor, Can they talk? But, Can they suffer?"
– Jeremy Bentham

"Those who, by their purchases, require animals to be killed have no right to be shielded from the slaughterhouse or any other aspect of the production of the meat they buy. If it is distasteful for humans to think about, what can it be like for the animals to experience it?"
– Peter Singer

"I do not like eating meat – because I have seen lambs and pigs killed. I saw and felt their pain. They felt the approaching death. I left in order not to see their death. I could not bear it. I cried like a child. I ran up a hill and could not breathe. I felt that I was choking. I felt the death of the lamb. I chose a mountain, where there were no people. I was afraid of being ridiculed."
– Vaslav Nijinsky

"I know what it feels like to be hurt, and I don't want to cause that pain to any other person or creature. But somehow, in society, we numb ourselves in order to make money or to feel better about ourselves, such as with cosmetics or food. We say to ourselves, 'I'm going to use this animal. I'm going to use this animal. I'm going to say it doesn't have much worth so that I can allow myself to do these cruel things.' And that just isn't fair."
– Alicia Silverstone

"One farmer says to me, 'You cannot live on vegetable food solely, for it furnishes nothing to make the bones with;' and so he religiously devotes a part of his day to supplying himself with the raw material of bones; walking all the while he talks behind his oxen, which, with vegetable-made bones, jerk him and his lumbering plow along in spite of every obstacle."
– Henry David Thoreau

"My experience with chickens for more than twenty years has shown me that chickens are conscious and emotional beings with adaptable sociability and a range of intentions and personalities. If there is one trait above all that leaps to my mind in thinking about chickens when they are enjoying their lives and pursuing their own interests, it is cheerfulness. Chickens are cheerful birds, quite vocally so, and when they are dispirited and oppressed, their entire being expresses this state of affairs as well. The fact that chickens become lethargic in continuously barren environments, instead of proving that they are stupid or impassive by nature, shows how sensitive these birds are to their surroundings, deprivations, and prospects."
– Karen Davis, United Poultry Concerns; UPC-Online.org

"Animals must be off the menu because tonight they are screaming in terror in the slaughterhouse, in crates, and cages. Vile ignoble gulags of despair.
I heard the screams of my dying father as his body was ravaged by the cancer that killed him. And I realized I had heard these screams before.
In the slaughterhouse, eyes stabbed out and tendons slashed, on the cattle ships to the Middle East, and the dying mother whale as a Japanese harpoon explodes in her brain as she calls out to her calf.
Their cries were the cries of my father.
I discovered when we suffer, we suffer as equals. And in their capacity to suffer, a dog is a pig is a bear… is a boy."
– Philip Wollen (see his speech on YouTube)

MYTHS AND TRUTHS ABOUT VEGANISM

"If anyone can show me, and prove to me, that I am wrong in thought or deed, I will gladly change. I seek the truth, which never yet hurt anybody. It is only persistence in self-delusion and ignorance which does harm."
– Marcus Aurelius

BY the term "meat," I mean all kinds of meat, including cow, hog, turkey, chicken, goat, lamb, deer, duck, ostrich, fish, shellfish, reptiles, amphibians, and any other creatures that people eat.

"Who can believe that there is no soul behind those luminous eyes?"
– Theophile Gautier

While some people consider not eating cows, pigs, and birds, but eating fish to be vegetarian, that is not vegetarianism. A woman told me, "I'm vegetarian, but I also eat fish." Oh? Of course. Everyone knows that brightly colored fish are fruits, and the other ones are vegetables. And flying fish are Frisbees, and catfish are vacuum cleaners.

Even consuming milk and eggs isn't vegetarian, because of the processes involved in obtaining milk (most of the baby bulls are killed), and in assuring that the chicken farms have female birds (the male baby chicks are killed). Also, since most cheese also contains rennet, which is the stomach lining of slaughtered animals, most cheese is clearly not vegetarian or vegan.

There are a variety of vegan foods with similar taste and texture of meat, cheese, milk, eggs, yogurt, kifir, cream, ice cream, creamer, sauces, and foods containing extracts of meat, milk, and eggs.

"When I met my first vegetarian, he told me he had not eaten meat for fourteen years. I looked at him as if he had managed to hold his breath that entire time. Today I know there is nothing rigorous or strange about eating a diet that excludes meat."
– Erik Marcus, author of the books *Vegan: The New Ethics of Eating*, and *Meat Market: Animals, Ethics, and Money*

MYTH: VEGANS DO NOT GET ENOUGH PROTEIN

TRUTH: Vegetarians, even strict vegetarians who do not eat dairy products or eggs, can very easily get enough protein from plant matter. (For more on protein, see page 180.)

Proteins are made up of chains of amino acids.

It is not necessary to eat animal protein to get the essential amino acids of the protein molecule. The amino acids needed to make protein in a human can easily be obtained by eating a variety of fruits and vegetables. All fruits and vegetables contain all of the essential amino acids.

It is **not** necessary to combine rice with beans to get protein. All fruits, vegetables, sprouts, nuts, beans, and seeds contain protein.

The protein found in meat, dairy, and eggs is much more concentrated than the protein found in plants. A diet that contains a lot of concentrated protein is a burden on the body, especially on the bones, joints, liver, blood system, digestive tract, brain, and kidneys.

In John McDougall's book *The McDougall Plan*, he tells of how the studies done to determine the protein requirements of humans were done on baby rats, not humans. Human protein requirements are much lower than the protein requirements of baby rats. McDougall explains how there are plentiful amounts of protein in plant substances to satisfy human protein requirements. (Access: DrMcDougall.com)

It is impossible to be deficient in protein while following a low-fat vegan diet advised in this book. This is because it includes a variety of plant substances rich in amino acids: These plant substances are raw fruits, vegetables, soaked nuts, seaweeds, and germinated or sprouted seeds. Even if the nuts and seeds aren't germinated, they still contain protein, but soaking them increases the nutrient value because they start to produce enzymes, which are rich in amino acids.

> "The meat industry has raised some alarm by suggesting that protein from plant sources may not be as 'complete' as that from animal sources. Fortunately, any essential amino acids that may be missing in grains are available in legumes or vegetables and vice versa. Our liver stores and redistributes the essential amino acids where they are needed. This is precisely how the animals raised for food get their 'complete' proteins."
> – Citizens for Healthy Options in Children's Education

43

MYTH: VEGANS DON'T GET ANY MINERALS

TRUTH: Many people believe that they have to eat meat and dairy to get quality nutrition, and especially minerals. The truth is that meat and dairy are not good sources of minerals.

When you look at the natural diet of cows, giraffes, gorillas, elephants, deer, and other large animals, you can understand that they obtain nutrition from eating green leaves and other vegetation. These animals are the substances of plants, water, air, and sunlight transformed through the miracle of life into living body tissues.

It is no coincidence that calcium is the primary mineral in leaves, and is also the chief mineral in the human body.

If you want to get high-quality minerals into your body, as well as an amazing assortment of other nutrients, be sure to regularly eat raw, green-leafed vegetables. The colloidal minerals that your body needs to construct and maintain your tissues are contained in raw plants. Leafy vegetables have a good balance of magnesium, manganese, and silicon, which are needed to assimilate calcium. Spinach is an ideal source of all these minerals, but spinach is only one of many leaves containing an excellent assortment of nutrients, including minerals. Water vegetables are especially rich in minerals.

Don't overlook fruit, including everything from tree fruit to vine fruit to berries, as fruit also contains minerals. Like raw green leafy and other vegetables, raw fruit also contains a variety of other nutrients, including vitamins that are assimilated into our tissues when accompanied by the very minerals in the fruits and vegetables.

Don't depend on supplements to obtain your minerals.

Do consume a variety of fruits, green leafy vegetables, and some sea vegetables, and you will get a spectrum of nutrients that eating meat, milk, and eggs, or taking supplements, could never, ever supply to you.

"How good it is to be well-fed, healthy, and kind all at the same time."
– Henry J. Heimlich

MYTH: VEGANS OFTEN BECOME ANEMIC BECAUSE THEY DO NOT GET ENOUGH IRON

TRUTH: Vegetables contain sufficient amount of iron. Many vegetables, such as bell peppers, broccoli, cauliflower, cucumbers, peas, spinach, and tomatoes have more iron per calorie than beef. Other vegan sources of iron include almonds, bok choy, Brazil nuts, cashews, chard, chia, garbanzo beans, currants, dried apricots, dulse, figs, flax, garlic, hazelnuts, kelp, lentils, leafy greens, millet, parsley, pine nuts, pistachios, poppy seeds, pumpkin seeds, quinoa, raisins, sesame seeds (including raw tahini/sesame seed butter), spirulina, sunflower seeds, and walnuts. Many types of fruit also are excellent sources of iron.

> "You would have to eat more than 1,700 calories of sirloin steak to get the same amount of iron as found in 100 calories of spinach."
> – Iron in the Vegan Diet, by Reed Mangels, Ph.D., R.D.; Vegetarian Resource Group, April 2006; VRG.Org/Nutrition/Iron.htm

The body uses vitamin C (ascorbic acid) to absorb and use iron. A lack of vitamin C can also result in anemia. Unlike some other creatures, humans do not synthesize vitamin C, so it must be obtained through food. Cooked meat, eggs, and dairy products do not contain vitamin C; raw vegetables, fruits, nuts, seeds, sprouts, and seaweeds do.

A partial list of natural vitamin C sources include the following raw foods: chard, kale, cabbage, cantaloupe, cauliflower, bell peppers, black currents, broccoli, Brussels sprouts, dandelion, grapefruit, guava, kiwi, red berries, rose hips, oranges, parsley, spinach, lemon, and tangerines.

Milk is *not* a good source of iron.

Meat is also *not* a good source of iron.

The iron in meat is heme iron (blood iron). A study conducted by researchers at the Harvard University School of Public Health found that high levels of heme iron raised the risk of heart disease. The iron found in vegetables is non-heme iron, does not lead to iron-loading, and is utilized by the body differently from the iron found in meat. (*Circulation*, 1994; 89:969-74)

It is pretty much impossible to be deficient in iron on a vegan diet right in raw fruits and vegetables, because it includes such a variety of plant substances that are both rich in iron and in vitamin C.

"Heme iron primarily from red meat has been positively associated with myocardial infarction and fatal coronary heart disease."

– Red Meat Consumption and Mortality, An Pan, PhD, Frank B. Hu, MD, et al; Harvard School of Public Health; *Archives of Internal Medicine*, March 12, 2012. Study tracked 37,698 men from the Harvard Health Professionals Follow-Up Study and 83,644 women from the Harvard Nurses Health Study for more than 20 years.

"In 1998, a collaborative analysis using original data from 5 prospective studies was reviewed and reported in the journal *Public Health Nutriton*. It compared ischemic heart disease-specific death rate ratios of vegetarians and nonvegetarians. The vegetarians had a 24 percent reduction in ischemic heart disease death rates compared with nonvegetarians. The lower risk of ischemic heart disease may be related to lower cholesterol levels in individuals who consume less meat."

– Nutrional Update for Physicians: Plant-based Diets, Dr. Michael Greger, NutritionFacts.org

"The United States spends more money per capita on health care than any country on earth, yet when the quality of our health care is compared with other industrialized nations, we rank near the bottom."

– T. Colin Campbell, in his book, *Whole: Rethinking the Science of Nutrition*. Campbell is Professor Emeritus of Nutritonal Biochemistry at Cornell University. He advises a low-fat vegan diet with no added (bottled) oils, no salt, no processed sugars, but with whole plant foods. He is also author of *The China Study*; TColinCampbell.org

"If one wants to live a long time, if one wants to see their grandchildren grow up – not just reach age 10 or 20, but reach age 50 – so you really find out what happens to them, you have got to survive, and you can't survive by blocking your intestinal tract with bovine muscle."

– Dr. William Clifford Roberts, Editor-in-Chief of the *American Journal of Cardiology*; Executive Director of the Baylor Cardiovascular Institute; former Head of Pathology section of the National Heart, Blood, and Lung Institute of the National Institutes of Health

"Heme iron intake from red meat sources is positively associated with the risk of type 2 diabetes."

– Dietary iron intake and blood donations risk in relation to risk of Type 2 diabetes in men: a prospective cohort study. *American Journal of Clinical Nutrition*, 2004.

MYTH: VEGANS DO NOT GET ENOUGH VITAMIN B-12

TRUTH: There is some truth in this, but only when you consider those who are limiting their diet to certain foods. A nonvegetarian diet can also provide insufficient amounts of B-12. Many nonvegetarians test low for B-12. Vegetarians and vegans are more likely to test low.

The broad claim that vegans and vegetarians don't get enough B-12 does not take into consideration that not all vegans and vegetarians follow the same diet. Some eat a lot of junk veggie food. Others don't.

The bacteria naturally living in the mouth, throat, and intestines supplies some B-12. Many foods found in natural foods stores where vegetarians often do their shopping are fortified with B-12. But eating processed or cooked foods is not necessary to obtain B-12.

Vegetarians who do not eat a balanced diet have the potential of experiencing nutritional deficiencies in the same way as people who are not vegetarians. A key to nutrition is to eat a variety of healthful foods, and not empty calories, or sugary, salty, bleached, refined, processed, fried, or cooked junk.

Some people believe that B-12 supplements are not needed when a person is following a healthy vegan diet that contains a variety of plant substances. Whether or not a diverse diet of plant matter is supplying enough B-12 depends on a number of factors.

Sources for B-12 in a healthy vegan diet include the following foods: raw (not pasteurized) fermented foods made in wood vats (raw kimchi, raw sauerkraut, etc.); nutritional yeast fortified with B-12 (not brewer's yeast); organically grown raw fruits and vegetables; rejuvelac, which is a raw fermented food; certain mushrooms, including white button mushrooms, which have been found to contain B-12; spirulina, chlorella, and other raw water vegetables; and grass juices and/or powders using grasses grown in organic soil.

Seaweeds may contain inactive B-12 analogs, and may be lacking in active forms of B-12. The analogs can take up the same receptor sites in cells, and also give a false positive on blood tests done to measure a person's B-12. Chlorella and spirulina are often given as examples of B-12-rich vegan foods, but they should not be held as the only source.

In 1996 the U.S. Department of Agriculture and the Department of Health and Human Services published a revised form of its *Dietary*

Guidelines for America. The guidelines are revised every five years and are used to create federal nutrition programs (such as for schools), nutritional labeling, and the *Food Guide Pyramid* (which is largely influenced by the meat, dairy, and egg industries that lobby heavily among elected officials and their associates to get the various government offices to promote the consumption of meat, dairy, and eggs, and to get government subsidies [corporate welfare] to keep flowing into the animal farming and associated industries [grain farming]). For the first time, the guidelines that were released in 1996 endorsed a vegetarian diet, but it included a message that vegetarians may need to supplement their diet with B-12.

Vegetarians and vegans often take B-12 supplements. These products are inexpensive and do not have to be derived from animal products. B-12 is chiefly made by bacteria. There are vegan vitamin supplements available in most natural foods stores. A person desiring to avoid animal products should make sure the label of the B-12 supplements indicates that the vitamin is derived from vegetable bacteria and not from beef liver, cod liver oil, or other part of a killed creature.

Many authorities in the vegan community encourage vegans to take a methylcobalamin B-12 supplement – not cyanocobalamin, which is a cheap form of B-12 that also contains cyanide, and is often used in processed foods. Methylcobalamine is a coenzyme form of B-12 that is more bioavailable, and is more easily absorbed into the system.

Expectant mothers, women who are breastfeeding, and those expecting to become pregnant should be sure to get sufficient B-12 (and a wide variety of other nutrients – especially those present in raw fruits and raw vegetables).

Those concerned about not getting enough B-12 can discard their concerns by taking a vegan B-12 supplement. There is no reason to lose sleep over this issue. (Access: VeganHealth.org.)

There is more about B-12 on page 330.

MYTH: VEGANS ARE SHORT

TRUTH: A 1991 study that appeared in the *European Journal of Clinical Nutrition* that involved 1,765 children found that those children who were mostly vegetarian (ate meat less than once per week) were taller than those who ate meat.

I started becoming a vegetarian when I was 10. I'm a hair under six feet tall. I know people who have been vegan their entire lives, and are taller than me.

There is no shortage of tall people in the vegan community.

People spewing such unfounded claims about vegans are often the very same people who don't understand the basics of nutrition, such as those who perpetuate misguided concepts about protein. They may also be the very same ones following the standard American diet that is rich in animal protein, heavily cooked foods, and the chemically saturated commercial foods that trigger disease. Depending on them for any sort of nutrition information is like depending on nutritonal supplements for the best nutrition.

Don't concern yourself with adjusting your diet everytime you hear a whim from misinformed persons who clearly don't know what they are talking about.

Avoid the chemical storm that is the common diet of people living in commercialized, industrialized, marketized society.

Follow a diet consisting chiefly of a variety of raw fruits and raw vegetables, and you will get the nutrients you need.

"Any food that requires enhancing by the use of chemical substances should in no way be considered food."
– John H. Tobe

"The only foods that contain immune-strengthening and cancer-fighting nutrients are plant foods."
– Mike Anderson

MYTH: VEGANS ARE WEAK

TRUTH: Tell that to 2012 welterweight boxing champ Timothy Bradley. Tell that to Mac Danzig, mixed martial arts champion. Tell it to boxer Keith Holmes. Tell it to Patrick Baboumian, Germany's 2011 Strongest Man winner. Tell it to Jane Wetzel, the U.S. National marathon champion. Tell it to running back Montell Owens. World champion discus thrower Ingra Manecki is vegetarian. Ridgely Abele, the winner of eight national championships in karate is vegan. Dave Scott, who won the Ironman contest six times, is a vegan. Stan Price, the world weight-lifting record holder in the bench press, is also a vegetarian. Scott Jurek, who won the Badwater race twice, is a vegan. Ironman triathlete Brendan Brazier is vegan. Bill Manetti, the power-lifting champion is vegetarian. In 2011, boxer Mike Tyson said he is on a vegan diet. Michael Arnstein, who won the Vermont 100-mile race in 2011, is vegan. As he cleaned up his act, in 2012, Lance Armstrong was training for a marathon while following a largely low-fat vegan diet.

"As a former world-class triathlete, I can assure you that athletes prosper on a plant-based diet. It's not just me who feels this way. So do the mixed martial arts fighter Mac Danzig, the Detroit Tigers home run slugger Prince Fielder, the golfer Phil Mickelson, the arm wrestler Rob Bigwood, the tennis greats Martina Navratilova and Billy Jean King and the boxer Mike Tyson, as well as the ultra-distance athletes Rich Roll and Scott Jurek."
– Rip Esselstyn, author of the low-fat vegan book, *The Engine 2 Diet: The Texas Firefighters' 28-Day Save-Your-Life Plan that Lowers Cholesterol and Burns Away the Pounds;* Farms2Forks.com

"Flesh, the muscle that we eat from pigs, cows, sheep, goats, fish, contains a lot of protein. And it turns out that the more protein we take in, the more calcium we lose from our bones. So, it is my understanding that osteoporosis, the thinning of the bones, which is so common in women in this country late in life – pure vegetarian fruit eaters infrequently get osteoporosis."
– Dr. William Clifford Roberts, Editor-in-Chief of the *American Journal of Cardiology*; Executive Director of the Baylor Cardiovascular Institute; former Head of Pathology section of the National Heart, Blood, and Lung Institute of the National Institutes of Health

MYTH: VEGANS DO NOT GET ENOUGH CHOLESTEROL

TRUTH: Cholesterol is made by human body cells, it helps the brains of babies to develop, and it is part of the cellular structure of the body. Babies benefit from the cholesterol in mother's milk – and their livers make it. Adults have no need for getting cholesterol through food.

As with babies, who get cholesterol from mother's milk, our system needs cholesterol, but all of the cholesterol we need is made by our liver. This self-generated cholesterol is called *blood cholesterol.*

Animal protein, as in all varieties of meat, dairy, and eggs, contains cholesterol and saturated fat. When we eat foods containing cholesterol, that cholesterol is *dietary cholesterol.*

When meat, dairy, or eggs are eaten by a human, the cholesterol ends up in their system, leading to an excess of cholesterol above what their liver makes for their needs. The excess cholesterol is what leads to plaque in the cardiovascular system, and that is disease that leads to heart attacks and strokes. *Dietary cholesterol* only comes from eating animal protein, never from eating plants. Fruits, vegetables, nuts, and seeds do not contain cholesterol.

The saturated fat in meat, dairy, and eggs triggers our liver to form more cholesterol than we need, and that also contributes to disease. While some plant substances contain saturated fats, plants also contain fiber that helps remove cholesterol from the system.

> "Fiber, found only in plant foods, has many health-promoting qualities. It binds with carcinogens, fats, and cholesterol and eliminates them in the feces. By eliminating carcinogens, it reduces your risk of developing cancer, and by eliminating fat and cholesterol, it reduces your risk of heart disease, atherosclerosis, and obesity. Fiber also improves the efficiency of insulin, so that we need less of it to maintain appropriate blood-sugar levels."
> – Dr. John McDougall, DrMcDougall.com

Strict vegetarians, those who abstain from animal products, have healthier cardiovascular systems than people who regularly eat mammals, birds, fish, or other animals, but also milk products, and eggs – which all contain saturated fat and cholesterol. People with high cholesterol also

51

experience higher rates of a variety of diseases, including diabetes, Alzheimer's, MS, and cancer.

However, vegetarians that eat an unhealthy vegetarian diet, such as one that includes dairy, including milk, butter, cream, ice cream, and cheese; fried and sautéed foods, processed sugars, salty foods, abundant bottled oils, bleached starches, and vegetarian junk food can develop cardiovascular disease. A fat-heavy diet triggers the body to create more cholesterol, and also can damage the endothelium, which is the lining in the cardiovascular and lymph systems. An unhealthy vegetarian diet can lead to heart attacks and strokes.

> "Cholesterol is a white, waxy substance that is not found in plants – only in animals. It is an essential component of the membrane that coats all our cells, and it is the basic ingredient of sex hormones. Our bodies need cholesterol, and they manufacture it on their own. We do not need to eat it. But we do, when we consume meat, poultry, fish, and other animal-based foods, such as dairy products and eggs. In doing so, we take on excess amounts of the substance. What's more, eating fat causes the body itself to manufacture excessive amounts of cholesterol, which explains why vegetarians who eat oil, butter, cheese, milk, ice cream, glazed donuts, and French pastry develop coronary disease despite their avoidance of meat."
> – Dr. Caldwell B. Esselstyn, author of *Prevent and Reverse Heart Disease*; HeartAttackProof.com

The main reason eaters of animal protein experience heart attacks and strokes is that their cardiovascular systems have been damaged by eating animals, dairy, and cheese, as well as transfats, processed sugars, and other junk. The majority of the people waiting for heart transplants are doing so because their hearts have been damaged from years of eating meat, dairy, egg products, transfats, processed sugar, salty foods, and junk food, and weakened by stress and lack of exercise.

Switching to a low-fat vegan diet consisting of mostly raw fruits and vegetables can help reverse damage an animal protein-, fat-, and sugar-rich diet has done to the cardiovascular system. A low-fat vegan diet will also lower the risk of experiencing diabetes, macular degeneration, cancer, and other chronic and degenerative diseases.

If you want to experience vibrant health, completely rid your body of dietary cholesterol, which means: Follow a vegan diet, and preferably one that is rich in raw plant matter, low in fat, and that does not contain an abundance of nuts, avocado, or bottled oils, and that contains no sautéed or fried oils whatsoever.

For more information on reversing heart disease through following a vegan diet and exercise regimen, see various books written by doctors Caldwell Esselstyn, Neal Barnard, Michael Klaper, T. Colin Campbell, Dean Ornish, and John McDougall.

"Cardiovascular disease kills about 45 percent of adults in the U.S. Heart failure is the biggest cause of hospitalization in the U.S. in people age 65 and over.

There is no question that if the U.S. became a vegetarian society, fruit-eating society, that the health of this nation would skyrocket.

Fish is flesh. Fish has cholesterol in it, just like cows, pigs, sheep, goats, chickens, turkeys. In actuality, for every 100 grams of cow muscle, or pig muscle, or chicken muscle, or fish muscle, there is about the same amount of cholesterol in there.

If you are purely thinking of it from the standpoint of cholesterol, it does no good to switch from cows to fish.

There's not as much fish in the oceans and lakes as there used to be, and when societies grow to 10 billion people, or 12 billion people, from 6 billion, there is not going to be enough fish.

Flesh, the muscle that we eat from pigs, cows, sheep, goats, fish, contains a lot of protein. And it turns out that the more protein we take in, the more calcium we lose from our bones. So, it is my understanding that osteoporosis, the thinning of the bones, which is so common in women in this country late in life – pure vegetarian fruit eaters infrequently get osteoporosis."

– Dr. William Clifford Roberts, Editor-in-Chief of the *American Journal of Cardiology*; Executive Director of the Baylor Cardiovascular Institute; former Head of Pathology section of the National Heart, Blood, and Lung Institute of the National Institutes of Health

"Could you look an animal in the eyes and say to it, 'My appetite is more important than your suffering?'"

– Moby

"So often, I hear people say, 'You do your thing, I'll do mine. You may choose to eat vegetables and fruit, and nuts and grains, I choose to eat meat and dairy.' That argument is basically and dangerously flawed, because the most interested party – the one being killed – is not party to the discussion."

– Marybeth Wosko

MYTH: VEGANS ARE DEFICIENT IN CHOLINE, ARACHIDONIC ACID, AND CARNITINE

TRUTH: Humans make arachidonic acid from the linoleic oils in plants. That is what herbivores do. Humans are herbivores – animals that do best on a plant-based diet. It is carnivores that do not, or do not easily, convert plant oils into arachidonic acid. Carnivores get arachidonic acid by eating meat. Humans naturally get their arachidonic acid by converting plant oils. When humans eat a diet rich in arachidonic acid, such as by eating meat, egg yolks, and oily fish, they are more likely to experience inflammation, including rheumatoid diseases.

There are dozens of types of rheumatoid diseases, which are largely autoimmune diseases in which the body attacks its own tissues. Some of the most common are rheumatoid arthritis, osteoarthritis, infectious arthritis, juvenile idiopathic arthritis, gout, lupus, Sjogren's syndrome, Ankylosing spondylitis, polymyalgia rheumatica, scleroderma, vasculitis, and fibromyalgia. One reason why people experiencing rheumatoid diseases respond very well to following a vegan diet is because the dietary arachidonic acid is eliminated, reducing inflammation.

"In *The Lancet*, a prominent British medical journal, researchers reported that a specially designed vegetarian diet could greatly reduce the signs and symptoms of arthritis. In the study, researchers found that a vegetarian diet lessened joint stiffness, swelling, and tenderness, and improved grip strength. The benefits lasted long after the study was over."
– Dr. Neal Barnard, author of *Foods That Fight Pain*

People with joint pain, connective tissue pain, back issues, tennis elbow, tendinitis, and other health issues relating to inflammation greatly benefit from eliminating dietary arachidonic acid, which means, following a completely vegan diet.

An abundance of arachidonic acid stimulates the production of pro-inflammatory prostaglandins and leukotrienes. This increases the likelihood of cancer as irritated cells are more likely to be susceptible to damage from free radicals, and to attract more blood flow and form capillaries. When cancer cells develop significant blood vessels, which is a process called angiogenesis – that is when the cells start to grow. Everyone has dormant cancer cells, and certain things either trigger those cancer cells to divide and grow, or work against the cancer, such as foods containing antiangiogenesis compounds.

The development of cancer is especially more likely if the diet contains dairy products and mammal meat, which contain the inflammatory neu5Gc molecule that can bind to cell walls, making cancer more aggressive. The neu5Gc molecule is a proangiogenesis compound, meaning that it promotes cancer growth.

As mentioned elsewhere in the book, neu5Gc is often found on human cancer cells and the only way it gets into the body is by eating dairy products or nonhuman mammal meat (humans are mammals, but they do not make the neu5Gc molecule). These are some of the reasons why people who have been diagnosed with cancer do well on a low-fat vegan diet rich in raw fruits and raw vegetables, even to the point of completely ridding themselves of cancer.

Diets rich in arachidonic acid, that is, diets rich in meat, eggs, and oily fish, also increase inflammation of the cardiovascular system, increase blood pressure, and increase risk of heart attacks and strokes. The increase in inflammation of the cardiovascular system is also partially caused by the free radical damage that is more likely to happen on a diet rich in arachidonic acid. This helps to explain why those with cardiovascular disease experience a reversal of their condition when switching to a low-fat vegan diet rich in raw fruits and vegetables.

Diets rich in arachidonic acid, which is an omega-6 fatty acid, interfere with cell membrane function, increasing the likelihood of toxins staying in the body, and nutrients not being absorbed easily through cell walls, which are made of lipids (fats) and lipid derivatives. This is one reason why people following a low-fat vegan diet rich in raw fruits and vegetables are more likely to experience a healthful weight.

Yes, arachidonic acid is a necessary nutrient. But humans do not need to get arachidonic acid from eating meat, eggs, or oily fish. Humans make the arachidonic acid that they need. Any additional arachidonic acid in the system can cause a variety of health problems, including autoimmune disorders, inflammation, and cancer.

> "Plasma TMAO levels predict the risk of incident major adverse cardiovascular events independently of traditional cardiovascular risk."
> – Intestinal microbial metabolism of phosphatidylcholine and cardiovascular risk, *New England Journal of Medicine*, April 25, 2013

The claim that vegans are deficient in carnitine is nonsense. The human body forms the carnitine that it needs. Eating meat to get carnitine, or taking carnitine supplements is problematic as the breakdown of carnitine by gut bacteria forms trimethylamine (TMA), which is then broken down by the liver, forming trimethylamine N-oxide (TMAO), which then enters the bloodstream. A high TMAO count in the bloodstream is one cause of the collection of cholesterol plaque in the veins, arteries, and capillaries, which is atherosclerosis. This increases the incidence of heart attacks and strokes. TMAO is also an inflammatory substance and plays a role in the incidence of cancer and autoimmune diseases. Meat, dairy, fish, and eggs all contain carnitine and eating them increases the TMAO content in the blood, increasing disease risk, including kidney disease as it is the kidneys that help filter out TMAO (see: Accumulation of trimethylamine and trimethylamine N-oxide in end-stage renal disease patients undergoing haemodialysis; *Nephrology Dialysis Transplantation Journal*, Vol. 21, issue 5, pp. 1300-1304).

Some sports drinks, energy drinks, and supplements contain carnitine. These should be avoided. There is a small amount of carnitine in fruits, vegetables, and grains. Beef is particularly rich in carnitine, 100 grams of beef contains 95 mg. 100 grams of pork contains 27.7 mg; 100 grams of chicken contains 9.9 mg; and 100 grams of cod contains 5.6 mg. One medium avocado contains about 2 mg, and 100 grams of other fruits, vegetables, nuts, and seeds contain less than 1 mg.

"Intestinal microbiota metabolism of choline and phosphatidylcholine produce trimethylamine, which further metabolized to a proatherogenic species, trimethylamine N-oxide."
– Intestinal microbiota metabolism of L-Carnitine promotes atherosclerosis; researchers at Cleveland Clinic, *Nature*; April 7, 2013.

"Malignant prostate cells have higher risk of choline concentration than do healthy cells, and choline kinase is overexpressed in prostate cancer."
– Intake of meat, fish, poultry, and eggs and risk of prostate cancer progression, *American Journal of Clinical Nutrition*, 2010.

Lecithin in eggs is broken down into choline, which has a similar chemical structure to carnitine. Eating eggs increases the level of TMAO in the blood, and has been identified specifically as increasing the risk of lethal prostate cancer (see: Choline intake and risk of lethal prostate cancer: incidence and survival, *American Journal of Clinical Nutrition*, 2012).

It is good to avoid foods with added lecithin, such as baked goods with lecithin as an ingredient. Don't use lecithin supplements.

A most interesting conclusion of these studies: Scientists have found that vegans lack the gut bacteria that breaks down carnitine and choline into TMA. The bacteria are associated with animal protein ingestion.

The choline in fruits, vegetables, nuts, and seeds is beneficial to health, and, on a vegan diet, does not play a role in the problematic rise of TMAO in the bloodstream.

MYTH: VEGAN DIETS ARE NOT HEALTHFUL

TRUTH: Meats, milk, and eggs contain saturated fat, cholesterol, and concentrated protein, have no fiber, contain no vitamin C, and are not a source of complex carbohydrates. Saturated fat, cholesterol, and animal protein trigger many health problems, such as obesity, gallstones, kidney stones, arthritis, osteoporosis, high blood pressure, heart disease, strokes, certain eye diseases, diabetes, Alzheimer's, Parkinson's, MS, erectile dysfunction, varicose veins, and hormone-dependent cancers.

Diabetics are more likely to suffer the ravages of diabetes if they consume meat and dairy products and follow a diet lacking in fresh fruits and vegetables. According to the American Academy of Pediatrics, "the avoidance of cow's milk protein for the first several months of life may reduce the later development of IDDM (insulin-dependent diabetes) or delay its onset in susceptible individuals."

Vegans have lower rates of cancers of the breast, lungs, colon, rectum, prostate, and the reproductive organs. They are more likely to avoid toxic farming chemicals, and they are not consuming the harmful mutagenic chemicals that form when meat, eggs, and dairy are cooked. They are also not consuming the Neu5Gc cell-surface molecule that exists in meat and dairy. This molecule (N-glycolylneuraminic acid) is synthesized in nonhuman mammals, such as cows, pigs, and lambs, but humans lack the enzymes needed to synthesize it. In humans, the Neu5Gc molecule can adhere to the surface of cells and trigger an immune response, causing inflammation and bringing more blood to the area, which can feed pre-cancerous cells. Neu5Gc is often found on the surface of human cancer cells, and it only gets into the human body through eating animal products.

"Recent research confirms a strong connection between impotence and cardiovascular disease. In December 2005, researchers reported on a study that followed 3,816 men with erectile dysfunction and 4,247 without over seven years. It turned out that the men who were impotent before the study began or who developed it during the study were 45 percent more likely to experience a cardiovascular event than those free of erectile dysfunction. Impotence, it turns out, is as robust a predictor of

cardiovascular disease as elevated cholesterol, smoking, or a strong family history of the diseases."
– Dr. Caldwell B. Esselstyn, author of *Prevent and Reverse Heart Disease*; HeartAttackProof.com

Men who consume animal protein are more likely to experience prostate cancer and erectile dysfunction than men who are vegan. There is no doubt about it, men who eat meat, milk, and eggs are more likely to experience problems downstairs. As T. Colin Campbell states in *The China Study*, "The totality and breadth of the evidence, operating through highly coordinated networks, supports the conclusions that consuming dairy and meat are serious risk factors for prostate cancer."

In other words, men, if you want to remain fit, strong, and keep the tools functioning and healthy, go vegan. Otherwise, you may be dealing with prostate cancer. Choosing to undergo the common medical treatments for prostate cancer, including surgery and radiation, if successful, can leave a man experiencing incontinence, radiation-induced bowel injury, nerve damage, infections, and impotence.

If it isn't clear to you by now, you should understand that a low-fat vegan diet rich in raw fruits and vegetables is also widely beneficial to women, including for the prevention of breast cancer.

Many women have been convinced that they are strongly predisposed to experiencing breast cancer, even to the point of undergoing mastectomies as a preventive measure when they have not been diagnosed with breast cancer. The National Cancer Institute refers to this procedure as *preventive mastectomy, prophylactic mastectomy*, or *risk-reducing mastectomy*.

What is the best preventive measure for reducing the risk of breast cancer? A clean, low-fat, plant-based diet along with regular exercise, and reducing or eliminating the use of products containing synthetic chemicals that have been linked to breast cancer (such as chemicals used in many widely used cosmetics, antiperspirants, and skin and haircare products). The genes increasing the likelihood of cancer may be there, but there are triggers that turn genes on, or off. Undergoing mastectomy as a preventive measure isn't going to reduce your risk of other cancers and health problems you may experience if you continue following a high-fat, junk diet rich in animal protein, and using toxic bodycare products.

"Countries with a higher intake of fat, especially fat from animal products, such as meat and dairy products, have a higher incidence of breast cancer. In Japan, for example, the traditional diet is much lower in fat, especially animal fat, than the typical western diet, and breast cancer rates are low. In the late 1940s, when breast cancer was particularly rare in Japan, less than 10 percent of the calories in the Japanese diet came from fat. The American diet is centered on animal products, which tend to be high in fat and low in other important nutrients, with 30 to 35 percent of calories coming from fat. When Japanese girls are raised on westernized diets, their rate of breast cancer increases dramatically. Even within Japan, affluent women who eat meat daily have an 8.5 times higher risk of breast cancer than poorer women who rarely or never eat meat. One of the proposed reasons is that fatty foods boost the hormones that promote cancer."

   – *Meat Consumption and Cancer Risk*, The Cancer Project, Physicians
   Committee for Responsible Medicine, CancerProject.org

Women who eat an abundance of vegetables have a 48 percent lower risk of breast cancer (*Journal of the National Cancer Institute*, January 18, 1995). The more meat a woman eats, the more likely she is to get breast cancer. A study led by doctors at Harvard Medical School, which was published in the November 13, 2006 issue of the *Archives of Internal Medicine,* concluded that women who eat more than 1½ servings of meat per day were nearly twice as likely to develop hormone-related breast cancer than those who ate fewer than three portions per week. The study used information being gathered by the ongoing Nurses' Health Study that began tracking the health and lifestyles of more than 90,000 women nearly two decades ago. Even after factoring the cigarette habits and obesity issues among the women in the study, it still concluded that those women who ate more meat experienced more breast cancer than those who ate less red meat. The study also mentioned that eating red meat greatly increases the risk of colorectal cancer.

Heavy people experience more health problems than those who are reasonably thin. Simply because fruits and vegetables contain fiber and more bulk, vegans are less likely to be overweight than the general population (Another Reason for Vegetarianism – Reduced Health Care Costs, *Vegetarian Journal*, July-August 1996).

"Meat and dairy products contribute to many forms of cancer, including cancer of the colon, breast, and prostate. Colon cancer has been directly linked to meat consumption. High-fat diets also encourage the body's production of estrogens, in particular, estradiol. Increased levels of this sex hormone have been linked to breast cancer. One recent study linked dairy products to an increased risk of ovarian cancer. The process of breaking down the lactose (milk sugar) into galactose evidently damages the ovaries.

Vegetarians avoid the animal fat linked to cancer and get abundant fiber and vitamins that help to prevent cancer. In addition,

blood analysis of vegetarians reveals a higher level of natural killer cells, specialized white blood cells that attack cancer cells."
– VegInfo.Org/Health

It is true that a person can claim to be a vegan and eat mostly junk food, but vegans are more likely to be nutritionally aware and to eat a more healthful diet than people who eat meat, eggs, dairy products, and junk food. People who eat a low-fat, raw or mostly raw vegan diet are more likely than the typical vegan to be aware of nutrition.

"Vegetarians have been reported to have lower body mass indexes than nonvegetarians, as well as lower rates of death from ischemic heart disease; vegetarians also show lower blood cholesterol levels; lower blood pressure; and lower rates of hypertension, Type-2 diabetes, and prostate and colon cancer."
– *Journal of the American Dietetic Association*; Vol. 103, No. 6; 2003

"Veganism gives us all the opportunity to say what we stand for in life. The ideal of healthy, humane living is now easy with modern transport bringing us vegan foods from all over the world. Join us and add decades of health to your life, with a clear conscience as a bonus."
– Donald Watson, who coined the word "vegan," and founded the Vegan Society

"The quantity of antibiotics and hormones that are given to the animals that we eat make the antibiotics less sensitive when used in humans with certain infections, so we use WAY too many antibiotics. We've got to diminish that. Now, some young girls, age 7, their bosoms are coming out. It may be related to all of these hormones that are put into the animals so that they (the animals) grow bigger and quicker." (Early pubescence is linked to higher rates of breast cancer.)
– Dr. William Clifford Roberts, Editor-in-Chief of the *American Journal of Cardiology*; Executive Director of the Baylor Cardiovascular Institute; former Head of Pathology section of the National Heart, Blood, and Lung Institute of the National Institutes of Health

"I now consider veganism to be the ideal diet. A vegan diet – particularly one that is low in fat – will substantially reduce disease risks. Plus, we've seen no disadvantages from veganism."
– T. Colin Campbell, Ph.D., Cornell University; author of *The China Study* and *Whole: Rethinking the Science of Nutrition*; TColinCampbell.org

MYTH: VEGANS LACK NUTRIENTS BECAUSE MEAT, MILK, AND EGGS CONTAIN MORE NUTRIENTS THAN FRUITS, VEGETABLES, NUTS, OR SEEDS

TRUTH: Let's do this as a question and answer: What has more nutrients per calorie than meat, milk, or eggs?

Answer: All of these raw fruits, vegetables, nuts, and seeds: germinated alfalfa seeds or sprouts, soaked almonds, arugula, artichokes, asparagus, apples, bell peppers, blackberries, blueberries, bok choy, broccoli, germinated or sprouted broccoli seeds, Brussels sprouts, germinated buckwheat, cabbage, cantaloupe, carrots, cauliflower, chard, cherries, germinated chia seeds, cilantro, collard greens, corn, cucumbers, dandelion greens, fennel, flax seeds, goji berries, seeded grapes, hemp seeds, kale, kidney beans, germinated lentils, mango, nectarines, oatmeal, oranges, parsley, peaches, peas, pineapple, pistachios, pomegranate seeds, germinated quinoa, romaine lettuce, sesame seeds, spinach, strawberries, sprouts, germinated sunflower seeds, sweet potatoes, tangerines, tomatoes, and many more fruits, vegetables, nuts, and germinated and sprouted seeds.

All of those fruits, vegetables, nuts, and seeds contain fiber. Meat, milk, and eggs do **not** contain fiber. One sesame seed, or flax seed, or chia seed, or hemp seed, or sunflower seed, or pomegranate seed contains more fiber than any amount of meat, eggs, or milk.

Meat, dairy, and eggs are **not** good sources of antioxidants, but **are** rich in free radicals, which damage tissues, including those of the cardiovascular system and the eyes. Raw plants contain an abundance of antioxidants, which prevent damage from free radicals.

"If there's anything I love more than rock and roll, it's animals. And when I learned how animals on factory farms are treated, I gave beef the boot and stopped eating pigs, chickens, turkeys, and fish. Cutting meat out of your diet is the best thing you can do for animals and your own health."

– Joan Jett

MYTH: ALL VEGANS ARE HEALTHIER THAN PEOPLE WHO EAT MEAT

TRUTH: Some vegetarians and vegans eat a lot of junk foods containing transfats, fried foods, and an abundance of fats, sugars, salts, and gluten grains, and also processed starches, corn syrup, and artificial sweeteners. Some nonvegetarians follow a low-fat diet that is more balanced, containing fresh vegetables and fruits, while avoiding junk food, synthetic chemicals, and added oils. In this case, the nonvegetarians following a more healthful diet may win – but not the animals.

"Two themes consistently emerge from studies of cancer from many sites: vegetables and fruits help to reduce risk, while meat, animal products, and other fatty foods are frequently found to increase risk. Consumption of dietary fat drives production of hormones, which, in turn, promotes growth of cancer cells in hormone-sensitive organs such as the breast and prostate. Meat is devoid of the protective effects of fiber, antioxidants, phytochemicals, and other helpful nutrients, and it contains high concentrations of saturated fat and potentially carcinogenic compounds, which may increase one's risk of developing many different kinds of cancer.

Vegetarian diets and diets rich in high-fiber plant foods such as whole grains, legumes, vegetables, and fruits offer a measure of protection. Fiber greatly speeds the passage of food through the colon, effectively removing carcinogens, and fiber actually changes the type of bacteria that is present in the intestine, so there is reduced production of carcinogenic secondary bile acids. Plant foods are also naturally low in fat and rich in antioxidants and other anticancer compounds. Not surprisingly, vegetarians are at the lowest risk for cancer and have a significantly reduced risk compared to meat eaters."

– *Meat Consumption and Cancer Risk*, The Cancer Project, Physicians Committee for Responsible Medicine, CancerProject.org

MYTH: YOU NEED TO EAT FROM THE "BASIC FOUR FOOD GROUPS"

TRUTH: The *Basic Four Food Groups* promoted by the animal farming industry interests were designed by the U.S. Department of Agriculture in 1956. The USDA largely functions as a public relations office and government concierge service for the meat, dairy, egg, and grain industries. With industry influence, they came up with the "four food groups" idea to increase the profits of the rapidly expanding animal farming industry. The colorful teaching materials used to convince children they need to eat meat, dairy, and eggs are supplied free in America by the animal farming industry. These promotional materials should not be allowed in schools. They promote a diet that greatly increases the likelihood of experiencing a variety of diseases, including cancers, diabetes, kidney disease, osteoporosis, Alzheimer's, Parkinson's, Crohn's, arthritis, MS, and cardiovascular disease.

> "The standard four food groups are based on American agricultural lobbies. Why do we have a milk group? Because we have a National Dairy Council. Why do we have a meat group? Because we have an extremely powerful meat lobby."
> – Dr. Marion Nestle, Professor, Department of Nutrition, Food Studies, and Public Health, New York University

Eating the meat, egg, and dairy promoted by the animal farming industry increases the incidence of osteoporosis, heart disease, cancers, diabetes, arthritis, strokes, high blood pressure, and other common health problems, including erectile dysfunction.

> "Vegetarian diets decrease the risk of cancer."
> – The World Cancer Research Fund and the American Institute of Cancer Research, 1997

Sunfoodists have their own basic eight food groups that are a recipe for health: fruits, vegetables, legumes, nongluten grains, germinated seeds, sprouted seeds, soaked nuts, and sea vegetables. These should be combined with an active life that includes exercise, the creating of a healthy atmosphere, and the utilization of talents and intellect to build a healthy and fulfilling existence.

63

MYTH: HUMANS ARE CARNIVORES; THEREFORE THEY NEED TO EAT MEAT

TRUTH: The teeth and mouths of humans are very different from the teeth and mouths of carnivores, such as animals in the cat, dog, and bear families. Carnivores have sharp teeth and wide mouths framed by snouts and can bite, lock, and tear at meat. Some people say the omnivore shape of human teeth suggests that humans are meant for a diet of both plant and meat content. Other people say that because human teeth are short and smooth, the human jaw swivels in a grinding motion, and the mouths are small and relatively weak, they therefore are more structured for eating plants. (Animals that eat plants are known as herbivores.)

> "Let's see one of these so-called meat eaters kill and strip the flesh with their 'canine' teeth and eat the meat raw. I bet nobody could do that without gagging and puking."
> – Chris Dobson

Carnivores eat meat when it is raw. Humans are not natural meat eaters. When humans do eat meat they do so only after it has been tenderized or ground, then softened even more by cooking with high temperatures – and then, at last, sliced with a knife – and often saturated with some sort of flavoring, like catsup, mustard, hot sauce, and/or herbs. Humans don't even like the taste of raw meat, and hide the flavor.

Even after preparing, cooking, and cutting meat, humans often have a hard time chewing and swallowing the stuff – sometimes losing teeth and gagging to death during the process (the animals' revenge?).

The human mouth structures are only part of the picture. Those who say humans are meant to eat a plant-based diet may have their beliefs verified by taking the human digestive tract into consideration.

Human bowels are very different from the smooth and relatively straight bowels of meat eating animals. The human digestive tract is more than 10 times body length. Carnivores have a digestive tract that may be as long as their body. The puckered, long, and curved structures of the human digestive tract indicate that humans are more attuned to eating a fiber-rich plant-based diet. The stomach acids of the human are also much weaker than those of carnivores, and are more in balance with the stomach acid levels of herbivores.

Humans need fiber to help digest food. Meat, dairy, and eggs do not contain fiber. Humans who do not eat enough fiber have higher rates of serious diseases, including cardiovascular disease, colorectal cancer, and kidney disease, and also are more likely to have strokes.

A vegan diet rich in raw fruits and vegetables easily contains sufficient amounts of fiber.

Unlike carnivores, humans do not have claws that can tear into another animal to kill it and rip it open.

> "You can't tear flesh by hand. You can't tear hide by hand. Our anterior teeth are not suited for tearing flesh or hide. We don't have large canine teeth, and we wouldn't have been able to deal with food sources that required those large canines."
> – Dr. Richard Leakey, anthropologist

Carnivores can survive perfectly well on raw meat and water. If a human consumed nothing but raw or cooked meat and water, they would become sick, and they would die.

> "A recent study by Smith found that high-fat, high-protein, low-carbohydrate (HPLC) diets (which are usually high in red meat, such as the Atkins and Paleolithic diets) may accelerate atherosclerosis through mechanisms that are unrelated to the classic cardiovascular risk factors. Mice that were fed an HPLC diet had almost twice the level of arterial plaque as mice that were fed a Western diet even though the classic risk factors were not significantly different between groups. The mice that were fed the HPLC diet had markedly fewer circulating endothelial progenitor cells and higher levels of nonesterified fatty acids (promoting inflammation) than mice that were fed the Western diet."
> – Dr. Dean Ornish, Holy Cow! What's Good For You Is Good For Our Planet: Comment on "Red Meat Consumption and Mortality," *Archives of Internal Medicine*, March 12, 2012. Ornish is the founder of the Preventative Medicine Research Institute, PMRI.org

Carnivores lack sweat glands and they pant. Humans, and other herbivores, have sweat glands, and they sweat.

Humans are not carnivores. Nor are they omnivores. They flourish in health on a low-fat vegan diet rich in raw fruits and vegetables. The human nutritional requirement for animal protein is absolute zero.

> "Just because we can doesn't mean we should. Just because we always have doesn't mean we always have to. Once we know better, we should choose better."
> – Colleen Patrick-Goudreah

"Most of us believe that eating meat is natural because humans have hunted and consumed animals for millennia. And it is true that we have been eating meat as part of an omnivorous diet for at least two million years (though the majority of the time, our diet was still primarily vegetarian). But, to be fair, we must acknowledge that infanticide, murder, rape, and cannibalism are at least as old as meat eating, and are therefore arguably as 'natural' – and yet we don't invoke the history of these acts as justification for them. As with other acts of violence, when it comes to eating meat, we must differentiate between natural and justifiable."
– Dr. Melanie Joy

"Humans do not eat like carnivores. Carnivores bring down living prey and eat it raw and most predators target the soft organs leaving much of the muscle for scavengers. Humans eat dead flesh and rarely eat the organs, preferring the muscle tissue. Most of the beef that people eat has been dead for months, and in many cases for years. The meat is disguised with bleach and dyes in many cases to hide the decay and the fact that the flesh is putrid. We are closer in our eating habits to vultures and jackals than wolves and lions.

Technically speaking, humans are not carnivorous hominids. Humans fall into the necrovore category, which means the eating of dead flesh. Humans do not kill their meat so much as they scavenge it. Even hunters do not kill and eat the hot living flesh of their victims. They wait for the meat to get cold and begin the putrification process before consumption."
– Captain Paul Watson of SeaShepherd.org

"When we use race to devalue human persons, we call it racism.
When we use sex to devalue human persons, we call it sexism.
When we use sexual orientation or preference to devalue human persons, we call it heterosexism.
When we use age to devalue human persons, we call it ageism.
When we use species to devalue nonhuman persons, we call it specism.
All these forms of discrimination are wrong. Please reject them all."
– Gary L. Francione

"People who eat meat are eating bits of dead body. No meat eater should ever be allowed to forget the source of the food on his plate."
– Vernon Coleman

MYTH: RAW VEGANS ARE FRUITARIANS

TRUTH: Some people who consume only raw foods limit themselves to fruit (including fruits of the vine, such as tomatoes, squash, grapes, melon, cucumbers, berries, and peppers). But all raw foodists, or sunfoodists, are not fruitarians.

Some say that eating only fruit is karmically better than eating plants that have had their roots destroyed in the harvesting process because a fruit diet does not kill the plant. Examples of plants that are killed when they are harvested include onions, garlic, beets, carrots, ginger, and whole-picked green-leafed vegetables, such as lettuce, cabbage, fennel and celery.

There are those who call themselves fruitarians who eat a more rounded diet than others. While some may seek to limit themselves to sweet fruit, which isn't something I would advocate, other fruitarians also consume cucumbers, olives, tomatoes, bell peppers, squash, beans, melon, avocadoes, berries, grapes, figs, dates, carob, goji, nuts, and coconuts. They might also include substances derived from these, such as olive oil, coconut oil, and grapeseed oil, but others avoid oil extracts (bottled oils). When considering that a fruitarian diet can contain a variety of plant substances, it is easy to recognize that is doesn't have to be limited to sweet fruit.

I wouldn't support a diet that consists wholly of fruits and nothing but fruit. I think it is better to include a variety of plant substances in the diet, including and especially green-leafed vegetables, and also sprouts, germinates, herbs, sea vegetables, and other edible plants, such as ginger and root vegetables.

The roots of plants seek nutrients. The nutrients travel into the highest and outermost areas of the plants – the leaves, flowers, seeds. and fruits. As the sun and air evaporate water from the leaves, the roots continually bring in more water, and within that water are more nutrients. The plant is also producing natural chemicals that protect it from wind, heat, cold, insects, and bacteria. Through this process the leaves, flowers, and fruits become amazing biospheres of nutrients. Within those leaves, flowers, seeds, and fruits are the substances that the human body needs to build healthy tissues. Considering that each plant mines a different spectrum of substances from the soil and creates its own formulation of nutrients, it is easy to understand that consuming an assortment of plant matter is the way to get a variety of nutrients.

The man who owns the Website, TheFruitarian.com, is Michael Arnstein, a raw vegan who follows a low-fat diet consisting of fruits and vegetables, including leafy greens. Arnstein runs and wins 100-mile races, and, with his wife, Victoria, he founded the Woodstock Fruit Festival (TheWoodstockFruitFestival.com).

Arnstein's diet style is more in tune with the 80/10/10 style of eating suggested in the book, *The 80/10/10 Diet*, by Douglas Grahem. It suggests a vegan diet that consists of 80 percent carbohydrates, 10 percent fats, and 10 percent protein. After Arnstein read Graham's book, and adapted the diet, he began winning races.

"Aim to get 80 percent of your caolories from carbohydrates, 10 percent from fat, and 10 percent from protein."
– T. Colin Campbell, in his book, *Whole: Rethinking the Science of Nutrition*. Campbell is Professor Emeritus of Nutritonal Biochemistry at Cornell University, and has been involved in the science and research of nutrition for several decades. He advises a low-fat vegan diet with no added (bottled) oils, no salt, no processed sugars, but with whole plant foods. He is also author of *The China Study*; TColinCampbell.org

MYTH: BREATHARIANISM (ALSO KNOWN AS INEDIA) IS THE ULTIMATE GOAL OF VEGANS, VEGETARIANS, AND RAW FOODISTS

TRUTH: That is nonsense.

There are those who promote breatharianism or say the body needs very little food. The truth of that statement depends on what they mean by "very little food." If they are saying that the body needs a lot less food than what the average American eats, the statement holds some truth. Many people eat way too many calories, and from the worst types of foods. They also don't engage in the physical activity needed to use up even a healthful amount of calories. Evidence of this is displayed in the obesity problem that is rampant in America, and an increasing detriment to the health of people in many parts of the world. There are more overweight people than starving people.

Some people fraudulently claim that the body needs no food at all.

That concept is seriously flawed. People who promote this baloney often say that if a person were spiritually enlightened he or she would not need any food. They say that a person can survive on the *prana*, which is a Hindu word that they misuse and that means "vital life force." They say this prana is available in the air and through the energy available in the light of sun. Or they describe the ultimate nourishment as "pranic light," which is the light of God within us, and that we can survive on without any additional nourishment. They claim that it is possible to survive on the nutrients in the air that include carbon dioxide, hydrogen, nitrogen, oxygen, and even pollen from plants, as well as other airborne substances.

It is true that there are nutrients in air, and that the lungs can be described as digestive organs because they take in nutrients. But it should be blatantly clear that it is impossible to depend on air and light to provide all the nutrients the body needs for experiencing the best of health.

Even wild animals, beings that couldn't be living a more natural and spiritual existence, regularly eat food and drink water.

The body needs the nutrients in unheated plant substances to build and maintain healthy tissues. At the very least, these nutrients include the basics of amino acids, essential fatty acids, enzymes, vitamins, minerals, trace elements, carbohydrates, biophotons, antioxidants, and water. When it is taken into consideration that scientists continue to discover substances in plants that benefit health, it is obvious that there are many undiscovered substances within plants that the human body utilizes and needs to maintain health.

There are those who argue that breatharianism is legitimate because Tibetan monks practice it. The monks do what could be better described as fasting, and they do it for a limited amount of time. They may also follow a frugal diet.

It is said that as a young ascetic monk we know as Buddha survived on one hemp seed per day for several years before his enlightenment. Hemp seeds are nutritious because they contain enzymes, amino acids, essential fatty acids, minerals, vitamins, fiber, and other nutrients. No human could survive on one hemp seed per day. Perhaps he ate one handful of hemp seeds per day – in addition to fruits and vegetables, and water.

The sadhus (men) and sadvis (women) of the Hindu religion also practice long fasts. They spend their time in devotion to deities and are said to renunciate their attachment to the world, including material possessions and sexual relations. Some give up wearing clothes and many include the smoking or consumption of some form of marijuana to get closer to Shiva. They generally live off of donations (alms). There are a wide variety of sadhus and sadvis. They are often given as examples of breatharians, but this is hardly accurate. Those I have seen appear to be quite well fed. A small number of them are said to eat human flesh as well as their own excrement, which is very far from any sort of ideal diet.

Responsible fasting and following a frugal diet of quality food can help the body to cleanse and to heal. But neglecting to provide the body with adequate nutrients for a lengthy period is unwise and dangerous.

People who promote the concept of breatharianism as a theory that the body can survive on only air, light, and/or the spirit within us are either lying, being irresponsible, delusional, severely misinformed, and/or displaying a lack of understanding for the basics of life. They are promoting what can lead to, and has led to starvation, dehydration, kidney failure, infections, and death.

There are people who promote breatharianism through Websites, publications, and seminars. Perhaps what they are best at is exposing themselves for what they are. Frauds.

Some may argue in favor of breatharianism by stating that the conclusion of many health studies show that those who ingest fewer calories tend to live longer and experience fewer health problems than overweight people. But the studies do not say that a person should eat nothing at all. The studies do not support the breatharianism concept.

Those who use such studies to promote breatharianism are stretching the conclusions of the studies beyond reason.

There are an amazing number of plants that form into or produce fruits, vegetables, nuts, seeds, sea vegetables, and flowers containing nutrients our bodies need if we are to experience vibrant health.

Food is a gift from nature, helps ground us, provides the substances for our health to blossom, and should be enjoyed.

MYTH: ADOLF HITLER WAS A VEGETARIAN

TRUTH: Hitler's favorite foods included Bavarian sausage as well as stuffed squab (pigeon or rock dove) and river fish in butter sauce. He outlawed vegetarian groups. He also ordered that the meat supply not be reduced, even though its production used up a tremendous amount of resources during those terrible years.

"A vegetarian diet has been advocated by everyone from philosophers such as Plato and Nietzsche, to political leaders such as Benjamin Franklin and Gandhi, to modern pop icons such as Paul McCartney and Bob Marley. Science is also on the side of vegetarianism. A multitude of studies have proven the health benefits of a vegetarian diet to be remarkable."
– VegInfo.Org/Health

"I became a vegetarian after realizing that animals feel afraid, cold, hungry, and unhappy like we do."
– Cesar Chavez

"If we so easily take the lives of animals, who are only a few evolutionary steps from us, what is to prevent us from doing the same to humans?"
– Peter Singer

"Words like humane, cage free, crate free, organic, free range are all ways to make people feel good about eating meat. The humane products are a perfect antidote for the guilt people feel about eating animal products, but humane labels make a mockery of an authentic movement of conscience.

The animal producers reached out to the animal (advocacy) industry leaders to colloabate on solving this problem together and turned the focus on how animals are treated, and not on the ethical question of, 'Is it right to eat them?' To me, this is like sitting down with Hitler trying to improve conditions for concentration camp victims."
– Jamie Cohen

FreeFromHarm.org	VeganOutreach.org	Vegan.org
GoVeg.com	VeganSociety.com	VRG.com
Vegan.com	VegInfo.org	PCRM.org
VeganHealth.org	VegSource.com	ForksOverKnives.com
VegetarianUSA.com	FatSickAndNearlyDead.com	

CANCER TRUTH: THE MORE MEAT, DAIRY, AND EGGS YOU CONSUME, THE GREATER YOUR RISK OF EXPERIENCING CANCER

"A number of studies have shown that cancer risk is lower and immune competence is higher in individuals who consume a vegetarian diet. Epidemiological studies almost unanimously report a strong correlation between a diet high in fruits and vegetables and low cancer risk."

– John Boik, in his book *Cancer & Natural Medicine: A Textbook of Basic Research and Clinical Research*

"I performed multiple regression analysis on breast cancer incidence. The highest correlation with breast cancer incidence was from animal source calories as compared to plant source calories. The saturated fat in meat and milk products increases the risk of breast cancer."

– Dr. William Harris, author of *The Scientific Basis of Vegetarianism*

As you have likely noticed, this book mentions cancer a lot. This is because there is no way to cover the issue of food-related illnesses without going into the topic of cancer.

Studies suggest that most cancers are largely related to food choices, and, apparently, less so with other factors, including genetics.

"Although fat is the dietary substance most often singled out for increasing one's risk for cancer, animal protein also plays a role. Specifically, certain proteins present in meat, fish, and poultry, cooked at high temperatures, especially grilling and frying, have been found to produce compounds called heterocyclic amines. These substances have been linked to various cancers including those of the colon and breast.[1]"

– Physicians Committee for Responsible Medicine, PCRM.org; Citing: Potter JD. Nutrition and colorectal cancer. Cancer Causes Control. 1996;7(1):127-146; Giovannucci E, Goldin B. The role of fat, fatty acids, and total energy intake in the etiology of human colon cancer. *Am J Clin Nutr.* 1997;66(6suppl):1564S-1571S; De Stefami E, Ronco A, Mendilaharsu M, et al. Meat intake, heterocyclic amines, and risk of

breast cancer: a case-control study in Uruguay. Cancer Epidem
Biomark Prev. 1997;6:573-881.

Causes of increased cancer risk in humans include eating foods
containing synthetic additives, eating foods containing farm chemical
residues, consuming meat, milk, or eggs from animals treated with
synthetic drugs and/or living in situations in which the animals were
exposed to any variety of synthetic chemicals; consuming meat, dairy,
eggs; eating foods containing heat-generated chemicals, such as
acrylamides, glycotoxins, heterocyclic amines, and polycyclic aromatic
hydrocarbons; eating foods containing nitrates; eating mammal meat,
because it contains the neu5Gc molecule; consuming nonhuman
mammal milk or foods made from nonhuman mammal milk, including
ice cream, butter, cheese, cream, yogurt, kifir, whey, and casein, because
they all contain the neu5Gc molecule; eating foods containing
arachidonic acid, which is in meat, egg yolks, and oily fish.

Eating meat infuses the system with androgens, which are hormones
that alter the function of the prostate gland. Without eating meat, dairy,
and eggs, the prostate functions healthfully, especially on a low-fat diet
rich in raw fruits and vegetables. Studies have concluded again and again
that diets rich in animal protein greatly increase risk of prostate and
other cancers.

To lower your cancer risk, don't consume meat, milk, or eggs, or
anything containing them, and stay away from foods containing
synthetic chemicals, including dyes, flavors, scents, emulsifiers, drugs,
and farming chemical residues. Avoid high temperature cooked foods.

"No single food or food component can protect you against
cancer by itself. But strong evidence does show that a diet filled with
a variety of plant foods such as vegetables, fruits whole grains, and
beans helps lower risk of many cancers."
– American Institute of Cancer Research

One common cancer in the U.S., and other countries where people
consume the most meat, dairy, and eggs is colorectal cancer.

"The most comprehensive and authoritative report on
colorectal cancer risk ever published has concluded that red and
processed meat increase risk of the disease and found that the
evidence that foods containing fiber offer protection against
colorectal cancer has become stronger.

This report shows that colorectal cancer is one of the most
preventable cancers,' said Elisa Bandera, MD, PhD, who served on
the World Cancer Research Fund/American Institute for Cancer
Research's Continuous Update Project (CUP) Expert Panel that

authored the report. 'AICR has estimated that about 45 percent of colorectal cancer cases could be prevented if we all ate more fiber-rich plant foods and less meat, drank less alcohol, moved more and stayed lean. That's over 64,000 cases in the U.S. every year.'

The report, released today as part of WCRF/AICR's groundbreaking Continuous Update Project, has examined the links between colorectal cancer risk and diet, physical activity and weight, and updated the colorectal cancer findings of the charity's 2007 Expert Report.

A systematic review of the evidence was carried out by WCRF/AICR–funded scientists at Imperial College London, who added 263 new papers on colorectal cancer to the 749 that had been analyzed as part of the 2007 Report. An independent CUP Expert Panel then analyzed the totality of evidence and made new judgments.

Meat Link Remains Convincing

For red and processed meat, findings from 10 new cohort studies were added to the 14 included in the 2007 Report. The CUP Expert Panel concluded that there is convincing evidence that both red and processed meat increase colorectal cancer risk."

– American Institute for Cancer Research, May 23, 2011; Most Authoritative Report on Colorectal Cancer and Diet Ever Conducted: Links with Meat, Fiber Confirmed

"Colorectal cancer is one of the leading cancers in the United States, attacking 140,000 Americans every year, with a mortality rate close to 50 percent. In 2007, the body of research on this disease, including nearly 60 independent studies, was deemed to provide convincing evidence – the highest possible level of scientific evidence – that hot dogs and other processed meats cause colorectal cancer. Americans eat 20 billion hot dogs a year. Per capita bacon consumption is 18 pounds a year.

Colorectal cancer is not the only processed meat danger. An NIH-AARP Diet and Health Study found that processed red meat was associated with an increased risk of prostate cancer. A study in Taiwan showed that consumption of cured and smoked meat can increase children's risk for leukemia. A study in Australia found that women's risk for ovarian cancer increased as a result of eating processed meats. A review in the journal *Diabetologia* found that those who regularly eat processed meats increase their risk for diabetes by 41 percent.

Adults have a right to take risks with their own health. But hot dogs and other processed meats are often fed to children, starting a lifelong habit that puts them at serious risk."
– Dr. Neal Barnard's blog, Processed Meat Is the Next Public Health Crisis; 2012; PCRM.org

In a study involving 27,000 men over 14 years, scientists at the University of California, San Francisco, found that men who consumed 2.5 or more eggs per week had an 81 percent higher risk of developing lethal prostate cancer compared to men who consumed fewer than half an egg per week on average. The study was published in the September 19, 2011 edition of the journal *Cancer Prevention Research*, and considered the possibility that the cholesterol and choline in eggs, which are also "highly concentrated in prostate cancer cells," played major roles in the incidence of the disease. The study also identified the consumption of meat, processed meat, and chicken as risk factors in the development of prostate cancer. The study also recognized that the men who consumed the most eggs also were more likely to smoke, to be overweight, to lack adequate exercise to keep fit, and to follow a poor diet, which all increase the risk of experiencing prostate cancer.

"Prostate cancer is one of the leading cancers among men in the U.S., and researchers have explored a number of possible dietary factors contributing to prostate cancer risk. These include dietary fat, saturated fat, dairy products, and meat, as well as dietary factors that may decrease risk, such as the consumption of carotenoids and other antioxidants, fiber, and fruit. As with breast cancer risk, a man's intake of dietary fat, which is abundant in meat and other animal products, increases testosterone production, which in turn increases prostate cancer risk. One of the largest nested case-control studies, which showed a positive association between prostate cancer incidence and red meat consumption, was done at Harvard University in an analysis of almost 15,000 male physicians in the Physicians' Health Study. Although this study primarily analyzed plasma fatty acids and prostate cancer risk, the authors found that men who consumed red meat at least five times per week had a relative risk of 2.5 for developing prostate cancer compared to men who ate red meat less than once per week. The most comprehensive dietary cohort study on diet and prostate cancer risk reported on nearly 52,000 health professionals in Harvard's Health Professionals Follow-Up Study, which completed food frequency questionnaires in 1986. The report, based on 3 to 4 years of follow-up data, found a statistically significant relationship between higher red meat intake and the risk of prostate cancer,

with red meat as the food group with the strongest positive association with advanced prostate cancer. These and other study findings suggest that reducing or eliminating meat from the diet reduces the risk of prostate cancer."
    – *Meat Consumption and Cancer Risk*, The Cancer Project, Physicians Committee for Responsible Medicine, CancerProject.org

"If you love your children, don't let them eat animals. You wouldn't let your children have cigarettes, yet meat-based diets cause more deaths from cancer each year than smoking."
    – EvolveCampaigns.org.uk

"A close look at the cultures with low rates of breast cancer showed an obvious common denominator: a low intake of dietary fat and correspondingly low cholesterol levels. The same was true for cancers of the colon, prostate, and ovary, and for diabetes and obesity."
    – Dr. Caldwell B. Esselstyn, author of *Prevent and Reverse Heart Disease*; HeartAttackProof.com

"As with breast cancer, frequent consumption of meat, particularly red meat, is associated with an increased risk of colon cancer. Total fat and saturated fat, which tend to be substantially higher in animal products than in plant-derived foods, and refined sugar, all heighten colon cancer risks. At Harvard University, researchers zeroed in on red meat, finding that individuals eating beef, pork, or lamb daily have approximately three times the colon cancer risk, compared to people who generally avoid these products. A review of 32 case-control and 13 cohort studies concluded that meat consumption is associated with an increase in colorectal cancer risk, with the association being more consistently found with red meat and processed meat. And, in the recently published Cancer Prevention Study II, involving 148,610 adults followed since 1982, the group with the highest red meat and processed meat intakes had approximately 30 to 40 percent and 50 percent higher colon cancer risk, respectively, compared to those with lower intakes. In this study, high red meat intake was defined as 3 ounces of beef, lamb, or pork for men and 2 ounces for women daily, the amount in a typical hamburger. High processed meat intake (ham, cold cuts, hot dogs, bacon, sausage) was defined as 1 ounce eaten 5 or 6 times a week for men, and 2 or 3 times a week for women – the amount in one slice of ham. In addition, earlier studies have also indicated that those consuming white meat, particularly chicken, have approximately a threefold higher colon cancer risk, compared to vegetarians.

Secondary bile acids are probably part of the problem. In order to absorb fat, the liver makes bile, which it stores in the gall bladder. After a meal, the gall bladder sends bile acids into the intestine, where they chemically modify the fats eaten so they can be absorbed. Unfortunately, bacteria in the intestine turn these bile acids into cancer-promoting substances called secondary bile acids. Meats not only contain a substantial amount of fat; they also foster the growth of bacteria that cause carcinogenic secondary bile acids to form."

– *Meat Consumption and Cancer Risk*, The Cancer Project, Physicians Committee for Responsible Medicine; CancerProject.org

The following is an interesting list of "Foods that Fight Cancer" and was compiled by the American Institute of Cancer Research. Here it is: Acai berries, apples, berries, blackberries, blueberries, broccoli and other cruciferous vegetables, cherries, chili peppers, citrus fruit, coffee, cranberries, dark green leafy vegetables, flax seed, garlic, grapefruit, grapes, green tea, kale, legumes (beans, peas, lentils), melon, mushrooms, nuts, onions, papayas, pomegranates, raspberries, soy, spinach, squash, strawberries, sweet potatoes, tomatoes, walnuts, watermelon, and whole grains.

Notice that there are no meats, dairy products, or egg products listed on the American Institute of Cancer Research's list of "Foods that Fight Cancer." This is because of the undeniable truth, which is that meat, dairy, and eggs increase the risk of cancer.

They may as well have kept listing every edible fruit, berry, green leafy vegetable, vegetable, and sprout.

It is interesting that, with as much evidence there is that meat, dairy, and eggs increase the risk of a varieties of cancers, and heart disease, kidney disease, arthritis, diabetes, Alzheimer's, Parkinson's, Crohn's, MS, macular degeneration, varicose veins, heart attacks, strokes, high blood pressure, and other health problems, the American Institute of Cancer Research and the World Cancer Research Fund don't tell people to avoid all animal products. Are they pussyfooting around a big fight with the well-financed milk, dairy, and egg industry lobbies?

"According to AICR/WCRF's second expert report and its updates, carrying excess body fat increases the risk of seven cancers (colorectum [rectum, colon], esophagus, endometrium, kidney, pancreas, post-menopausal breast cancer, gall bladder). Vegetables and fruits are low in calories, which help us to get to and stay a healthy weight. Whole grains and beans are rich in fiber and

moderate in calories, which also help in weight management efforts."
  – American Institute of Cancer Research, World Cancer Research Fund

What will significantly reduce your chances of experiencing cancer is to avoid foods containing proangiogenesis compounds, and to include foods that contain antiangiogenesis compounds. In relation to cancer cell growth, angiognesis is the growth of capillaries, bringing more blood flow to cancer cells that would otherwise remain dormant and be obliterated by the natural processes of the immune system.

Foods containing proangiogenesis compounds are: meat, milk and milk products, eggs and eggs as ingredients, foods that are rich in free radicals, and foods that have been cooked to high temperatures, creating acrylamides, glycotoxins, heterocyclic amines, and polycyclic aromatic hydrocarbons. Also to be avoided are foods containing nitrates, such as processed meats. Avoid all foods containing synthetic chemicals.

Does this sound repetitive? Maybe it should be. People often learn better when things are repeated. Reduce cancer risk: go vegan.

Foods containing antiangiogenesis agents are good. Antiangiogenesis agents are the opposite of proangiogenesis.

Foods that are antiangiogenesis include raw, organic, non-GMO fruits, vegetables, nuts, seeds, and seaweeds. Certain types of tea, herbs, and spices, such as green tea, white tea, jasmine tea, Earl Grey tea, nutmeg, turmeric, ginseng, and ginger, have also been identified as containing antiangiogenic agents. Fresh berries are rich in anti-angiogenesis compounds. Pretty much whatever raw fruit, vegetable, herb, and spice you can think of, from pumpkins and pumpkin seeds to pears, oregano, pineapple, citrus fruit, watermelon, dill, hemp seed, lychee fruit, cumin, bell peppers, cherries, currants, cucumbers, chard, fennel, blackberries, spinach, apples, tomatoes, broccoli leaf, bok choy, mango, kale, broccoli, papaya, and camu camu berries, contain anti-angiogenesis compounds.

Raw marijuana leaves put through a wheatgrass juicer produce a juice that is rich in antiangiogenic compounds. Raw marijuana will not get you high, only heated, cooked, or smoked marijuana will get you high. All cancer patients should have safe access to raw marijuana juice.

Some of the drugs used to treat cancer are known as anti-angiogenesis drugs, or drugs that prohibit the growth of blood vessels. But if you are still eating foods containing proangiogenesis substances, it seems to defeat the purpose of taking the antiangiogenesis drugs.

Any cancer patient would be wise to cut out all foods containing proangiogenesis substances, and to follow a raw or mostly raw, organic, non-GMO vegan diet rich in raw fruits and raw vegetables, and with no highly heated foods (fried, grilled, baked, smoked, roasted, toasted, sautéed, broiled, or microwaved).

To greatly reduce your chances of experiencing cancer, do these things:

- Eliminate all animal protein from the diet. Animal protein, and not plant protein, increases the liver's production of IGF-1 (insulin growth factor), which has been found to play a role in cancer growth. As Dr. Michael Greger of NitritionFacts.org explains in his article, *Animal Protein and the Cancer Promoter IGF-1*, "For years, we didn't know why eating a plant-based diet appeared to so dramatically improve cancer defenses within just a matter of weeks. But researchers recently figured it out: eating healthy lowers the level of the cancer-promoting growth hormone, IGF-1… Studies have found no association between total protein intake and IGF-1 levels. But that's because they didn't take into account animal versus plant protein. It took a study comparing meat eaters to vegans to show that higher IGF-1 levels were only associated with animal protein intake. In fact, plant protein seemed to decrease IGF-1 levels. Animal protein appears to send a much different signal to our livers than most plant protein. Even vegans eating the same amount of protein as meat eaters still had lower levels of IGF-1, so it's apparently not about excessive protein in general, but about animal protein in particular."

- Don't eat meat, including beef, pork, lamb, deer, and other land animals. The tissues from fish, birds, frogs, and other small animals are also meat. Don't eat them. The human nutritional need for meat is absolute zero.

- Eliminate foods containing meat extracts, such as chicken broth, beef broth, lard (beef fat, pork fat, chicken fat, etc.), rennet (the stomach lining of a slaughtered animal and used in cheese), gelatin, and other meat "products" and extracts.

- Don't eat eggs, including anything containing eggs, such as mayonnaise, meringue, some mustards, and other foods that may contain egg as an ingredient, such as baked foods, some breads, crackers, cookies, sauces, creams, soups, and even some types of beer. If choosing to consume these items, look for products that are labeled as "vegan."

- Don't drink milk from another animal.
  The only milk you need during your life is breast milk from your mother when you are a baby and up until you reach toddler stage.

Milk is baby food. Cow milk is for baby cows and baby bulls. Dog milk is for baby dogs. Cat milk is for baby cats. Elephant milk is for baby elephants. Deer milk is for baby deer. Human milk is for baby humans. You get the idea.

Avoid all dairy products, including milk, chocolate milk, cheese, creamer, yogurt, cottage cheese, ice cream, butter, kifir, whey, and casein, and foods containing milk or milk extracts.

Typical dairy products sold in the U.S. are from cows treated with rBGH and rBST, which are GMO growth hormones that manipulate the cow's mammary glands to produce more milk. These artificial hormones also increase the likelihood that the cow will experience infected udders, painfully swollen mammary glands, and infertility. As Jayson Calton, Ph.D., author of, *Rich Food, Poor Food*, explains, "The milk is supercharged with IGF-1 (insulin growth factor-1), which has been linked to breast, colon, and prostate cancers."

Milk and all milk products contain the neu5Gc molecule, which is pro-inflammatory and is a proangiogenesis compound, meaning that it can trigger dormant cancer cells to become active, develop capillaries, grow, and spread throughout the body.

There are a variety of vegan alternatives to dairy, including nut and seed milks and cheeses; coconut yogurt and kifir; and sauces and creams from a variety of nuts, seeds, and other plant substances.

For information on how to make vegan alternatives to dairy products, do an Internet search for vegan milk recipes. It is better to make your own vegan milk, and avoid those sold in the boxes that are lined with plastic = petroleum = carcinogenic substances. Boxed milks also may contain rice syrup sweetener, carrageenan, and other substances that are not healthful.

- Avoid added sugars, including white sugar, brown sugar, agave, corn syrup, rice syrup, and products labeled as "fruit sweetened."

Yes, agave is a garbage sweetener, and can cause similar health problems as corn syrup.

Products labeled as "fruit sweetened" shouldn't be considered "healthful foods." Concentrated fruit sweetener is a processed sugar that is heated and has the pectin/methanol bind fractured.

If you want something sweet, eat fruit.

If you must use a sweetener, try dates. Learn how to make date paste. And, if you want a processed sugar, consider maple syrup or coconut crystals – reading up on them to learn if they are something you would want in your diet.

Sugars really can help the growth of cancer. To find out more, research "processed sugar and cancer."

- Avoid artificial sweeteners. These synthetic chemicals can alter brain function; cause brain lesions; damage the lining of nerves; increase the incidence of asthma; interfere with nutrient absorption and transfer; and increase the risk of seizures, tumor growth, cancer, and fertility issues. For more information, do an Internet search for "artificial sweeteners and health problems."

- Avoid synthetic preservatives, such as BHA and BHT. These are made from petroleum, and have been identified as being carcinogenic.

- Avoid other synthetic chemical food additives, including coloring, scents, flavors, emulsifiers, and preservatives.

   These toxins are made from a variety of substances, such as coal tar extract. Some countries ban them, but the U.S. has not. Chemical additives are found in many packaged and processed foods, and in some cafeteria and restaurant foods. A variety of studies have identified synthetic food additives as being carcinogenic. They also may contribute to such health conditions as asthma, sleep disorders, nerve disorders, learning disabilities, and seizures.

- Avoid bleached foods, such as bleached rice and bleached gluten grains (including wheat, rye, and barley, and all forms of wheat).

   Bleached grains are not as healthful as whole grains, can contribute to digestive and sugar level issues, and are more likely to drain some nutrients from the system. Consider no grains.

   One way grains may be bleached is by using azodicarbonamide, a bleaching agent that can also be used to make foamed plastics, like those in yoga mats and shoe soles. According to Jayson Calton, Ph.D., in his book *Rich Food, Poor Food*, this agent can also trigger asthma.

- Don't eat margarine, including soy margarine, palm oil margarine, or other margarines.

- Follow a plant-based diet rich in raw fruits and raw vegetables.

   "Vegan proteins may reduce risk of cancer, obesity, and cardiovascular disease by promoting increased glucagon activity.
   Amino acids modulate the secretion of both insulin and glucagon; the composition of dietary protein therefore has the potential to influence the balance of glucagon and insulin activity.

Soy protein, as well as many other vegan proteins, are higher in non-essential amino acids than most animal-derived food proteins, and as a result should preferentially favor glucagon production. Acting on hepatocytes, glucagon promotes (and insulin inhibits) cAMP-dependent mechanisms that down-regulate lipogenic enzymes and cholesterol synthesis, while up-regulating hepatic LDL receptors and production of the IGF-I antagonist IGFBP-1. The insulin-sensitizing properties of many vegan diets – high in fiber, low in saturated fat – should amplify these effects by down-regulating insulin secretion. Additionally, the relatively low essential amino acid content of some vegan diets may decrease hepatic IGF-I synthesis. Thus, diets featuring vegan proteins can be expected to lower elevated serum lipid levels, promote weight loss, and decrease circulating IGF-I activity. The latter effect should impede cancer induction (as is seen in animal studies with soy protein), lessen neutrophil-mediated inflammatory damage, and slow growth and maturation in children. In fact, vegans tend to have low serum lipids, lean physiques, shorter stature, later puberty, and decreased risk for certain prominent 'Western' cancers; a vegan diet has documented clinical efficacy in rheumatoid arthritis. Low-fat vegan diets may be especially protective in regard to cancers linked to insulin resistance – namely, breast and colon cancer – as well as prostate cancer; conversely, the high IGF-I activity associated with heavy ingestion of animal products may be largely responsible for the epidemic of 'Western' cancers in wealthy societies. Increased phytochemical intake is also likely to contribute to the reduction of cancer risk in vegans. Regression of coronary stenoses has been documented during low-fat vegan diets coupled with exercise training; such regimens also tend to markedly improve diabetic control and lower elevated blood pressure. Risk of many other degenerative disorders may be decreased in vegans, although reduced growth factor activity may be responsible for an increased risk of hemorrhagic stroke. By altering the glucagon/insulin balance, it is conceivable that supplemental intakes of key nonessential amino acids could enable omnivores to enjoy some of the health advantages of a vegan diet. An unnecessarily high intake of essential amino acids – either in the absolute sense or relative to total dietary protein – may prove to be as grave a risk factor for 'Western' degenerative diseases as is excessive fat intake."

– US National Library of Medicine, National Institutes of Health; PMID: 10687887; [PubMed - indexed for MEDLINE]; *Med Hypotheses*, Dec. 1999; McCarty MF. Source, Nutrition 21/AMBI, San Diego, CA, USA. Abstract. PubMed.gov

- Aim for a diet that is organic and non-GMO.

    The best way to guarantee that your food is organic and non-GMO is to obtain and collect quality seeds, and grow an organic food garden with soil enriched with compost from your own kitchen scraps.

    You can also locate the organic farmers in your region, and support them, such as through you-pick farms, organic food co-ops, farmers' markets, and becoming a member of a CSA (community supported agriculture group).

- Follow a low-fat diet, with few or no added oils.

    This means limiting or completely avoiding all processed oils, including olive oil, canola oil, palm oil, cottonseed oil, corn oil, and other bottled oils marketed or perceived as health foods.

    Don't simply believe in the distortions of "the Mediterranean diet."

    If you do choose to use oil in your foods, choose raw coconut oil and raw hemp seed oil. Is them sparingly, not every day.

    Read Campbell's books *The China Study* and *Whole*, and Esselstyn's *Prevent and Reverse Heart Disease*. Research the points made in the books relating to dietary fat intake. Read the studies cited in the books, and consider what this might mean for adjusting your diet to be as healthful as you can make it.

- Include berries in your diet.

    Raw berries are rich in a variety of nutrients, and are especially abundant in antioxidants.

    If possible, grow some berries. Research which berries are local to the region where you live, and plant some – either on your land, or on nearby wildland.

- Include green leafy vegetables in your daily diet.

    While chlorophyll is in other plants, green leafy vegetables, like spinach, kale, chard, parsley, cilantro, basil, lettuce, beet leaves, broccoli and broccoli leaves, celery, mint, dandelion, thyme, oregano, chives, fennel, leeks, turnip greens, green beans, asparagus, Brussel's sprouts, cabbage, peas, cauliflower leaves, and other greens are also rich in chlorophyll, which helps the plant absorb and convert sunlight.

    Chlorophyll is responsible for the green coloring in plants, including sea vegetables. It has been identified as an interceptor molecule, which means that it intercepts and binds with mutagentic and carcinogenic molecules before they can bind with the our DNA. By binding with mutagens and carcinogens, chlorophyl helps to prevent certain cancers from forming.

The chemical structure of chlorophyll is similar to that found in our red blood cells. But, while the chemical structure of blood is centered around an atom of iron, the chemical structure of chlorophyll is centered around an atom of magnesium. When plants are cooked, an atom of hydrogen replaces the atom of magnesium, a process that also changes the color of the plant from vibrant to dull, and the chlorophyll is changed to pheophytins. It is best to avoid cooking plants so much that the complete chlorophyll structure is lost. That is why, if you choose to heat them, you should only briefly steam or boil vegetables. Clearly, the biggest benefit is in eating them raw, unheated.

• Include cruciferous vegetables in your daily diet.

Cruciferous vegetables include: collard greens, kale, broccoli, broccoli leaves, cabbage, Brussels sprouts, kohlrabi, cauliflower, cauliflower leaves, bok choy, rapini, turnips, rutabaga, mustard seed, mustard greens, arugula, radish, radish sprouts, daikon, watercress, maca, and tatsoi. Grow some!

• Include a variety of sprouts in your diet.

While all fresh sprouts are rich in a variety of nutrients that benefit health and prevent cancer, broccoli sprouts are strong in anticancer agents.

Sprouts are easy to grow. Most natural foods stores sell organic seeds for sprouting, and also sell sprouting jars. You can also grow them in a screen bag, making it easy to rinse the sprouting seeds two or three times per day.

• In addition to sprouts, all organically grown raw fruits and vegetables, and any fruits, vegetables, nuts, and seeds that you grow yourself using organic methods, there are susbances which have been labeled as "superfoods," which include:

◊ Amla (Indian gooseberrys) powder. A traditional Indian medicine berry used for treating a variety of health issues. It is rich in a variety of anticancer, antimutagenic, antioxidant, and anti-inflammatory properties.

◊ Ashwaganda herb

◊ B-12 and other B-vitamins (from vegetarian sources)

◊ Chlorella (a freshwater algae)

◊ Vitamin D. In a vegetarian supplement form based on mushrooms. Mushrooms exposed to sun form vitamin D. The best form of vitamin D is what your body creates when your skin is exposed to sunlight. Don't overdo sun exposure. There is no need to burn or even get tan. Even a dozen minutes a day of sunlight on a large area of skin can increase vitamin D levels. Some D supplements are derived from wool.

◊ Digestive enzymes (in a vegetarian supplement form)

◊ Dulse powder (a seaweed)

◊ Essential fatty acids (they are contained in raw vegetables, fruits, berries, nuts, seeds, and water plants, and in germinated buckwheat and chia seeds)

◊ 5-hydroxytryptophan, also known as 5-HTP (in veg caps)

◊ Gamma-aminobutyric acid (also known as GABA)

◊ Goji berries (and all edible and organically grown berries, including blueberries, raspberries, blackberries, and mulberries)

◊ Hemp seeds (raw and organically grown)

◊ Kelp powder (a variety of seaweed that grows in a variety of forms)

◊ Lions mane mushrooms

◊ Mesquite powder

◊ MSM powder

◊ Mucana prureins

◊ Pomegranate

◊ Probiotic powder (from a vegan source)

◊ Pumpkin seeds (raw and organically grown)

◊ Red cabbage. Raw red cabbage is rich in a variety of nutrients, including antioxidants, and is a cruciferous vegetable containing compounds identified as cancer preventers and cancer fighters

◊ Sesame seeds (raw and organically grown)

◊ Silibinin herb, an extract of milk thistle

◊ Spirulina (an algae)

◊ Green powder, such as Infinity Greens, which can be blended into orange juice, green smoothies, vegetable juices, and used in recipes such as hummus, raw/dehydrated crackers, and salad dressings. (InfinityGreens.com)

- Some studies have concluded that drinking green tea can protect against cancer. Some people are very sensitive to caffeine, and don't do well on green tea. However, green tea does have far less caffeine than coffee, cola, and energy drinks.

- Avoid alcohol. Many studies have identified a link between the amount of alcohol a person drinks and the risk of experiencing cancer, including breast cancer in women.

     If you do drink alcohol, drink red wine, which also contains the beneficial substance, resveratrol.

     If you have any problems with alcohol at all, please completely avoid it.

- Don't use Teflon kitchen products.

- Avoid canned foods, as the cans are lined with extracts of petroleum, known carcinogens.

- Exercise daily to break a sweat.

- Follow a regular sleeping pattern.

- Use nontoxic cleansers that are free of synthetic chemicals

- Avoid cosmetic products containing parabens and synthetic chemicals

- Plant and maintain a food garden, and compost your organic food scraps into soil for the garden

- Support local organic farmers, such as through local farmers' markets and u-pick farms.

- Locate a local co-opportunity that sells organic produce.

- Consider getting deliveries of organic fruits and vegetables from a local CSA (Community Supported Agriculture) group.

     "You can never eat enough cruciferous vegetables. These vegetables are very potent in reducing the risk of numerous types of cancer. They have very potent compounds and they need to be crushed and chewed to let the reaction occur that releases the most potent anticancer agents."

     – Donald Abrams, MD, Chief of Hematology and Oncology, San Francisco General Hospital; Professor of Clinical Medicine, UCSF Osher Center for Integrative Medicine

CARDIOVASCULAR TRUTH: HEART ATTACKS AND STROKES ARE GREATLY REDUCED BY FOLLOWING A LOW-FAT VEGAN DIET RICH IN RAW FRUITS AND VEGETABLES

"I believe that coronary artery disease is preventable, and that even after it is under way, its progress can be stopped, its insidious effects reversed. I believe, and my work over the past twenty years has demonstrated, that all this can be accomplished without expensive mechanical intervention and with minimal use of drugs. The key lies in nutrition – specifically, in abandoning the toxic American diet and maintaining cholesterol levels well below those historically recommended by health policy experts."
– Dr. Caldwell B. Esselstyn, author of *Prevent and Reverse Heart Disease*; HeartAttackProof.com

"We spend incredible amounts of money annually to get the best health care we can afford. With all the money we throw at it, we should expect to be some of the healthiest people in the world. Sadly, that is not the case. We keep spending more money, only to find ourselves getting sicker. It feels at times like we are paying to become ill.

Chronic illnesses, and acute illnesses for that matter, are primarily due to biochemical and physiological imbalances. Studies have shown that chronic illnesses are the direct result of our poor lifestyle choices, the most damaging of which are our food choices. We eat too many unnatural, processed foods that are toxic to our bodies, in place of foods that are natural and supply what our bodies need.

We need a paradigm shift in our approach to healthcare. Our efforts need to start with removing unnatural foods from our diet, and replacing those foods with ones that are 'natural,' as a way of reversing illness and facilitating health. This new approach would be a shift away from the standard approach of using medical and surgical interventions as our primary protocols."
– Dr. Baxter Montgomery of the Houston Cardiac Association, DrBaxterMontgomery.com

"Particles of cholesterol – from eating meat, dairy, and eggs – enter the artery wall and they cause artery blockages to gradually grow. And that causes heart attacks, and we have 4,000 of them every day. And if we went on a vegetarian diet, collectively, that would not happen with that kind of frequency."
– Dr. Neal Barnard, 2004; NealBarnard.org

W̱E know very clearly that the average American diet of junk food, processed salts, bleached grains, clarified sugars and oils, fried food, and sautéed food, along with dairy, meat, and eggs damages the heart, creates arthritis, promotes diabetes, increases the incidence of cancers of the colon, prostate, breasts, bladder, and kidneys, and increases the risk of macular degeneration, asthma, stroke, heart attack, kidney stones, attention disorders, and obesity. It is a fact. Meanwhile, if you go into school cafeterias, hospital cafeterias, military cafeterias, prison cafeterias, and other institutional eating establishments and popular restaurants and grocery stores, you will see that they are selling the very foods that cause heart disease, cancer, diabetes, and a variety of common health problems.

"I don't understand why asking people to eat a well-balanced vegetarian diet is considered drastic, while it is medically conservative to cut people open and put them on cholesterol-lowering drugs for the rest of their lives."
– Dr. Dean Ornish

"I cut out meats and dairy. After two months, my cholesterol shot down 83 points. That's enough proof to me that it works. (Before becoming vegan) I existed on cigarettes, Coca-Cola, and coffee, and I got away with that for a while. And I never used to exercise. I think you begin to look and feel lousy the older you become, so now I eat really well. I don't smoke and I'm learning meditation."
– Michelle Pfeiffer

A study conducted at McMaster and McGill universities in Canada, and published on October 11, 2011 by the *PLoS Medicine* journal (published by Public Library of Science) reported that a diet rich in raw fruits and vegetables favorably modified the chromosome 9p21 region genetic variant, which had been identified as a marker for heart disease. The study, titled The Effect of Chromosome 9p21 Variants on Cardiovascular Disease May Be Modified by Dietary Intake: Evidence from a Case/Control and a Prospective Study, included data of over 27,000 people from a variety of ethnic ancestries, including Chinese, European, Latin American, and Arabian. The study authors concluded that the people with the genetic variant could, if they followed a diet rich in raw fruits and vegetables, reduce their risk of heart disease to the level experienced by those who do not have the genetic variant. The authors of the study concluded, "The risk of myocardial infarction and cardiovascular disease conferred by chromosome 9p21 SNPs appears to be modified by a prudent diet high in raw vegetables and fruits."

Scientists have known that certain chemicals that form in cooked food, including acrylamides, glycotoxins, polycyclic aromatic hydrocarbons, d-Nitrosodiethanolamine, and heterocyclic amines, can damage DNA and trigger the growth of cancer cells. But the McMaster and McGill study identified how a diet rich in raw plant matter favorably alters human genes to prevent disease. This was no surprise to me. I have read many studies concluding that dietary choices certainly can trigger genes to express favorable or unfavorable health events.

That being said, I should mention that the vast variety of degenerative diseases are not initialized by genes, but are triggered by bad diet, lack of exercise, toxins, and substance abuse, including cigarettes and drugs. In his book *The China Study*, T. Colin Campbell reinforces the fact that genes are a lesser part of the puzzle when it comes to common diseases, and as little as 3 percent of common diseases can really be blamed on genes. Even among those diseases that are triggered by genes, there is something that sets the genetic expression in motion, such as an environmental toxin, horrible dietary choices, cigarettes, and otherwise, an unhealthful lifestyle. As Campbell states, "The genes that you inherit from your parents are not the most important factors in determining whether you fall prey to any of the ten leading causes of death." What matters most for disease prevention and reversal? A clean diet, and especially one that is low-fat and free of synthetic chemicals and of animal protein – as in, low-fat vegan.

Some of the best things you can do for your heart, brain, and health include getting daily exercise, and follow a plant-based diet that is largely or completely organic, and free of processed salts, clarified sugars (including agave), preservatives of any kind, MSG, synthetic chemicals, fried substances, heated oils, and bottled oils. Even better if the diet contains a variety of raw fruits and fresh greens, and is rich in omega-3s (such as from raw green vegetables, freshly ground flax seeds, fractured or ground raw hemp seeds, unheated walnuts, and germinated chia and buckwheat). It isn't a maybe or a kind-of, it is an absolute.

"By eating these whole foods, and getting away from processed foods, getting away from the dairy, and anything with a mother, anything with a face – meat, fish and chicken – it's incredible how powerful the body can be. If we are going to have a seismic

revolution of health in this country, which is really right at our fingertips, then the major behavior that has to change is our food (intake). That is absolutely the key card, it trumps everything."
    – Dr. Caldwell B. Esselstyn, author of *Prevent and Reverse Heart Disease*

For those who advocate taking fish oil for heart health, I strongly advise that you avoid taking fish oil, because:

1) We don't need to kill fish. The fish and sea life populations have suffered greatly because of industrial fishing, and from pollution. Sea life around the planet has been decimated and is at a fraction of what it was just a few decades ago.

We also don't need to be harvesting krill from the seas for its oil. Krill is a shrimp-like crustacean and is the food for sea life, such as baleen whales, mantas, and whale sharks, which are suffering from what humans have done to the seas.

2) Ingesting fish and extracts of sea creatures increases your exposure to mercury, PCBs, and other environmental toxins from industrial pollution the creatures are exposed to in the increasingly polluted lakes and oceans. Consuming these contaminates leads to an accumulation of them in your cells, which then increases your risk of cancer and other health disorders.

Some may say that the fish oil products they get are from uncontaminated waters free of industrial pollution. Unfortunately, there is no longer such a thing. Industrial pollution flows into lakes and rivers and into the oceans, and it also ends up in the air, which is then absorbed into the rivers, lakes, and oceans around the world. Mercury from coal-fired electric generating plants and cement kilns travels in the atmosphere, and is absorbed into the oceans thousands of miles from where it was released into the air. The main reason polar bears are now so contaminated with industrial pollution, such as fire retardants and heavy metals, is because they are getting these toxins by eating fish. It is impacting polar bears to such an extent that it is affecting their bones, their nerves, and their ability to reproduce.

3) The benefit of taking fish oil is to obtain the omega-3 essential fatty acids. Instead of taking fish oil to get omega-3s, you can take algae supplements (which is where the fish get the omega-3s), and/or also include things like hemp seed powder, germinated chia, germinated buckwheat, soaked flax seeds, and other plant sources rich in essential fatty acids in your diet, including raw fruits and vegetables. All raw fruits and all raw vegetables contain sufficient amounts of omega-3 fatty acids.

The eggs that are advertised as being rich in omega-3s are simply from chickens that have been fed raw flax seeds and/or fed fish meal. Skip the eggs, eat the flax, and eat raw greens.

You may hear people say that they get their omega-3s by eating grass-fed beef. They may say that grass-fed cows are healthier. The beef that is marketed as rich in omega-3s is from cattle that have grazed in meadows, eating raw greens. The only way the omega oils exist in the cow is because the cow ate food containing those omega oils. Skip eating the cow, simply eat fresh green salad, as raw greens are rich in omega-3s. You will get far more omega oils by eating a meal consisting of raw plant matter than you would by eating a meal of meat.

Grow a garden. Become a garden-fed human. Garden-fed humans are healthier, you know. By doing so, you will have no worry about getting enough omega-3s.

A friend of mine in his 30s had a cerebral hemorrhage that doctors attributed to his use of fish-oil supplements. To those who understand the risks of fish-oil supplements, this is not a surprise. Hemorrhage is one of the very real risk factors of taking fish-oil supplements. His doctors looked up studies concluding this and showed the studies to my friend.

My friend was in the hospital for three months. He was left with a $140,000 hospital bill, in addition to the cost of a variety of pharmaceuticals. He spent months going through physical therapy to regain his muscle coordination and strength, and the experience devastated his life.

The fish-oil supplements are being marketed like crazy. It has nothing to do with health, and everything to do with money. It also is helping to deplete the seas of medium-sized fish that are relied on as food for other creatures, including other fish, sea mammals, and birds. The massive amount of fish being removed from the seas every month to make fish-oil supplements is one of the reasons many types of sea creatures are struggling to survive.

In addition to ending up being used for oil to make supplements for humans, massive quantities of fish end up as fish meal for feeding farm animals, including hogs, cows, goats, lambs, horses, chickens, and turkeys. These farm animals are creatures that would never eat fish. Yet, supplying fish to animal feed manufacturers is now one of the leading causes of overfishing, which, in addition to ocean acidification, is threatening to cause the collapse of life in the oceans.

The fish do not form the omega-3s. They accumulate them from what they eat, such as by eating algae.

There is no reason to kill fish to get omega-3 fatty acids from algaes. You can purchase algaes at any natural foods store. The stores usually sell chlorella, spirulina, and blue-green algae. Not that you really must have those, but they do contain a variety of nutrients, in addition to omega-3 fatty acids.

We can skip taking fish oil, skip participating in the depletion of the seas, skip helping to cause the extinction of species, skip the serious side effects of fish-oil supplements, and skip making the fish oil companies rich, and instead eat raw fruits and vegetables, nuts, and seeds, which contain the oils we need to obtain from food, and our bodies will manage from there, converting what is needed for our health and well being. (See the documentary: Sea The Truth: SeeTheTruth.nl/en)

There is no reason to eat animal products to get omega-3 fatty acids. The animals are getting the omega-3s by eating plant substances, or by eating animals that eat plants.

"Men dig their graves with their own teeth, and die more by those instruments than by all weapons of their enemies."
– Pythagoras

"We know that 9p21 genetic variants increase the risk of heart disease for those that carry it. But it was a surprise to find that a healthy diet could significantly weaken its effect."
– Dr. Jamie Engert

"We observed that the effect of a high risk genotype can be mitigated by consuming a diet high in fruits and vegetables. Our results support the public health recommendation to consume more than five servings of fruits or vegetables as a way to promote good health."
– Sonia Anand

"Since we know that these foods are injuring people, why would we ever want to have them on the menus for our schoolchildren? Why wait until people do have heart disease? We know, for instance, that if we do autopsies on our guys who died in Korea and Vietnam, roughly eighty percent of young GIs will already have gross evidence of coronary heart disease that you can see without a microscope. If we are ever going to make a breakthrough in this epidemic of cardiac disease, we really have to start when it's young."
– Dr. Caldwell B. Esselstyn, author of *Prevent and Reverse Heart Disease.*

"When it comes to heart healthy eating, fresh fruit and vegetables are essential. A natural plant-based diet can not only help prevent heart disease and other chronic illnesses, but help to reverse it, even in its most advanced forms."
– Dr. Baxter Montgomery

Books of Interest:
- *Becoming Raw: The Essential Guide to Raw Vegan Diets*, by Brenda Davis, RD, Vesanto Melina, MS, RD, and Rynn Berry
- *The Engine 2 Diet: The Texas Firefighter's 28-Day Save-Your-Life Plan that Lowers Cholesterol and Burns Away Pounds*, by Rip Esselstyn. This is the son of Dr. Caldwell Esselstyn of the Cleveland Clinic. Rip is a firefighter who persuaded his Austin, Texas firehouse workers to go vegan.
- *The McDougall Program for a Healthy Heart: A Life-Saving Approach to Preventing and Treating Heart Disease*, by John McDougall, MD, and Mary McDougall
- *Prevent and Reverse Heart Disease: The Revolutionary, Scientifically Proven Nutrition-Based Cure*, by Caldwell B. Esselstyn, Jr., MD
- *The Raw Cure*, by Jesse Jacoby
- *The Spectrum: A Scientifically Proven Program to Feel Better, Live Longer, Lose Weight, and Gain Health*, by Dr. Dean Ornish
- *Whole: Rethinking the Science of Nutrition*, by T. Colin Campbell
- *Wild Edibles: A Practical Guide to Foraging*, by Sergei Boutenko

Dr. Mary Clifton, Traverse City, MI; DrMaryMD.com
Dr. Joel Fuhrman, DrFuhrman.com
Dr. Michael Greger, DrGreger.org
Dr. John McDougall, DrMcDougall.com
Preventative Medicine Research Institute, Sausalito, CA, USA; pmri.org. Dr. Dean Ornish has proved that heart disease and narrowing of the arteries can be reversed through a vegan or near vegan diet combined with exercise, stress reduction, and lifestyle changes.
Dr. Baxter Montgomery, Houston Cardiac Association, 10480 Main St., Houston, TX; DrBaxterMontgomery.com
True North Health, 1551 Pacific Ave., Santa Rosa, CA 95404; HealthPromoting.com. Staffed by vegan and vegetarian doctors. The food is all vegan. The facilities include yoga classes. Howard Lyman of Mad Cowboy fame has stayed here. He was a Montana cattle rancher who went vegan, greatly improving his health. He wrote the books *Mad Cowboy* and *No More Bull*.

BRAIN AND HEART NUTRITION TRUTH

B RAIN nutrition begins before birth as billions of brain cells are forming. Because of this, women who are planning on becoming pregnant, and those who are pregnant, would benefit their babies by striving for the most excellent nutritional foods available to them.

Excellent prenatal nutrition is beneficial in many ways. Women who consume a variety of fresh fruits and vegetables during pregnancy are found to have babies with more healthful lung function, less susceptibility to asthma, and fewer complications. It should be obvious that the mother benefits in many ways by following a healthy diet prior to and during pregnancy, and during the breast-feeding stage.

> "Either it is appropriable material for tissue building – a food, or it is not. If not, then it is a foreign substance – a poison – and as such can only damage and cannot possibly ever benefit the organism."
> – Dr. Hereward Carrington

Substances in fresh fruits and vegetables are particularly beneficial to brain function. It is known that the neurotransmitter acetylcholine is key to cell communication and a healthful memory. That brain chemical tends to decline with age. Antioxidants in raw, dark-colored fruits and vegetables, and especially in apples, apricots, broccoli, cantaloupe, chard, kale, mangos, blueberries, goji berries, spinach, and watermelon, help to preserve a healthful level of acetylcholine.

Blueberries are often mentioned as a brain-friendly food because they contain anthocyanins, which stimulate neural regeneration and improve neural connections. Because they are rich in antioxidants, blueberries have been mentioned in various studies as being particularly beneficial for maintaining long-term memory, and also for reducing the chances of Parkinson's and Alzheimer's diseases. If you are able, plant and maintain some blueberry bushes so that you will have access to the freshest blueberries at the lowest cost.

Goji berries are especially brain-friendly. Gojies contain even higher levels of antioxidants than blueberries, and more of the antioxidant beta-carotene than in carrots. Gojies contain sesquiterpenoids, which stimulate the pineal and pituitary glands. The amino acids l-glutamine and l-arginine in gojies increase the production of human growth hormone, which protects against aging. Gojies contain polysaccharides, which are long-chain sugars that help to feed the brain. The berries also stimulate the production of choline, which combats free radicals attributed to neurological degeneration. The zeaxanthin in gojies is beneficial to the eyes. Zeaxanthin is also found in the highly nutritious fresh water algae, spirulina. Goji berries grow in a variety of terrains. Perhaps you can grow some in your garden, or on nearby wildland.

Among other nutrients, bananas contain vitamin B6, potassium, and tryptophan. B6 helps to maintain blood sugar, which is the brain's food. Potassium regulates blood pressure, protecting the fine blood system in the brain. The tryptophan in bananas is used to create serotonin in the body, including in the intestines and brain cells. Serotonin is a neuro-transmitter that stabilizes the mood and improves attention. Serotonin also helps a person to sleep better, which helps the brain to function at a higher level.

Flax seeds are known for containing essential fatty acids, and are a particularly excellent source of alphalinolenic acid (ALA). This omega-3 fatty acid has been shown to aid in the function of the cerebral cortex, the area of the brain involved in processing sensory information, such as pleasure. Many people purchase flax seed oil and use this in their foods. Instead of using clarified flax oil, I purchase whole flax seeds, soak them in water, dry them, and then grind them in a coffee grinder. It is good to grind the seeds after soaking them in water for several hours or over-night, and letting them mostly dry at room temperature for a day (spread a quarter cup of them on a ceramic tray or plate), as this will ignite the enzymes and other nutrients in the seeds. The ground flax powder, which is also rich in fiber, can be used in salads, added to juices and smoothies, mixed in with hummus, pesto, and dips, used as an in-gredient in vegetable pâté, and included in dehydrated vegetable crackers made with the antioxidant-rich pulp left over from juicing vegetables. By consuming the freshly ground flax seeds, you will be consuming not only the oil, but also the other nutrients in the seeds.

Some people mix together raw flax oil, hempseed oil, and pumpkin seed or grapeseed oil for a particularly nutrient-rich oil combo they use in salad dressings and other raw foods. However, there is no sense in go-ing overboard with consuming oils. No added oils are necessary when consuming a diet rich in raw fruits and raw vegetables. The heart-health expert, Dr. Caldwell B. Esselstyn, advises against adding any oils to the diet, and instead to eat the whole plant foods. Many people have found they do much better by **not** using bottled oils, and only eating the whole foods that contain the oils, such as raw flax, pumpkin seeds, hemp seeds or hemp seed powder, raw walnuts, germinated buckwheat and germinated chia, and raw greens, such as chard, kale, spinach, lettuces, and cilantro, and wild purslane. As I mention elsewhere, all raw fruits, vegetables, nuts, seeds, and seaweeds naturally contain some essential fatty acids in every cell, and getting enough calories in a raw food diet rich in fruits and vegetables easily provides a sufficient amount of both essential fatty acids and amino acids – and a load of other nutrients.

Raw sesame seeds are rich in the brain, neuron, heart, and bone nutrients methionine, tryptophan, other amino acids, vitamin E, B6, folic acid, riboflavin, thiamine, niacin, zinc, potassium, magnesium, manganese, copper, phosphorous, calcium, iron, and essential fatty acids, and contain more omega-6 than omega-3 (best to get sesame seeds raw, unheated, and organic). Sesame seeds are rich in fiber, and the phytosterols contained in the seeds lower blood cholesterol. The sesamin lignan in sesame seeds is an antioxidant phytoestrogen that has been identified as having anti-cancer properties. The delicate polyunsaturated fats in sesame seeds are particularly easy to damage by heating.

When raw, unheated sesame seeds are rinsed in a fine mesh strainer and kept wet for a few hours, it allows for the nutrients in the seeds to multiply. These soaked seeds can be used in various raw recipes, tossed into salads, and also used to make raw tahini, which is commonly used in raw hummus, dips, dressings, and desserts. Raw sesame seeds are also used in raw piecrust, dessert truffles, gomashio, halvah, baba ghanoush, and dehydrated sesame cracker recipes found in many of the popular raw food recipe books. One way of making raw vegan ice cream is to blend two frozen bananas with a tablespoon each of raw tahini and vanilla, and then spoon mixing in one or more of the following: berries, sliced soft fruit, raw walnuts, cinnamon, or raw carob powder.

Sesame seeds have been a common food throughout history, including for oil, and especially in the Middle East, parts of Africa, and India. The sesame plant is probably native to the sub-Saharan Africa or the East Indies. The Romans ground sesame seeds with herbs to make a spread. Buddhist monasteries in Japan commonly use sesame oil in many of their foods. Raw sesame oil has been used as a skin moisturizer for thousands of years. Ancient Chinese used sesame seed oil as an ingredient in ink. According to Assyrian legend, the gods drank sesame wine the night before they created Earth. African slaves are said to have brought sesame seeds to the Caribbean and the Americas. Sesame grows easily in many parts of the world.

Raw sesame seeds can be purchased in the bulk sections of many natural foods stores. I don't use sesame oil, but if you choose to do so, look for oil that is cold-pressed (raw), organically grown, and does not contain other oils. It is good to keep sesame seeds stored in glass bottles in a cool, dry, dark place. Because the hull protects and preserves the seed, dehulled sesame seeds tend to go rancid within months, so it is good to purchase only what will be used within three or fewer months. They can also be frozen.

Another source of essential fatty acids are germinated buckwheat seeds, which are about 10 percent oil, including omega-3 essential fatty acids. Buckwheat seeds are also known as buckwheat groats. The raw seeds can be purchased at most natural foods stores. Similar to sunflower seeds, buckwheat has a thick outer hull. Before they are sent to markets, the hull of the seeds is removed. The seeds should be kept in a cool, dry, dark place, and in an airtight container to preserve the delicate polyunsaturated fatty acids. Glass bottles work best. Because the oils naturally contained in buckwheat are subject to degradation, buckwheat isn't good for long-term storage, but can be frozen.

Buckwheat seeds contain the minerals calcium, copper, iron, magnesium, manganese, phosphorus, potassium, and zinc. Like all fruits, vegetables, nuts, seeds, and seaweeds, they also contain the eight amino acids essential for human health. Buckwheat seeds are especially rich in lysine and arginine. Lysine and cystine are two of the amino acids that are easily damaged or destroyed by heat.

It is easy to germinate buckwheat seeds by soaking them in water for a few hours, then draining the water, transferring them to a clean bowl and keeping them slightly wet by using a screen strainer to rinse them two to three times per day for two or three days. Germinating buckwheat for two or three days greatly increases the presence of linolenic acid, and also triggers the production of enzymes. As with other seeds, germinating buckwheat more than quadruples the amino acid content, which means that buckwheat is an excellent source of protein. Germinated buckwheat is also a source for vitamins B1, B6, and C.

Because buckwheat is free of gluten, it is safe for those who have been diagnosed with celiac disease and irritable bowel syndrome, and those with a history of anxiety, depression, bipolar disorders, and autism.

Buckwheat is also rich in fiber, and has been shown to absorb cholesterol from the digestive tract, which means it is excellent for cardiovascular health. Buckwheat is also beneficial to coronary health because the seeds contain alpha tocopherol, delta tocopherol, and gamma tocopherol, which protect against cardiovascular disease.

Trace nutrients in buckwheat include the polyphenols rutin and quercitin, which are beneficial in lowering blood plasma cholesterol (and are also heart-friendly nutrients present in red wine). Rutin helps to strengthen capillary walls while improving circulation. The cholesterol-lowering substances in buckwheat also reduce the incidence of gall stones.

The chlorogenic acid in buckwheat protects health because it is anti-bacterial, antifungal, and antiviral. Chlorogenic acid also helps to slow the release of glucose into the bloodstream.

The D-chior-inositol in buckwheat helps to maintain the balance of insulin, which means that germinated buckwheat is an excellent food for those with blood-sugar issues, which can also affect brain function.

In very rare cases, some people are allergic to buckwheat. In rare cases, buckwheat can trigger asthma-like symptoms. I know one person who has experienced a mild reaction to eating germinated buckwheat, including itching mouth and slight and temporary problems swallowing.

Boiled porridge made of buckwheat and/or hemp seeds has been a common breakfast food in Asia and Eastern Europe. In the raw food diet, freshly germinated buckwheat is a common breakfast food. Freshly germinated buckwheat can be used in fruit salad as a breakfast food, which is more healthful than common packaged cereals. However, although buckwheat resembles a grain, it is not a cereal, a grain, or a grass, but has been defined as a fruit. Typically this salad includes a heaping spoonful of germinated buckwheat mixed with a chopped apple, bananas, and/or berries, a squeeze of lemon, and a dash of cinnamon.

Germinated buckwheat seeds can also be dried, which is used as kasha. Traditionally, kasha is roasted buckwheat. In the raw food diet, kasha consists of buckwheat that has been germinated and then dried, either at room temperature by spreading it out on a clean, dry cloth, or in a dehydrator. This kasha can be used in raw granola, and for adding crunch to raw piecrust, raw carob treats, and dehydrated vegetable crackers, and mixing in banana or mango whip (frozen bananas and/or mangos put into a high-speed blender or in a food processor until whipped [peel the ripe bananas and mangos before freezing!]).

Chia seeds also contain brain and heart nutrients. Chia were cultivated along with beans and corn by the Nahuatl culture (Aztecs). Chia are more than 25 percent oil, and raw chia are another excellent source of essential fatty acids. Similar to hemp, chia are particularly rich in omega-3 fatty acids. Chia oil contains about 64 percent omega-3 fatty acid, which is more than what is in flax seeds. Chia are rich in amino acids, quickly absorb water, and form an enzyme-rich gel coating. Germinating chia greatly increases their amino acid content, which means that they are an excellent source of protein. Chia are rich in the antioxidants caffeic acid, chlorogenic acid, kaempferol, myricetin, and quercetin, which make chia seeds excellent protectors of cellular and neural health. They are also rich in soluble fiber, making them a heart-healthful food. Similar to buckwheat, chia are free of gluten, making them safe for those who are sensitive to that protein, including those with celiac disease, and for those with bipolar disorders, anxiety, a history of depression, and autism.

When consumed, germinated chia seeds are a slowly digested form of carbohydrate, which prevents the sugar rush that can be experienced after eating other forms of carbohydrates, such as wheat and rice. Many raw foodists include chia in their smoothies and nondairy mylks, such as hemp mylk. (Blend water, hemp powder, dates, banana, vanilla, chia. Optional: lucuma powder, mesquite powder, and/or berries.)

> "Chia seed is a superfood that resembles black sesame seed and is nutty to the taste. It is an excellent source of minerals and antioxidants. According to the U.S. Department of Agriculture, 2 tablespoons of chia seeds provide approximately 100 milligrams of calcium, 7.5 grams of dietary fiber, and 3 grams of protein. Chia seeds are also high in alpha-linolenic acid, an omega-3 fatty acid, with 3.5 grams of alpha-linolenic acid in 2 tablespoons."
> – Julia Driggers, RD, *Vegetarian Journal*, VRG.org

Similar to buckwheat, germinated chia seeds can be used in a breakfast salad with chopped fruit; tossed into salads; used as an ingredient in vegetable burgers and dehydrated vegetable pulp crackers; and dried for use in raw granola and raw piecrust. A pudding that is similar to tapioca can be made from chia seeds, and this is also popular among raw foodists. In Latin America, chia fresca is made of chia seeds soaked in water and fruit juice. Some raw foodists stir chia seeds into kombucha juice. Because chia seeds absorb water, fruit juice, or coconut water so quickly, it only takes less than a half hour to make recipes containing them.

There is such a wide assortment of edible plants from around the world containing varieties of health-giving substances that it would be difficult, or impossible, to include them all in one book. But it would be beneficial to know which ones you can include in your diet so that you may experience vibrant health.

While we can speak of the relatively few antioxidants that have been identified and named, humans don't actually know how many chemicals are found in plants, or how those chemicals benefit health. There are clearly many thousands of various plant chemicals in a simple raw vegan meal – such as a salad or green smoothie. Among the reasons so many plant chemicals have not been identified is that many of them have been identified by those working for or funded by companies interested in making synthetic copies of the chemicals in the form of patented pharmaceutical drugs. Many of the drugs that are out there are synthetic versions of some substance identified in a plant. But, drugs do not contain beneficial co-substances that may be in the plant. It is interesting that people who take patented drugs but who don't clean up their diet don't do as well as people who clean up their diet and don't take patented synthetic pharmaceutical drugs. Coincidence? I don't think so. The most basic things that you need for health are not found in pill form, or in a syringe, but they are in plants – including biophotons, amino acids, fiber, enzymes, essential fatty acids, and an unknown variety of antioxidants and unidentified phytochemicals.

The brain is over 50 percent fat and benefits from healthful oils naturally present in raw fruits, vegetables, sprouts, nuts, seeds, and seaweeds. Oil in raw hemp seeds, grape seeds, flax seeds, sunflower seeds, sesame seeds, and pumpkin seeds are often used in the raw diet. Instead of purchasing the oil from these seeds, purchase the actual raw seeds, and use those as food. Eating these whole raw plant substances, or including them as ingredients in raw recipes, especially if the raw seeds and raw nuts have been soaked in water to enliven them, also provides the beneficial brain nutrients of amino acids, enzymes, vitamins, and minerals, including magnesium, which is important for brain health.

Scientists have discovered that pregnant women who consume healthful quantities of high-quality essential fatty acids are more likely to have babies with higher IQs and that possess better language comprehension and eye-hand coordination. This reveals that it is especially important that pregnant women, and women planning on becoming pregnant, totally eliminate low-quality fats from their diet, including fried and sautéed oils, and also lard, mayonnaise, margarine, shortening, corn oil, other bottled oils, and heated tropical fats. They would benefit by making sure to include raw fruits and raw vegetables, especially raw green vegetables, in their daily food choices.

Raw nuts are beneficial to both heart and brain health. Raw nuts contain monounsaturated fats, which can lower LDL (bad) cholesterol levels while boosting HDL (good) cholesterol levels. It is good to soak raw nuts in water for an hour or so to deactivate their enzyme inhibitors and activate their enzymes. After they become dry, store them in bottles and refrigerate, or place in a cool, dry, dark place.

Raw walnuts contain high-quality dietary oils. Walnuts also contain a substance called uridine, which has been found to improve memory retention. Uridine also aids in the growth of the branches on brain cells called neurites, improving the connection between neurons. Many people make note of the similarities between the shape of the walnut and the shape of the human brain.

Nuts only become damaging to health when they have been heated, such as broiled, roasted, sautéed, fried, microwaved, or otherwise exposed to high temperatures, and/or when they are coated with unhealthful substances, such as processed salt, sugar, artificial dyes, flavors, or preservatives, milk chocolate, or other low-quality chocolate; or candy substances, such as caramel.

Because nuts contain a lot of calories, it is best to limit your intake of nuts to less than one-third cup per day. Some people completely avoid nuts, and that is absolutely fine. Dr. Caldwell Esselstyn advises patients with cardiovascular disease to avoid all nuts. If you are on a weight-lowering program, aim for consuming fewer nuts and more vibrant fruits and also fresh greens, such as kale, broccoli, chard, celery, dandelion, spinach, purslane, collards, cilantro, and parsley, which all contain some essential fatty acids. All raw fruits, including citrus fruits, and avocados are also sources of essential fatty acids. Figs are another source because their tiny seeds are rich in quality fat, rich in fiber, and contain a number of vitamins, minerals, and antioxidants (avoid figs that have been treated with sulfur, other drying agents, or preservatives, or that are cooked, such as in fig cookies [which usually also contain corn syrup or other unhealthful ingredients]).

Essential fatty acids act as doorways on the cell membranes to exchange nutrients, enzymes, and electrical currents. They also allow for the output of cellular waste. Healthful cell membrane function is one of the many reasons it is good to maintain a diet rich in raw fruits and vegetables to obtain fresh essential fatty acids.

The white matter in the brain is a fatty substance that plays a role in the speed of information processing. The nerves are coated with a fatty material called myelin.

The quality of nutrients in your diet plays out in the level of your thinking, including in your reasoning, judgment, and decision-making.

To get your brain to function at its highest level, avoid cooked and other low-quality fats.

Again, to stress the issue of fat in the diet: You do not need a large amount of oil in your diet. Less oil is better. It is beneficial to brain health to follow a diet rich in natural, plant-based omega-3 fatty acid sources, not fish, and not eggs, or other animal protein advertised as rich in omega-3s.

While it is true that meat from grass-fed cattle is higher in omega-6 fatty acids than meat from grass-fed cattle, its also true that all meat contains substances damaging to human health, so meat should not be considered as a good dietary source of essential fatty acids. Unlike plants, meat, eggs, and dairy contain no fiber, but are rich in free radicals that negate health. Unlike meat, dairy, and eggs, plants are rich in antioxidants that promote health by working against free radicals. Unlike meat, plants do not contain arachidonic acid (AA), which is found in animals, is a source of omega-6 fatty acids, and can trigger mood swings. Omega-3 fatty acids help to combat the effects of AA.

Some people say that you need to eat fish and other animal products to get essential fatty acids. This is not true. Excellent sources of essential fatty acids exist in the plant sources mentioned above, and in sea vegetables. There is no need to kill and eat fish or sea creatures, or oils derived from killed sea creatures, to obtain essential fatty acids.

Some people will say they need the long-chain omega-3 fatty acids from fish, including docosahexaenoic acid (DHA) and eicosapentaenoic acid (EPA). Like other omega-3s, which are long-chain fatty acids, DHA and EPA help to combat the effects of arachidonic acid (AA), protecting the brain and nerves from what can play out as mood swings and stress symptoms. Consuming fish does not guarantee that the body will function at a better level with the benefit of the DHA and EPA in the system – but fish oil may cause malfunction, as in: bleeding problems.

"The proportions of plasma long-chain n–3 fatty acids were not significantly affected by the duration of adherence to a vegetarian or vegan diet. This finding suggests that when animal foods are wholly excluded from the diet, the endogenous production of EPA and DHA results in low but stable plasma concentrations of these fatty acids."
– *American Journal of Clinical Nutrition*, Vol. 82, No. 2, 327-334; August 2005

The human system makes EPA and DHA from alpha-linolenic acid (ALA), an omega-3 fatty acid found in all raw fruits, vegetables, sprouts, germinates, nuts, and seaweeds. As mentioned elsewhere in this book, purslane, which is a common weed, is a source of eicosapentaenoic acid (EPA). Because the body makes DHA from ALA and EPA means that you don't need to include purslane, or fish oils, in the diet. A vegan diet rich in raw fruits and vegetables manufactures what the body needs to function healthfully, including protecting the brain and nerves.

Today much of the fish on the planet live in water contaminated by industrial pollution, such as mercury, which is damaging to human health. Mercury is particularly damaging to brain function. In addition to mercury, the oil from fish may contain other heavy metals and industrial pollutants. This is because the oil is typically from the liver of the fish, and the liver is the detox center of the body – it filters pollutants.

"Contrary to the slick advertisements of the fish industry, or the misinformed American doctors who only receive around three hours of nutrition information during their eight-year medical programs, fish is not a health food. With mercury, dioxin, and PCBs, fish meat is the most contaminated food product available.

Additionally, a 3.5-ounce serving of fish meat has twice the amount of cholesterol as a single hot dog."
– Gary Yourofsky, ADAPTT.org

Mercury occurs naturally in the environment, but the increase in mercury in the tissues of waterlife is largely the result of industrial pollution, and much of that consists of pollution from coal-burning electric generating plants and from kilns used to process cement that is used in construction of buildings, walls, sidewalks, and roads.

The high levels of mercury and other heavy metals in sea life are among the many reasons it is unhealthful to eat fish. Sea creatures are exposed to all sorts of toxins in the water. The toxins are also the result of poisoned rivers emptying into the lakes, marshes, and oceans; of pollution directly flowing into the oceans from coastal cities, military operations, and industries; from toxic chemical fertilizers and "pest control" chemicals spread on the greens of golf courses, lawns, farms, schools, and corporate campuses; from the shipping and oil industries; from cruise ships; and from air pollution, including from cars, trucks, airplanes, restaurants, coal-fueled electric generating plants, and cement kilns. Human exposure to the toxins in seafood can lead to nerve damage, miscarriages, learning disabilities, birth deformities, skin problems, and various types of cancer.

Another problem with fish liver oil is that when people are taking more than 5 grams or 5,000 milligrams per day, it can cause excessive bleeding, from simple skin wounds to brain hemorrhaging.

Then there are all of the damages being done to the oceans by the fish oil industry, such as in the Atlantic Ocean, where menhaden are so depleted that it is damaging the populations of other creatures that feed on them. The menhaden of North America's Atlantic coast are being fished to supply oil to the omega-3 nutrition market, and to supply oil and fishmeal for farmed fish, hog farms, egg farms, chicken and turkey farms, and cow farms, including on other continents. And they are being fished to supply bait for shellfish traps. And, they are being fished to sell as fertilizer, including for growing grains to feed farmed animals that end up being killed, cut up, and cooked.

"Menhaden are going bust, according to a highly vocal coalition of scientists, conservationists, and fishermen. Whereas they were once abundant along the entire Atlantic seaboard, the fishery has shrunk to an area from Virginia to New Jersey, and the annual catch has plummeted by almost 80 percent since the 1950s. Omega Protein executives like to point out that the commercial fishery leaves enough menhaden in the water to produce 18.4 trillion menhaden eggs annually. It sounds like a big number, and in theory it's almost double what's needed to maintain the species at target levels. But the 18.4 trillion is down from a peak of 117 trillion in 1961. Moreover, something in the process of turning those eggs into grown-up fish has gone badly awry in recent decades. Conservationists say overfishing is the problem, and they liken the collapse of the menhaden to the decimation of the great bison herds and the extinction of the passenger pigeon in the nineteenth century.

Three-quarters of the remaining catch now goes to Reedville (Virginia), which has the East Coast's last surviving reduction plant [which extracts the oil of the fish to sell as supplements for humans and also for farmed animals, such as farmed hogs and fish in the U.S. and in other countries, including China].

Hence Reedville's split reputation. Depending on your point of view, it is a manufacturing center for what has lately become one of the healthiest and most highly prized products on the planet – omega-3 fatty acids in the form of fish meal and fish oil. Or it is the Death Star for marine species on the entire Atlantic seaboard.

… Striped bass in the Chesapeake Bay are starving. They are starving, he said, because the reduction [omega-3 industry] has fished the menhaden almost down to nothing.

Many of the most familiar Atlantic Coast predators, from bluefish to humpback whales and from pelicans to bald eagles depend on menhaden."

– Oiliest Catch, by Richard Conniff, *Conservation* magazine, University of Washington; winter 2012/13

What is going on with the menhaden fish of the North American Pacific Coast is similar to what is going on in other parts of the world, because of sea life being overfished to supply nutritional oils for humans and oil and meal for farmed fish and farmed mammals being raised for slaughter. The sea creatures that are heavily relied on by a variety of fish, shellfish, sea mammals, and sea birds are being overfished, endangering a variety of forms of wildlife. Because so many other forms of wildlife, including coastal animals and forests, are dependent on those ocean-based creatures, the fish oil and fish meal market is part of the group of human activities that is endangering all forms of life on the planet, and causing some to go extinct – with many more being forced in line to do so.

While fish is not a good source of omega fatty acids, water plants, such as chlorella and spirulina, are good sources – as are unheated leafy greens you can grow in your garden, including spinach, chard, kale, cilantro, collards, basil, parsley, broccoli leaf, fennel leaf, and others – and the common weed, purslane.

The fish that people eat to get omega-3s, including menhaden, sardines, and anchovies, don't create the omega-3s in their systems. Instead, they get the omega-3s by eating algae, and the omega-3s store as fat in the tissues of the fish.

Chlorella is a fresh-water algae. It is often consumed in small amounts by vegans as a supplement, such as in compressed tablets, or in powder form added to salads and smoothies, and as an optional ingredient in other dishes. In addition to the nutrients B-6 and beta-carotene, the minerals iron, magnesium, phosphorus, and potassium, and a variety of amino acids, chlorella contains porphyrins and sporopollenim, which bind with heavy metals, including mercury, and help remove them from the body.

While fish and crustaceans do contain substances that are damaging to health, they *do not* contain something necessary to maintain health, which is fiber.

The soluble fiber in a vegan diet consisting largely of fruits and vegetables is excellent for protecting the brain and heart, because soluble fiber helps to prevent heart disease and strokes.

A raw food diet may include plant substances containing soluble and insoluble fiber. These include raw oats, germinated quinoa, germinated buckwheat, soaked millet, sprouted barley, and whole nongluten grains; fresh or dried apples, pears, figs, and other fruits, including fresh citrus; germinated beans and germinated bean and vegetable pâtés; soaked raw nuts; and a variety of fresh vegetables including cucumbers, broccoli, celery, fennel, and Brussels sprouts. Fiber helps to maintain a healthful balance of cholesterol in the system, which is important for brain health.

Some raw food recipes contain psyllium seed husks, which are also an excellent form of soluble fiber. Psyllium husk collects moisture, and it is best accompanied by adequate water or other hydration to help it move through the digestive tract.

Many people take psyllium husk for its beneficial impact on cholesterol levels. A healthy level of cholesterol is beneficial to brain health, but too much is not good. The body will make adequate amounts of cholesterol needed for maintaining brain and nerve health. There is absolutely no need to obtain cholesterol from food.

"Typical high-protein diets are extremely high in dietary cholesterol and saturated fat. The effect of such diets on blood cholesterol levels is a matter of ongoing research. However, such diets pose additional risks to the heart, including increased risk for heart problems immediately following a meal. Evidence indicates that meals high in saturated fat adversely affect the compliance of arteries, increasing the risk of heart attacks. Adequate protein can be consumed through a variety of plant products that are cholesterol-free and contain only small amounts of fat."

– Physicians Committee for Responsible Medicine, PCRM.org; Citing Nestle PJ, Shige H, Pomeroy S, Cehun M, Chin-Dusting J. Post-prandial remnant lipids impair arterial compliance. *Journal of the American College of Cardiology.* 2001;37:1929-1935.

Because the body makes the necessary cholesterol, there is no need to include cholesterol in the diet, such as from meat, dairy, or eggs. For those who have high cholesterol, it would be beneficial for them to eliminate all animal protein from their diet, to eliminate bottled oils (including foods containing them, such as fried and sautéed foods), and to include a variety of fresh fruits, vegetables, whole grains, and sprouted beans. These edible plants will help to remove excess cholesterol. This is because in the intestines, soluble fiber attaches to cholesterol and bile acids, and then carries them out of the body through the natural digestive process.

Bile acids are made from cholesterol and are necessary for fat digestion. When the digestive system needs more bile acids, the body will take cholesterol from the bloodstream to form more bile acids, thus lowering cholesterol levels.

A low-fat plant-based diet helps to remove cholesterol plaque from the body. This is why a vegan diet is particularly beneficial for those who have experienced serious health problems, such as a heart attack or stroke.

"My message is clear and absolute: coronary artery disease need not exist, and if it does, it need not progress. It is my dream that one day we may entirely abolish heart disease, the scourge of the affluent, modern West, along with an impressive roster of other chronic illnesses."

– Dr. Caldwell B. Esselstyn, author of *Prevent and Reverse Heart Disease*; HeartAttackProof.com

The sterols and stanols (phytosterols and phytostanols) found in a plant-based diet provide additional benefits to maintaining heart and brain health. This is because these natural plant chemicals help maintain cholesterol levels.

In the intestines, sterols and stanols block the reabsorption of cholesterol that has been removed from the digestive tract by soluble fiber. They do this by replacing cholesterol, or filling in for cholesterol in mixed micelles, which are composite molecules containing substances that are fat- and water-soluble. When the stanols and sterols end up in the micelles, the cholesterol instead gets put out of the body through the regular digestive process.

Micelles exist in the bloodstream, where they carry beneficial fats transporting nutrients, including fat-soluble vitamins. Sterols and stanols are in unheated plant oils. Lower amounts of them are in whole plant foods, such as raw fruits, vegetables, nuts, seeds, sprouts, and seaweeds.

In a person following a low-fat vegan diet rich in raw fruits and vegetables, the micelles are healthful because they contain stanols and sterols. But in a person following an unhealthful, meat-, dairy-, and egg-laden diet, the micelles contain cholesterol that ends up as plaque throughout the body.

If you are a person who shops at typical supermarkets, you may notice that some processed food products contain information on the labels that sterols and stanols have been added to the food, and thus the food companies have labeled the food as "heart healthy." But what the processed foods may also contain are cooked fats; bleached and gluten grains; processed salts; clarified and processed sugars, such as corn syrup; synthetic chemical preservatives, dyes, flavors, and scents; MSG (monosodium glutamate), which is a neurotoxin; and traces of fossil fuel-based farming chemicals from low-quality, nonorganic farming processes. The better choice would be to stick with a low-fat, raw or mostly raw vegan diet. The plant substances will provide the heart-healthy nutrients that are truly beneficial to maintaining vibrant health.

Because a low-fat vegan diet does not contain transfats, fried foods, heated nuts, processed salts, processed sugars, or MSG or other excito-toxins, it is all that more beneficial for protecting the heart and brain.

Raw fruits and vegetables containing the B vitamin folate also feed the brain. Folate improves brain memory and also appears to reduce the occurrence of Alzheimer's disease. Folate is found in oranges, dark greens, and in legumes. (Sprouted or germinated [slightly sprouted for two or three days] legumes, such as lentils, are used in a variety of live food recipes.) Other B vitamins help to protect the neural cell sheaths, so it is important to eat foods containing B vitamins. Raw, fermented foods, such as sauerkraut, kimchi, and fermented nondairy seed cheeses, especially those containing nutritional yeast, are sources of B vitamins, enzymes, and amino acids. Those concerned with not getting enough B-12 can put their worries to rest by simply taking a vegetarian B-12 supplement.

Many people have heard that wine is particularly beneficial to brain health. Red wine and the skins of red grapes contain substances called polyphenols. The polyphenol that has been recognized as most beneficial in the skin of red grapes is resveratrol. This phytochemical has been found to lower cholesterol while also improving blood circulation to the brain. Because resveratrol brings more nutrients into the brain, it has a positive effect on memory. Resveratrol prevents the formation of the plaques in the brain that interfere with neural communication. Resveratrol may help to prevent Alzheimer's disease because it prevents the formation of beta-amyloid protein, an ingredient in the plaque found in the brains of Alzheimer's patients. Within plants, resveratrol helps to ward off fungal growth and bacterial infection.

Wine happens to be a raw food. But you don't have to drink red wine to get resveratrol. It is also found in berries and peanuts. Some stores and Internet sites selling raw food products also sell raw "jungle peanuts" which do contain resveratrol. I have grown peanuts in my garden, which is one way to get fresh, raw peanuts.

To those who drink wine to obtain the health benefits, such as from resveratrol, I suggest that they seek out wine that is made from organically grown grapes, and preferably from the continent you live on, or are closest to, so that you are supporting local organic farmers. Pinot noir seems to be the most beneficial wine in the health-benefits category, and white wine is the least.

Some people have a problem with alcohol, so they should stay completely away from it, as it can become an addictive and ruinous substance. Many people, including some raw foodists, also stay away from alcohol because they consider it to be a neurotoxin.

Snacking on fresh seeded grapes, or blending whole seeded grapes into orange and apple juice with hemp seed and flax seed powders provides a variety of brain nutrients. If you don't have access to seeded grapes, find a place where you can grow some. You may also want to contact a local organic farm that may be growing seeded grapes, or encourage them to do so. A local food co-op or CSA may also carry or have access to seeded grapes.

There are a variety of nutrients found in live foods that the brain and nerve cells rely on. Vitamin C, which is in oranges, tomatoes, strawberries, dandelion greens, and other fruits and vegetables, works in combination with vitamin E as antioxidants that prevent the oxidation of cells. Vitamin E is found in green leafy vegetables, raw nuts, and raw vegetables and their oils.

Vitamin C also works in combination with iron in a number of ways, including in transporting oxygen to the tissues, including the brain.

Most animals form vitamin C in their bodies. Some animals don't, including fruit-eating bats, guinea pigs, certain birds, and humans and other primates. Many foods that modern people consume have been so processed through canning, cooking, fermenting, pickling, milling, clarifying, and frying that they contain no or very little vitamin C. A plant-based diet that is rich in variety and mostly or all raw contains plentiful amounts of vitamin C.

When you consume fruits and vegetables, consider that what you use on your foods, including any oils, salts, sweeteners, or condiments, should also be of high-quality. Consider not using any oils, salts, sweeteners, or condiments.

Processed salts are not good for brain health. In the live food diet, those who use salt use unprocessed sea salt, pink salt, and powdered sea vegetables, such as dulse and kelp. Processed salts have been heated to temperatures that change their structure, may contain additives, and are harsh and damaging to the body tissues, including nerve cells, the kidneys and liver, and the walls of the veins, arteries, and capillaries. Processed salts can help cause varicose veins.

Dietary minerals are essential to the brain's ability to function, including the ability to memorize and recall. The sunfood diet includes highly mineral-rich foods, including sea vegetables, which are particularly abundant in both minerals and the nutrients that help transport the minerals in the body.

Minerals work in combination with other nutrients, such as vitamins, amino acids, essential fatty acids, antioxidants, and trace nutrients. If you don't have a wide spectrum of nutrients in your diet, other nutrients can't be metabolized, and truly vibrant health is less likely to blossom.

In other words, when selecting food, use your brain – especially if you want your brain and heart to function at the highest level.

"In previous generations, how we ate appeared to be a personal and private matter. Our food choices didn't seem to contribute much, one way or the other, to the well-being or suffering of other people, let alone animals, plant life, and the carrying capacity of the entire plant. But even if that were ever true, it no longer is. What we eat, individually and collectively, has repercussions far beyond our waistlines and blood pressure readings. No less than our future as a species hangs in the balance."

– T. Colin Campbell, in his book, *Whole: Rethinking the Science of Nutrition*. Campbell is Professor Emeritus of Nutritonal Biochemistry at Cornell University, and has been involved in the science and research of nutrition for several decades. He advises a low-fat vegan diet with no added (bottled) oils, no salt, no processed sugars, but with whole plant foods. He is also author of *The China Study*; TColinCampbell.org

BRAIN FUNCTION

As the popularity of junk food has risen, so has the use of prescription antidepressant medication. According to the August 2009 issue of *Archives of General Psychiatry*, 27 million Americans were taking antidepressants in 2005. That was double the number of people on antidepressants in 1995. From the late 1980s to 2008, the use of antidepressants increased by over 400 percent. In 2011, antidepressants were the third most prescribed group of medications in the U.S. When the National Center for Health Statistics considered data from 2005 to 2008, they found that eleven percent of Americans over age 12 were taking antidepressants, and that women were more than twice as likely to take antidepressants than men. The study, released by the Centers for Disease Control on October 19, 2011, identified risk factors of depression as isolation, lack of exercise, and diets rich in processed foods.

It is clear that an astounding number of people are popping antidepressants. A large number of them are women and children. It is highly likely that the vast majority of the people popping the toxic happy pills also are consuming junk foods and diets rich in meat, milk, dairy, gluten, fat, salt, sugar, and synthetic chemicals. It is no doubt that their diets are also NOT rich in raw fruits and vegetables. It is no wonder why there are so many pharmacies in every city and town of the U.S. – often sharing the same rooftop with supermarkets and fast-food joints selling exactly the types of foods a person needs for experiencing cardiovascular disease, obesity, diabetes, asthma, osteoporosis, cancer, and low-quality brain and nerve function. All of this reveals why drug companies are making so much money, and why they spend so much money to promote the use of their patented chemical drugs that carry serious risks.

What I strongly advise for those who feel they are experiencing mood swings, depression, emotional instability, and/or general brain fatigue is to eliminate all unhealthful fats from their diet, including fried and sautéed foods, bottled oils (including olive oil), dairy, meat, bottled salad dressings, and heated nuts. Also, eliminate bleached grains, gluten grains, processed sugars and salts; artificial sweeteners and other synthetic food chemicals; and MSG. Then, follow a plant-based diet rich in raw fruits and raw vegetables, sprouts, germinates, and some sea vegetables. Green smoothies, salads, and some blended foods, such as oil-

111

free hummus, vegan and oil-free pestos and soups are also fine. If something heated is desired, do boiled foods, such as quinoa, lentils, brown rice, wild rice, beans, oats, and millet, and steamed vegetables, and no-oil vegan soups. As they remain on a healthful diet while getting daily exercise and maintaining a regular sleeping pattern, they will likely experience a more stable state of mind.

Those experiencing or with a history of depression may benefit from reading a book by Gabriel Cousens and Mark Mayell titled *Depression-free for Life: A Physician's All-natural, 5-step Plan*. Cousens is a psychiatrist and family therapist. He founded the Tree of Life Rejuvenation Center in Patagonia, Arizona, which is a raw foods health retreat. Mark Mayell was the editor-in-chief of *Natural Health* magazine.

I don't typically advise people to take supplements. However, to overcome depression, and especially if someone is transitioning from an unhealthful lifestyle and low-quality diet, there are certain supplements and "superfoods" that may help fuel the change toward better brain and neural function. This is why, in addition to following a fresh plant-based diet rich in green vegetables, getting daily morning exercise, following a list of goals, and getting into a habit of positive thinking and intentional living, I also encourage those with a history of depression to research the following natural amino acids, berries, herbs, mushrooms, foods, supplements, and vitamins to identify those that may be of benefit: ashwaganda herb; B-12 and other B-vitamins (from vegetarian sources); chlorella (a freshwater vegetable); vitamin D (in a mushroom supplement form); digestive enzymes (in a vegetarian supplement form); dulse powder (a seaweed); essential fatty acids (they are contained in raw vegetables, fruits, berries, nuts, seeds, and water plants, and in germinated buckwheat and chia seeds); 5-hydroxytryptophan, also known as 5-HTP (in veg caps); gamma-aminobutyric acid (also known as GABA); goji berries (and all edible and organically grown berries, including blueberries, raspberries, blackberries, and mulberries); hemp seeds (raw and organically grown); kelp powder (a seaweed); l-glutamine; lions mane mushrooms; mesquite powder; MSM powder; mucana prureins; pomegranate; probiotic powder (from a vegan source); pumpkin seeds (raw and organically grown); red cabbage; sesame seeds (raw and organically grown); spirulina (an algae); taurine; and tyrosine. Also, consider adding a green powder to your daily intake, such as Infinity Greens in salad dressing or blended in a green smoothie.

While I may mention steamed veggies, boiled foods (quinoa, lentils, brown rice, wild rice, beans, millet, and oats), and oil-free vegan soups, for those who desire heated foods, by a plant-based diet, I mean one that consists of fresh, raw, unheated fruits, vegetables, berries, nuts, seeds, seaweeds, and sprouts, and absolutely no meat, dairy, eggs, processed sugars (including corn syrup and agave); processed salts; synthetic food chemicals, or MSG. If there is anything that people don't eat enough of, it is fresh, uncooked fruits, and vegetables – and especially raw, organically grown green leafy vegetables, cruciferous vegetables, juicy fruits, and berries.

It can be especially helpful to those suffering from depression to follow a lower-fat diet, and *not* one that contains a lot of nuts and bottled oils (oil is fat). Any fat should also be raw, from a plant source, and preferably organic, such as unheated green vegetables, organic walnuts, hemp seeds, sesame seeds, Brazil nuts, germinated buckwheat, germinated chia seeds, seeded grapes, pumpkin seeds, and sprouted sunflower seeds. As I mention elsewhere, all raw fruits and all raw vegetables contain sufficient amounts of essential fatty acids, and there is no need to add oil to the diet.

As I write this there are many millions of people taking prescription medications for sleep, mood, and psychological disorders while they are at the same time consuming the lowest-quality foods and trying to get more energy by consuming coffee, cola, soda, and caffeine "energy drinks," and even diet pills and addictive street drugs. To experience better psychological health they would greatly benefit by getting their diet in order while following a daily morning exercise regimen, and avoiding in-gesting chemical food additives and artificial sweeteners, or using chem-ical drugs.

How is society supposed to progress to a more healthful state if the brains of the people can't function at a healthful level because the people are eating health-depleting, brain-numbing junk food and popping pre-scription chemical pills and/or other substances at every turn of the day to control their brain function?

All parts of you, including your brain, run on some sort of fuel. If your brain is bogged down by useless thought processes, stagnation, and clutter, you are not going to be able to function at your highest level. With the wrong brain and body fuel you will have limited use of your power. If you follow the typical lifestyle of low-quality foods and junk media thoughts, you will not be able to accomplish the goals through in-tentional living that you would otherwise be capable of if you thought, exercised, ate, and communicated better.

The brain grows in a way consistent with the quality of our thoughts and actions, and the nutrients in our food choices. As a person remains focused on a certain thought or action over a period of time, the brain grows more neurons in the area of the brain that is being used to con-duct those thoughts and actions. What a person does, says, sees, and otherwise experiences, creates patterns of thoughts, which result in pat-terns of connections between neurons.

The processes involved with thoughts and actions trigger certain genes on the brain neurons to be turned on or off. The patterns of activities being conducted among the brain's hundred billion or so neurons, including how the synaptic connections between the neurons take place, are what we call "thinking."

While not all of your thinking can be controlled by you, a significant amount of it can, and you can think on a higher level if you feed your brain better-quality nutrients and engage in worthwhile activities that train your brain to act and respond more to your liking.

What you are doing, saying, seeing, hearing, and feeling, and what you are eating, is affecting the neurons in your brain. Your brain is continually either engaging already formed synapses, or creating new ones.

Activity, social interaction, and intellectual stimulation are good for the brain. Slothfulness is not. People who stare at the television, screen games, or Internet, and/or do not engage in daily activities that utilize their skills, talents, and intellect are doing their brain no favors. Isolating yourself from social and intellectual stimulation also degrades your brain.

Vigorous exercise is beneficial to the brain because it increases the flow of information through the neurons while also increasing blood flow and releasing endorphins, which relieve stress. Exercise works the brain to produce more cells, especially in the hippocampus region of the brain, which helps to manage retention and organization of information.

People who regularly exercise have more healthful amounts of gray matter in their brains. This is proof that exercise protects against age-related brain degeneration.

Anxiety and psychological stress have a negative effect on the brain. Regular exercise and quality nutrition are most effective in reducing stress and anxiety.

Physical activity and intellectual and social stimulation engage the brain in ways that stimulate it to form new neural pathways. It also triggers the brain to release neurotrophin molecules, which are beneficial to maintaining cellular health.

Those wanting to maintain brain health should remain active on several levels, including physically, socially, and intellectually while following a diet rich in raw plant matter. Everything you do and eat has an impact on the brain. If one part of the brain is not used as often, the activities of that part of the brain will diminish and a certain amount of atrophy will take place. Like a muscle, the brain needs activity combined with quality nutrients to stay strong. A diet consisting largely of raw, unheated plant matter is rich in biophotons, which are tiny fields of light that play a part in cellular communication. The brain is rich in photoreceptor proteins, which work as light sensors in the cells.

"Each of us has that right, that possibility, to invent ourselves daily. If a person does not invent herself, she will be invented. So, to be bodacious enough to invent ourselves is wise."
– Maya Angelou

You are continually forming new brain cells while also, through your thoughts, actions, relationships, and nutrition helping to form the way the brain is wired and rewired. Realize that you have some control over how your brain forms. You can build neural pathways that correspond to what you want to think, feel, and do. Or you can build neural pathways that correspond to what you don't want. For these reasons, it is important to be involved with what you love – every day.

A growing concern about brain health is the incidence of Alzheimer's disease. In the U.S., more than 55,000 people a year die of Alzheimer's.

Diets rich in beta-carotene and vegetables, and with little or no animal protein, have been found to greatly reduce the incidence of Alzheimer's. Beta-carotene is found in many fruits and vegetables, including basil, beet greens, broccoli, butternut squash, cantaloupe, carrots, chard, cilantro, collard greens, dandelion greens, grape leaves, kale, lettuce, mustard greens, red peppers, parsley, pumpkin, spinach, and sweet potatoes, and in turnip greens.

"People eat meat and think they will become as strong as an ox, forgetting that the ox eats grass."
– Pino Caruso

As mentioned in the next chapter, the world's leading expert on Alzheimer's disease, Dr. Rudolph Tanzi has said that there is a clear connection between Alzheimer's disease and meat consumption. Because of what he has learned about the connection between the consumption of animal protein and Alzheimer's disease, Dr. Tanzi has become a vegetarian.

In other words, if you want a healthy brain, follow a low-fat vegan diet rich in a variety of raw fruits and vegetables, and get daily exercise, regular sleep, and keep your brain active through intellectual stimulation and goal-oriented activities that utilize your talents, skills, and other graces.

THE RISE OF ALZHEIMER'S DISEASE AND TYPE-2 DIABETES

HETEROCYCLIC amines, which form in cooked meat, have been identified as playing a role in the development of neurological disorders, and specifically tremors, or the shaking that people often associate with old age, a condition called *kinetic tremor* or *essential tremor*. People experiencing this are more likely to develop dementia. Other diseases of dementia include Alzheimer's and Creutzfeldt-Jakob disease. In cows, the related disease is Bovine Spongiform Encephalopathy (BSE), also known as *mad cow disease*. Mad cow disease can be transferred to humans through the consumption of meat. How many cases of Alzheimer's may actually be a misdiagnosis of Creutzfeldt-Jakob disease? We don't know, because the U.S. does not test for CJD in autopsies. We wouldn't want to damage the meat and dairy industries, would we?

The incidence of Alzheimer's disease in the U.S. has grown in relation to how much meat the U.S. population has been eating. It is reflective of how Alzheimer's is also becoming more common in other countries that also have been increasing their consumption of animal protein. Alzheimer's, like diabetes and obesity, has grown into a tremendous health problem in the U.S., and rising costs relating to it threaten to collapse the government health systems.

Years after the invention of mechanized refrigeration, and soon after the mass expansion of refrigerator use, which greatly increased meat consumption, Alzheimer's was identified in Europe. Since then, the incidence of the disease has increased dramatically – especially in countries that consume the most meat.

"In the coming decades, science will probably be able to ascribe a cause to Alzheimer's with the same certainty that it can now ascribe a cause to heart disease. And I firmly believe that it will be the exact same cause: meat... Studies have shown that between five and 14 percent of those diagnosed with Alzheimer's actually suffered from CJD. The amyloid plaques – waxy clumps of protein called beta-amyloid – discovered at autopsy in the brains of Alzheimer's victims are not terribly unlike the plaques to be found in the brains of victims of CJD. In both cases, abnormal protein buildup in the brain is involved."

– Former Montana cattle rancher Howard Lyman, in his book *No More Bull: The Mad Cowboy Targets America's Worst Enemy: Our Diet*; MadCowboy.Com

The world's leading expert on Alzheimer's disease, Dr. Rudolph Tanzi has stated that there is a clear connection between Alzheimer's disease and meat consumption. Tanzi is a professor of neurology at Harvard Medical School, Massachusetts General Hospital, and is Director of Genetics and Aging. He is the person who originally discovered two of the four genes related to Alzheimer's disease. It can be said that there is nobody more centric to the study of Alzheimer's disease than Tanzi.

Tanzi is now a vegetarian. He concluded that carnivores are the ones that experience diseases of dementia. Tanzi advises that to greatly reduce your chances of experiencing Alzheimer's disease, you should eliminate all meat from your diet.

In the U.S., Alzheimer's affects approximately one in ten people over age 65. Over 600,000 Americans under age 65 are living with the disease. For those over age 85 the chance of having Alzheimer's is nearly 50 percent. In 2006 approximately 4.5 million people had been diagnosed with the disease. As of 2005 the medical expense of Alzheimer's was estimated to be more than $100 billion.

From where did the protein misfolding disease called Alzheimer's originate? It appears that nobody knows. It has only been a recognized disease since a German psychiatrist and neuropathologist, Aloysius Alois Alzheimer, first identified it as "presenile dementia." In 1901 Alzheimer noticed the curious behavior and short-term memory loss of a 51-year-old patient, August Deter, at the Frankfurt Asylum. After she died in April 1906, Alzheimer studied her brain and identified the amyloid plaques and neurofibrilary tangles that became the identifiable physical characteristics of the disease. On November 3, 1906, Alzheimer gave a speech identifying the pathology and clinical symptoms of presenile dementia. His colleague, Emil Kraepelin, later referred to the condition as "Alzheimer's disease." Back then it was considered rare. But now, millions suffer with it, and it is expected to become more prevalent and a huge burden on society. Over 100 times more Americans have it today than just 25 years ago.

Elevated levels of homocysteine have been linked with a greater incidence of Alzheimer's disease. Homocysteine is an amino acid formed by the liver from the ingestion of methionine. Animal protein contains two to three times more methionine than vegetable protein. So, an easy way to reduce methionine is to avoid consuming animal protein.

Many studies have concluded that the more animal protein you consume, the more likely you are to experience Alzheimer's. It is interesting that the more animal protein you consume the more likely it is that you will develop Type-2 diabetes. Is there a connection?

In Alzheimer's it is found that there is a buildup of amyloid protein in the brain. In Type-2 diabetes there is a buildup of amyloid protein in the pancreas. Like Alzheimer's disease, Type-2 diabetes is on the rise.

"Glucose, a simple sugar, is the body's main fuel. It is present in the bloodstream, but in people with diabetes it cannot get into the cells where it is needed. In Type-1 diabetes (which was once referred to as childhood-onset diabetes), the problem is an inadequate supply of insulin, the hormone that ushers sugar into the cells of the body. Without insulin, the cell membranes keep sugar out. About 5 to 10 percent of people with diabetes have this type.

The more common type of diabetes, Type-2, usually does not occur until adulthood. In this form, there may be plenty of insulin in the bloodstream, but the cells are resistant to it. Glucose cannot easily get into the cells, and it backs up in the bloodstream. Over the short run, people with uncontrolled diabetes may experience fatigue, thirst, frequent urination, and blurred vision. In the long run, they are at risk for heart disease, kidney problems, disorders of vision, nerve damage, and other difficulties."

– Dr. Neal Barnard, *Dr. Neal Barnard's Program for Reversing Diabetes: The Scientifically Proven System for Reversing Diabetes without Drugs*; PCRM.org

The heavier you are, the more likely you are to have Type-2 diabetes. People that consume animal protein are more likely to be obese than those that follow a vegetarian diet. Those that follow a vegan diet are even less likely to be overweight.

In the past 50 years, the percentage of overweight children has risen dramatically. The number of younger people becoming afflicted with Type-2 diabetes is increasing at the same rate.

On January 26, 2011, the United States Centers for Disease Control released updated facts about diabetes:
- Diabetes affects 25.8 million people in the U.S.
- 8.3 percent of the U.S. population has diabetes
- 18.8 million people with diabetes are diagnosed
- An estimated 7.0 million people with diabetes have not been diagnosed
- Among U.S. residents aged 65 years and older, 10.9 million, or 26.9 percent had diabetes in 2010
- About 215,000 people younger than 20 years had diabetes (Type 1 or Type 2) in the U.S. in 2010

- About 1.9 million people aged 20 years or older were newly diagnosed with diabetes in 2010 in the U.S.
- In 2005-2008, based on fasting glucose or hemoglobin A1C levels, 35 percent of U.S. adults ages 20 years or older had prediabetes (50 percent of adults aged 65 years or older). Applying this percentage to the U.S. population in 2010 yields an estimated 79 million American adults aged 20 years or older with prediabetes.
- Diabetes is the leading cause of kidney failure, nontraumatic lower-limb amputations, and new cases of blindness among adults in the U.S.
- Diabetes is a major cause of heart disease and stroke
- Diabetes is the seventh leading cause of death in the U.S.

By the year 2000, epidemiologists were estimating that about one in three babies born in the U.S. would develop Type-2 diabetes. As those children become adults and continue to eat an unhealthful diet, it is likely that they increase their chances of having Alzheimer's.

As the consumption of meat and the number of people eating junk food is on the rise throughout the world, the number of children and young adults being diagnosed with Type-2 diabetes is on the rise. It is estimated that there were about 30 million people with Type-2 diabetes in the early 1980s. Today that figure has surpassed 225 million.

"A 2006 study, conducted by the Physicians Committee for Responsible Medicine with the George Washington University and the University of Toronto, looked at the health benefits of a low-fat, unrefined, vegan diet (excluding all animal products) in people with Type-2 diabetes. Portions of vegetables, grains, fruits, and legumes were unlimited. The vegan diet group was compared with a group following a diet based on American Diabetes Association (ADA) guidelines. The results of this 22-week study were astounding:

- Forty-three percent of the vegan group and 26 percent of the ADA group reduced their diabetes medications. Among those whose medications remained constant, the vegan group lowered hemoglobin A1C, an index of long-term blood glucose control, by 1.2 points, three times the change in the ADA group.
- The vegan group lost an average of about 13 pounds, compared with only about 9 pounds in the ADA group.
- Among those participants who didn't change their lipid-lowering medications, the vegan group also had more substantial decreases in their total and LDL cholesterol levels compared to the ADA group.

This study illustrates that a plant-based diet can dramatically improve the health of people with diabetes. It also showed that

people found this way of eating highly acceptable and easy to follow."
– Dr. Neal Barnard, *Dr. Neal Barnard's Program for Reversing Diabetes: The Scientifically Proven System for Reversing Diabetes without Drugs*; PCRM.org

Also to be considered in relation to Alzheimer's disease is Creutzfeldt-Jakob disease.

Not only the future, but also the present-day holds the promise that the more animal protein you consume, the more likely you are of ingesting the mutant proteins, or infectious prions, related to Creutzfeldt-Jakob disease, the human form of mad cow disease (bovine spongiform encephalopathy [BSE]).

As Howard Lyman points out in his book, *No More Bull*, the brains of those with the human form of mad cow disease are found to have a buildup of protein plaque in their brain in a similar manner to those with Alzheimer's disease. We don't know how many people in the U.S. may be dying from CJD rather than Alzheimer's disease, because the U.S. does not test for CJD in autopsies. Why? Consider that the powerful multibillion-dollar U.S. beef and dairy industries would collapse if CJD were found to be rampant in the U.S. Because the pharmaceutical industry also makes loads of money by selling drugs to the animal farming industry, they would also not welcome a collapse of the beef industry.

In April 2012, a cow that had died at a dairy in Hanford, California, tested positive for bovine spongiform encephalopathy, which is commonly known as mad cow disease. Within days, major supermarket chains in South Korea halted sales of U.S. beef. That move was considered a huge threat to the U.S. beef industry. South Korea held place as the world's largest importer of U.S. beef. In 2011, South Korea imported 107,000 tons of beef worth $563 million.

Of course, the cattle industry was quick to point out that the contaminated cow was never any threat to the nation's food supply. Scientists reported that the cow had tested positive for "atypical BSE," which is considered to be a form of the disease resulting from a random mutation of proteins. The state government concierge service for the animal farming industry, the California Department of Food and Agriculture, issued a statement saying that BSE "is not transmitted through milk," and that "milk and beef remain safe to consume." Knowing how few animals they actually test for the disease, and that they just happened to identify this cow's condition by chance, I certainly would not consider the assurance by the California Department of Food and Agriculture very reassuring. In fact, I think they are full of bull.

"Safe" is a matter of perception. People have reason to doubt the words of government workers engaged in protecting the financial interests of the beef industry. They also have reason to consider avoiding all meat and dairy – especially if they want to protect their health from degenerative and chronic diseases. Even without BSE, meat and dairy always contains a number of substances not good for human health, and meat and dairy are continually at risk of hosting a number of other harmful substances. If you eat meat or dairy, you may want to consider that you are also eating E. coli, salmonella, cholesterol, saturated fat, hormones, uric acid, purines, farming chemicals, Neu5Gc (N-glycolylneuraminic acid), polycyclic aromatic hydrocarbons, pesticides, the pharmaceutical drugs used to treat farm animals, and so forth.

A person consuming the meat or substances extracted from the meat or bones (lard, gelatin, bullion, etc.) of a cow infected with bovine spongiform encephalopathy can experience the human form of the disease, Creutzfeldt-Jakob disease. It is a debilitating and progressive condition that causes holes to form in the brain and leads to the loss of motor skills, and eventually to death

As of April 2012, U.S. authorities had only admitted to having found four other cows that tested positive for BSE. Previous to 2012, the last cow publicly identified in the U.S. as having mad cow was in 2006. As part of a screening process, in 2012 the USDA claims it had been testing approximately 40,000 cows each year. That is only a fraction of the approximately 34 million ranch cattle, dairy cows, and baby bulls killed every year to be cut up and sold as food for humans. But also, a lot of meat, and products that contain substances from meat and bones, is imported into the U.S. from other countries. Because the meat from so many different cows is mixed together in meat that is sold in restaurants and supermarkets, one hamburger, or other meat dish, may contain the meat from many dozens of cows.

In 2012 cattle ranching was taking up 38 million acres of land – and that was just in California. For decades, the number-one use of water and fuel in the state, and the number-one cause of air pollution and environmental destruction have all been related to feeding, raising, and slaughtering millions upon millions of farm animals (cows, cattle, chickens, turkeys, pigs, lamb, goats, and ducks), and cooking the meat and boiling the bones. To feed those animals, a tremendous amount of food needs to be grown, and an increasing amount of it is coming from the oceans, as in: fish. So, the animal farming industry is playing an increasingly bigger role in the destruction of the oceans and the collapse of species. The California Cattleman's Association and the California Beef Council reported that California had 620,000 beef cattle and 1.84 million dairy cows. In 2008, the sale of calves and cattle was a $1.82-billion industry in California. If you think that California had a lot of cows, consider that Kansas, Nebraska, and Texas had more. Consider that the cow population in the U.S. fluctuates around 85 million, and that there are something like ten billion chickens and about 250 million turkeys killed in the U.S. every year, and that the U.S. has about 60 million pigs, and you start to get an idea of how much resources and land are used and how much pollution is created to produce, market, and cook meat that we *do not* need for good health.

When I first heard of mad cow disease and what it does to the human brain and body, I thought that perhaps there would be a link between mad cow and Alzheimer's disease. In 1995 I wrote about it in my book, *Surgery Electives*. I was hardly the first person to make the connection. In his book, *The Food Revolution*, John Robbins mentions studies concluding that many presumed U.S. Alzheimer's victims were instead victims of CJD. If those studies represent current statistics, then there are likely several hundred thousand Americans suffering from CJD.

In the book *Dying for a Hamburger: Modern Meat Processing and the Epidemic of Alzheimer's Disease*, by Murray Waldman, the Toronto coroner, and his co-author, Marjorie Lamb, presents a convincing argument that Alzheimer's is related to infectious prions. Stanley Prusiner, who discovered prions, considered that prions might be causing Alzheimer's.

Another book that would likely be of interest to anyone wanting to know details about America's food supply is *Brain Trust: The Hidden Connection Between Mad Cow and Misdiagnosed Alzheimer's Disease*, by Colm A. Kelleher. Among the books that may be of interest on this matter is *How the Cows Turned Mad: Unlocking the Mysteries of Mad Cow Disease*, by Maxime Schwartz, a molecular biologist and former head of the Pasteur Institute in Paris, and Edward Schneider.

What will most certainly guard you from CJD? Not eating meat, milk, or eggs, or anything made with them or containing extracts of them (including gelatin, bouillon, and lard).

"Experimental animal studies have convincingly shown that a high-cholesterol diet will promote the production of the beta-amyloid common to Alzheimer's. In confirming these experimental animal results, a study of more than 5,000 people found that greater dietary fat and cholesterol intake tended to increase the risk of Alzheimer's disease specifically, and all dementia in general.

In another study on Alzheimer's, the risk of getting the disease was 3.3 times greater among people whose blood folic acid levels were in the lowest one-third range and 4.5 times greater when blood homocysteine levels were in the highest one-third. What are folic acid and homocysteine? Folic acid is a compound derived exclusively from plant-based foods, such as green and leafy vegetables. Homocysteine is an amino acid that is derived primarily

from animal protein. This study found that it was desirable to maintain low blood homocysteine and high blood folic acid. In other words, the combination of a diet high in animal-based foods and low in plant-based foods raises the risk of Alzheimer's disease."
– T. Colin Campbell, Ph.D., Cornell University; author of *The China Study* and *Whole: Rethinking the Science of Nutrition*; TColinCampbell.org

What will decrease your chances of becoming a member of both the Alzheimer's disease and the Type-2 diabetes clubs? It very clearly appears that avoiding animal protein while following a vegan diet that is abundant in fruits and vegetables and other plant substances while staying physically fit and intellectually engaged are the most promising ways to avoid those dreaded diseases.

It is well documented that following a healthy, balanced, low-fat vegan diet free from junk food while getting plenty of physical activity will greatly reduce your chances of experiencing cancer, obesity, arthritis, osteoporosis, cardiovascular disease, and other degenerative diseases, including diabetes and Alzheimer's.

"There's a problem. Could this be a case of 'Don't look, don't find'? Nearly 34 million cattle are slaughtered every year in the U.S. Of those, only 40,000 are tested for BSE. That's about one in every thousand animals. If we tested 80,000, would we find two? If we tested them all, would we find 1,000 cases a year? One cow can make its way into many thousands of burgers. So then, how many burgers might be contaminated?"
– John Robbins, Pink Slime and Mad Cow Disease: Coming to a Burger Near You, *Huffington Post*, April 26, 2012

The human nutritional need for animal protein is absolute zero. Humans flourish in health on a low-fat vegan diet rich in raw fruits and vegetables. Even better if the foods are locally grown and organic.

"Plant-based diets may offer advantages over those that are not plant-based with respect to prevention and management of diabetes. The Adventist Health Studies found that vegetarians have approximately half the risk of developing diabetes as nonvegetarians. In 2008, Vang et al reported that nonvegetarians were 74% more likely to develop diabetes over a 17-year period than vegetarians. In 2009, a study involving more than 60,000 men and women found that the prevalence of diabetes in individuals on a vegan diet was 2.9%, compared with 7.6% in the nonvegetarians."
– Nutritional Update for Physicians: Plant-based Diets, by Dr. Michael Greger, NutritionFacts.org

FOOD AS ENTERTAINMENT

"We are indeed much more than what we eat, but what we eat can nevertheless help us to be much more than what we are."
– Daisie Adelle Davis

POP culture treats food as a form of entertainment. Food is no longer eaten for nutritional needs, but is eaten for want and for some sort of imagined enjoyment. It has been turned into a hip adventure. And it has become all so dangerously silly. Food commercials feature talking pizzas, dancing cupcakes, gangsta' burritos, and people who fall in love at the bite of a potato chip. Selling food has turned into a pile of putrid nonsense. And people are buying it.

The processing, packaging, marketing, and consumption of unhealthful food products have become something more serious than simple blatant commercialism. From the commercials to the packaging, from the theme restaurants to the product giveaways, the marketing of food is something that causes an enormous amount of pollution and environmental damage all over the planet. The consumption of the very same mass-marketed foods paves the way for gluttony and illness at rates and in ways humanity has never experienced.

"Poor countries sell their grain to the West while their own children starve in their arms. And we feed it to livestock. So we can eat a steak? Am I the only one who sees this as a crime? Every morsel of meat we eat is slapping the tear-stained face of a starving child. When I look into her eyes, should I be silent?

The Earth can produce enough for everyone's need. But not enough for everyone's greed.

We are facing the perfect storm.

If any nation had developed weapons that could wreak such havoc on the planet, we would launch a pre-emptive military strike and bomb it into the Bronze Age.

But [the meat industry] is not a rogue state. It is an industry.

The good news is we don't have to bomb it. We can just stop buying it.

George Bush was wrong. The Axis of Evil doesn't run through Iraq, or Iran, or North Korea. It runs through the dining tables. Weapons of Mass Destruction are our knives and forks."
    – Philip Wollen, KindnessTrust.com

The most popular restaurants, those that can be found in every city in the US, along freeway exits, and often very close to schools and on many school and medical campuses, are marketing the most toxic concoctions of food and drink that they can get away with selling, and especially to children. The fast food industry spends huge amounts of money to advertise their toxic foods to children. If you can get the children in there, the parents come along and also chug down disease-inducing drinks and eat what amounts to the exact foods that pave the way for obesity, cardiovascular disease, diabetes, Alzheimer's disease, Parkinson's disease, Crohn's disease, kidney disorders, arthritis, osteoporosis, MS, macular degeneration, and other diseases that we call *chronic, degenerative* and *autoimmune*. Fast food restaurants sell foods containing exactly what your body needs for the development of cancer and for you to experience strokes and heart attacks.

"As a culture, we've become upset by the tobacco companies advertising to children, but we sit idly by while the food companies do the very same thing. And we could make a claim that the toll taken on the public health by a poor diet rivals that taken by tobacco."
    – Kelly Brownell, Yale University professor of psychology

"There is no question that advertising and entertainment are shaping countless people's minds – especially children. In western society, the subconscious mind of the individual is often subject to a number of heavy influences, through entertainment mediums especially. Television, movies, music, and of course, advertisements, create a profound subconscious effect on the human mind that influences and helps to dictate the choices that they will make."
    – Elizabeth Renter, Imprinted: Kids' Brains 'Branded' with Fast-Food Logos; NationOfChange.org

"Some research finds that children identify the golden arches for McDonald's before they know the letter M."
    – Dr. Amanda Bruce.

As I am writing this, McDonald's is selling a "McDouble Mighty Kids Meal with Fat-Free Chocolate Milk Jug" that packs a whopping 765 calories, 30 grams of fat, and 1,215 mg of sodium. Saturated, trans-, and sticky fried fats come with the package, as do bleached gluten grains, a variety of synthetic chemicals, and the carcinogenic substances casein, acrylamides, glycotoxins, heterocyclic amines, polycyclic aromatic hydro-carbons, and N-glycolylneuraminic acid. If you don't understand by now about how these carcinogens risk your health, I don't know how much more simpler I can explain it.

"The United States is currently facing a health crisis of unprecedented proportions. Unhealthy diet is a major cause of health problems such as obesity and chronic disease, which are now increasingly beginning in childhood.
- The youth of today are the first generation predicted to have a lower life expectancy than their parents.
- Children as young as seven years old have diseases formerly classed as those of adulthood, such as heart disease, Type-2 diabetes, and many forms of cancer.
- The number of children who are overweight or obese has more than tripled since 1980, being now more than 16 percent – that's over 9 million U.S. children. As adults, over 30 percent of Americans are obese; 60 million people.
- The U.S. spends more on health care than any other industrialized country, yet has one of the highest rates of life-threatening disease. This cost totaled $1.5 trillion in 2002 and is still rising at an alarming rate.

The impact of chronic disease is not restricted to the U.S. – it is global in reach.
- 60 percent of deaths are due to chronic disease and 80 percent of these deaths are now thought to occur in low- and middle-income countries.
- An estimated 1 billion people worldwide are overweight; that includes 22 million children under the age of five.
- Each year, 2.6 million people die as a result of being overweight or obese; 4.4 million due to raised total cholesterol levels; and 7.1 million due to raised blood pressure – many of these deaths could be avoided with improvements to diet."
– The Food Studies Institute, Dr. Antonia Demas' plant-based nutrition for children; FoodStudies.org.

It isn't only McDonald's that is selling disease-inducing foods, it is the entire fast food industry, the supermarkets, the "convenience" stores, the snack machines, and the school food and government food programs.

Most of the packaged products being sold as food contain labels listing the nutrients, the fats, the sodium, and measurements of some other substances they are required to list. Much of this is based on government standards set not by nutritionists, but by lobbyists working for the meat industry, the dairy industry, the egg industry, the sugar industry, and other corporate food interests. This is something that many people don't know. The recommended daily nutrition requirements and limits of various food substances, including the famous "food pyramid," are based on a lot of nonsense, and were not set by those with training in nutrition, or those with interest in your health. They were developed to sell meat, dairy, eggs, sugar, grains, and other products of various industries. The food pyramid, with its advice to consume lots of meat, dairy, and eggs will lead you not to health, but to sickness. That pyramid was created to increase the sales of industrial food products, and it has done a very good job at that – at the expense of health and the environment.

Relying on the government for nutrition information and health is thrusting yourself into a den of nutritional ignorance festering with common degenerative and chronic diseases.

> "Everybody has read 'Endorsed by Uncle Sam,' 'In Accordance With the Pure Food Law,' and 'Guaranteed Under the Food and Drug Act.' These are a few of the innumerable commercial ruthless suggestions which catch the ignorant, the credulous, and those who pay the doctor to think for them."
> – George Julius Drews, in his 1912 raw food book *Unfired Foods and Tropho-Therapy*

On average, those people who watch television are heavier than those who do not watch television. Probably the chief reason for that is, in addition to being a sedentary activity, watching television exposes a person to an enormous number of images of processed and cooked foods that are made to look appealing, exciting, filled with flavor, and sexy. The majority of the products featured in the commercials shouldn't be considered food. Most of it has significantly less nutritional content than edible garden weeds.

> "We know how to flavor food with salt and condiments, and how to wash it all down with wine, beer, coffee, and tea. In short, we have elevated the practice of eating to an intensely pleasurable art form in which eating is encouraged as much by a craving for addictive tastes, such as sugar and salt, as it is by genuine hunger, thus leading to the over-indulgence that overloads our vital organs, pollutes our blood, and diminishes our vitality. Our cells get sick and we get sick."
> – Ross Horne, author of *Cancerproof Your Body*

When the money spent on corporate food is taken into consideration, the consumers are paying about 80 percent of their food dollar for processing, packaging, shipping, and other marketing-related costs. In 2000 the U.S. Department of Agriculture estimated that less than 15 percent of a dollar spent on food goes to the farmer. In other words, what most people are eating from the supermarket barely consists of real food, and what they spend on it is also not for food, but for the commercialism – the supermarketing.

> "The average American child sees 20,000 junk food ads per year on television. That is their nutritional education. That is how children are being taught about food."
> – Eric Schlosser, author of *Fast Food Nation: The Dark Side of the All-American Meal,* and *Chew on This: Everything You Don't Want to Know About Fast Food,* appearing in *McLibel;* SpannerFilms.Net

Corporate food is not an efficient use of resources, and does not provide a body with what it needs to experience vibrant health.

> "Food is an important part of a balanced diet."
> – Fran Lebowitz

Commercials are designed to stimulate passions, to play with emotions, and to entice people to feel a need or a want for a product or service. Commercials are created to seduce money out of pockets and into cash registers to satisfy stockholders.

Food commercials promote substances that you have no need for. Other than a very few commercials that promote fruits and vegetables, the vast majority promote foods that are damaging to health. Commercialized foods contain saturated fats, fried oils, transfats, cholesterol, processed salts and sugars, and synthetic dyes, flavors, and preservatives, and other chemicals and additives that degrade health. From burgers to sodas to desserts and fast food and TV dinners, the vast majority of the foods in the commercials are not healthful – even if the commercials say the products are healthful. Advertising lies.

> "Our poor eating habits and lack of activity are literally killing us, and they're killing us at record levels."
> – US Health and Human Services Secretary Tommy G. Thompson; March 9, 2004

A study released in 2003 by the Santa Monica-based Rand Corporation predicted that within 20 years the diseases related to unhealthful food and lack of exercise would cancel out health improvements seen in other areas. This is because the extent of obesity being experienced in industrialized countries is unlike any that has been experienced in human history. It is leading people down a path toward heart disease; high blood pressure; hardening of the arteries; cirrhosis of the liver; macular degeneration; cataracts; arthritis; cancers of the colon and other organs; skin problems; kidney disease; bone structure and joint injuries; immune system disorders like MS, diabetes and diabetes-related nerve damage; and early death.

Americans and others living in an industrial society are watching more television than ever, spending a large chunk of their time in front of the TV or computers, and many times in front of numerous TVs that are stationed in various rooms of their homes. Even when they get outside, they are increasingly occupied with smaller techno screens, on laptops, computerized pads, and cell phones.

"I think we risk becoming the best informed society that has ever died of ignorance."
– Reuben Blades

Television is collectively a negative and greed-based energy that provides almost nothing worthy of watching and it has a negative impact on society. The television news and magazine show producers dig up the freakiest stories of the day to keep people tuned in, add an alarmist spin on terrible events, work the shows to play with viewer emotions, titillate, instill fear, and create havoc, and they rarely offer solutions. Television and other pop media are mostly tools for companies to advertise their products to turn people into consumers. A majority of the advertising has to do with unhealthful foods sold in supermarkets and restaurants, and those advertisements are followed by commercials for over-the-counter and prescription drugs promising to make you feel better.

When you consider the ingredients, nutritional value, and advertising of foods that people purchase in supermarkets, they are often not buying food. They are buying entertainment. They don't need the fancy packaging and the sugar coating, synthetic dyes, scents, and flavors, and the pop sexiness to feed their bodies. All they really need are pure foods that are highly nutritious, such as raw fruits and vegetables. But instead they are buying cookies and cakes, chips, candy, processed dinners and snacks, and fried foods, and generally foods that squash health. A large number of the foods in supermarkets and restaurants not only contain chemical dyes, flavors, scents, preservatives, and emulsifiers, but also the residue of toxic farming chemicals. All of this garbage works against health. It clogs body tissues, interferes with brain and nerve function, wastes money, and causes health problems that limit and shorten lives.

"Advertising is the art of making whole lies out of half truths."
– Edgar A. Shoaff

What drives the purchase and consumption of commercial foods is the emotion the marketers have successfully attached to the products. People eat sugarcoated breakfast toasty things because that is what they ate in the morning when they were little. They eat potato chips because the commercial tells them how crunchy and desirable the chips are. They drink soda because that is what cool people drink, but the caffeine and processed sugars and salts are addictive and damage tissues, including their bones (which are also damaged by the phosphoric acid and other substances in the sodas). They fill themselves with cooked starches because cooked starches are dense and give them that filled feeling that replaces the emptiness they have in their lives from the disconnection from nature and the lack of love that they may not even know they are experiencing. Children stuff themselves with all sorts of junk associated with marketing tie-ins of their favorite films and TV shows.

> "We often forget that we are nature. Nature is not something separate from us. So when we say that we have lost our connection to nature, we've lost our connection to ourselves."
> – Andy Goldsworthy

In about 2006, Disney finished a ten-year business relationship with McDonald's to familiarize children with various Disney film characters. After the pact with Disney ended, in 2006 McDonald's signed a deal with another film studio, DreamWorks Animation. Another fast-food chain, Burger King, signed a deal with Warner Brothers. But fast foods are not the only foods being used to market to children. Makers of the most unhealthful breakfast cereals often have business arrangements with major studios to market films on cereal boxes. What better time to get into the minds of children than by having them see your cartoon and super hero characters on their cereal box every morning? When the children go to school they are likely to see a vending machine on their school campus. On the labels of the junk snacks there are likely to be more images associated with film or TV characters.

Want kidney and bone damage with that? In June 2010 McDonald's recalled 12 million drinking glasses being sold as promotional tie-ins with the "Shrek" animated film. The glasses, which had been sold for several weeks, were found to contain the toxic heavy metal cadmium in the paints used on the images of the cartoon characters. Cadmium is a carcinogen that can also damage kidneys and bones – not exactly things a consumer is likely to expect from using a glass. As the recall was announced, stock shares in McDonald's fell 51 cents.

"I am amazed when I see young people eating meat. It seems to me so much a thing from other times. The carnivore youth is not with the times, it has a stomach of the nineteenth century."
– Guico Ceronetti, Italian poet and philosopher

Taking into consideration that the foods with which the film studios align in advertising are of the worst types of foods children can eat, it appears that the film studios don't care about the health of children. What seems to be the only concern of the studios is that the stockholders stay happy with the returns on their investments. Let the environment suffer and the rates of obesity, diabetes, and heart disease in young people rage – the greedy film studios need to make money! (For information about plant-based nutrition education for school children, access: FoodStudies.org)

"We pray on Sundays that we might have light. To guide our footsteps on the path we tread. We are sick of war, we don't want to fight, and yet we overeat ourselves upon the dead."
– George Bernard Shaw

It is strange that cigarette packaging and tobacco advertising is required by law to contain warnings of the diseases they cause, including asthma, emphysema, and cancers, but food sold at fast food restaurants don't have to carry such warnings when they clearly cause similar health problems, and perhaps a wider variety of health problems than what are caused by regular exposure to tobacco smoke.

If the fast food restaurants were going to have truth in advertising, their packaging and advertising would state that consuming the food increases the risks of obesity, diabetes, kidney disease, kidney stones, stroke, heart attacks, cardiovascular disease, high blood pressure, colorectal cancer, prostate cancer, breast cancer, pancreatic cancer, arthritis, asthma, depression, and erectile dysfunction. The polycyclic aromatic hydrocarbons, heterocyclic amines, acrylamides, glycotoxins, d-Nitrosodiethanolamine, synthetic chemicals, and other cancer-causing substances, and the corn syrup (aka corn sugar), processed salts, cholesterol, saturated fats, transfats, fried oils, artificial substances, farming chemical residues, bleached grains, and other unhealthful ingredients found in the foods being sold at these restaurants should be listed as hazardous to health on packaging, in advertising, at the doorways, and at the cash registers. It doesn't mean that people can't eat them, but if they do, they will have some idea of what they may be doing to themselves.

"The scientific evidence of risk to your heart from eating the standard American diet rivals in depth, breadth, and uniformity the evidence that smoking causes cancer...

People who merrily eat their cheeseburgers and pepperoni pizzas while putting their faith in drugs and medical technology to keep them alive might as well cheerfully beat themselves over the head with an anvil while keeping a first-aid kit handy."

– Former cattle rancher Howard Lyman, in his book *No More Bull: The Mad Cowboy Targets America's Worst Enemy: Our Diet;* MadCowboy.Com

After people eat commercial processed foods for months and years, they end up going to the doctor to deal with all the health problems they have when their body doesn't function right because it can't function healthfully when all of the cells in their body are saturated with toxic junk food residues. But the doctor doesn't tell them to stop eating junk. Instead, the doctor prescribes medications made of toxic chemicals that some international drug company is selling successfully, filling their stockholders' pockets with money. The doctor may also suggest risky surgeries that bring money into the hospitals and medical centers.

All pharmaceutical drugs end up in the environment, in the aquifers, streams, rivers, lakes, marshes, oceans, and soil. Fish in the oceans, birds in the sky, and bears in the Arctic all have been found to contain residues of pharmaceutical drugs. The pharma drug industry profits by selling enormous amounts of drugs to the animal farming industry, and also by selling to people suffering from degenerative illnesses related to their consumption of meat, dairy, eggs, and junk food. Go to your local hospital cafeteria and look at the foods they are selling and serving. It's absolutely absurd and pathetic. Illness-inducing foods from the sickly animal farming industry, and foods rich in processed sugars, salts, oils, and synthetic chemicals. The hospital, animal farming, and corporate food industries are money machines for the pharmaceutical industry.

"Modern hospitals offer almost nothing to enhance public health. They are cathedrals of sickness."

– Dr. Caldwell B. Esselstyn, author of *Prevent and Reverse Heart Disease;* HeartAttackProof.com

As far as a business, the prescription drug industry is very successful, and they are successful across the planet as more people turn to the toxic chemical drugs in an attempt to ward off health problems or to "maintain health." Pharmaceutical companies consistently earn billions of dollars every year, get huge tax breaks while also benefiting from enormous amounts of government subsidies, and own the patents on drugs for which they can charge whatever they wish. All of the chemicals they manufacture end up in the environment, in rivers, in lakes, in wetlands, in marshes, in aquifers, in oceans, and in wildlife. They are also in our drinking water, our farmland, our food, and our bodies.

Hospitals, surgery equipment manufacturers, hospital supply companies, and the drug companies – and companies serving those companies – are all making more money as more people are eating more unhealthful food. Allopathic (typical Western medical) doctors aren't so poor, either. The medical field continues to grow as people experience health problems associated with diet and lack of exercise – and it is growing in many countries.

Meanwhile, people in industrial and high-tech societies throughout the world keep eating massive amounts of junk food, increase their consumption of factory farmed meat, dairy, and eggs, and continue to gain weight, and persistently experience record numbers of diet-induced health problems known as _degenerative diseases_. The average weight of people living in commercial society has increased so much that furniture, automobile, and airplane manufacturers are creating wider seating to accommodate the plumper bodies.

I can go on and on and quote all sorts of studies and statistics about how fat people are getting, and the subsequent health problems. The point is that obesity is a problem, and it is getting worse. The problem is tied in with the spiritual health of the culture in which we are living; in the damage people are doing to the planet; and in their disconnection from nature and from natural foods that nature supplies in the form of raw fruits and vegetables.

"Here are the facts. Coronary artery disease is the leading killer of men and women in Western civilization. In the United States alone, more than half a million people die of it every single year. Three times that number suffer known heart attacks. And approximately three million more have 'silent' heart attacks, experiencing minimal symptoms and having no idea, until well after the damage is done, that they are in mortal danger. In the course of a lifetime, one out of every two American men and one out of every three American women will have some form of the disease."
– Dr. Caldwell B. Esselstyn, author of _Prevent and Reverse Heart Disease_; HeartAttackProof.com

Eating a bad diet perpetuates a vicious circle of human disease and environmental destruction. The diets people in modern society are following are ruining their health, damaging the environment, using vast quantities of natural resources, and playing a major role in disrupting wildlife to the point that reginal or complete extinction of many species is accelerating.

"If you allow the media to guide your food choices, the next step will be to ask *your* doctor is if *this drug* is right for you."
– Brigitte Mars, in her book *The Sexual Herbal: Prescriptions for Enhancing Love and Passion*; BrigitteMars.com

There is some hope in a healthier society as statistics are showing that average meat consumption in the U.S. is falling. In 2011, the average American was eating 171 pounds of meat. That was down from the peak of 184 pounds in 2004. People are realizing how unhealthful eating meat is for human health and how terrible the production of it is for the environment, how tremendous resources of land, water, food, and fuel are used to produce meat, and how horrible it is to mass breed and contain billions of animals for slaughter and dismemberment. Other factors are also playing into the reduction of meat consumption. Heat waves and drought have wreaked havoc on grain and hay production, reducing the amount of hay and grain available for feeding farm animals. As of 2011, there were fewer cattle in the U.S. than at any time since the early 1960s.

"Attitudes about meat are changing. Rather than considering meat requisite at every dinner or an indication of wealth, many people are deliberately choosing to eat less meat than before, often citing concerns about health, the environment, and the ethics of industrial meat production."
– Janet Larsen, Peak Meat: U.S. Consumption Falling; Earth Policy Institute; March 7, 2012; Earth-Policy.org

"I believe that moving toward a more plant-based diet was a major reason that I was able to continue playing professional tennis through my 40s. It made me mentally sharper, and made it possible for me to endure the physical conditioning that is required to compete at that level."
– Martina Navratilova, record-setting nine-time Wimbledon singles tennis champion and a vegan; MartinaNavratilova.com

"For every pound of beef produced in the industrial system, it takes two thousand gallons of water. That is a lot of water and there is plenty of evidence that the Earth cannot keep up with the demand. Here in the United States I am told one acre is lost to development every minute of every day, which means that since 1982 an area the size of Indiana has been built over. Again, in the U.S., soil is being washed away ten times faster than the Earth can replenish it."
– Prince Charles, May 2011, Future of Food conference at Georgetown University.

"This process of atherosclerosis, this hardening of the arteries that comes from a lifetime of eating beef and other high-fat foods, it doesn't just cause heart attacks, it can also make you impotent."
– Dr. Neal Barnard, 2004; NealBarnard.org

"I brainwashed youngsters into doing wrong. I want to say sorry to the children everywhere for selling out to people who make millions by murdering other living creatures."
– Geoffrey Guiliano, actor who played Ronald McDonald in the 1980s

"I was three years old, to this day it is a vivid memory. My family and I were on a boat, catching a fish. As one fish was caught, he was writhing, then he was thrown against the side of the boat. You couldn't disguise what it was. This was what we did to animals to eat them. The animal went from a living, vibrant creature fighting for life to a violent death. I recognized it, as did my brothers and sisters."
– Joaquin Phoenix

"We need, in a special way, to work twice as hard to help people understand that the animals are fellow creatures, that we must protect them and love them as we love ourselves."
– Cesar Chavez

"I know it's hard sometimes to face reality and instead to try to ignore the pain that we inflict by living out our daily lives, but it doesn't have to be that way. Like waging a war to create peace doesn't make sense, we don't need to kill other sentient beings in order to live. In fact, it's healthier for us to not eat animal products at all."
– Elizabeth Kucinich

"Animal factories are one more sign of the extent to which our technological capacities have advanced faster than our ethics. We plow under habitats of other animals to grow hybrid corn that fattens our genetically engineered animals for slaughter. We make free species extinct and domesticate species into biomachines. We build cruelty into our diet."
– Jim Mason

THE EXPERIMENT

"How many times has a doctor told you to change your diet before they tried to sell you on toxic medications?"
– Dr. John McDougall, DrMcDougall.com

"I have come to the conclusion that when it comes to health, government is not for the people, it is for the food industry and the pharmaceutical industry at the expense of the people. It is a systemic problem where industry, academia, and government combine to determine the health of this country. Industry provides funding for public health reports, and academic leaders with industry ties play key roles in developing them. A revolving door exists between government jobs and industry jobs, and government research funding goes to the development of drugs and devices instead of healthy nutrition. It is a system built by people who play their isolated parts, oftentimes unaware of the top decision makers and their ulterior motivations. The system is a waste of taxpayer money and is profoundly damaging to our health."
– T. Colin Campbell, Ph.D., Cornell University; author of *The China Study* and *Whole: Rethinking the Science of Nutrition*; TColinCampbell.org

A great and unfortunate experiment has been taking place in modern society. It's like a race and it involves hundreds of millions of people, trillions of prescription pills, billions of dollars to study where diseases come from, and trillions of dollars in medical costs to "treat" environmentally- and diet-induced diseases. To support this activity there are nearly 100,000 drug salespeople sent forth from the pharmaceutical companies to get American doctors to prescribe chemical pills. Other pharmaceutical representatives focus on medical schools to make sure the students are familiar with the various drugs available to prescribe to their future patients. Doctors are also employed by the drug companies to work as "consultants" to convince other doctors to prescribe drugs. Hundreds of millions of dollars are spent to advertise pills to the public while other millions are spent to advertise the drugs in medical journals that are read by doctors. There have been thousands of "drug stores" built throughout cities and towns to dispense the drugs; some of these drug stores are located in supermarkets, on college campuses, and in shopping malls. Thousands more structures have been built to carry out medical experiments, often involving hundreds of caged animals. In other structures we call "hospitals" and "medical centers," ailing people are turning to doctors who prescribe drugs and perform surgery to "treat" the ills people get from eating horrible food, not getting enough exercise, and living in unhealthful ways that are distant from the ways of nature. In the hospital cafeterias, much of the food is the same food that, when consumed, helps cause the very ailments and diseases the patients are suffering from. To get laws passed and subsidy programs funded benefitting the medical industry, according to the Center for Responsive Politics, the doctor, hospital, pharmaceutical, and medical device industries spend almost double the amount on lobbying than what is spent by the oil, gas, and defense industries combined.

"Discovery consists of looking at the same thing as everyone else and thinking something different."
– Albert Szent-Gyrogyi

The experiment is a big failure and nobody is winning. People keep getting more obese and sickly; cholesterol-lowing, diabetes, arthritis, and pain drugs are making more money every year; pharmaceutical shares continue to be the stock market's most profitable area; the medical lobby is the most well funded in Washington; and the environment continues to suffer from the junk diet and the disposable and wasteful lifestyle choices of humanity. But instead of changing their eating and exercise habits, people often turn to drugs and surgery to try to improve their health. Meanwhile, the cause of their problems, as well as the answers to them, may be sitting right in front of their eyes – on their dinner plates.

"Dietary contributors to disease are easily swept aside, as our culture assumes it's normal to be chronically medicated to regulate cholesterol, blood pressure, and blood sugar."
– Dr. Neal Barnard, Physicians Committee for Responsible Medicine, PCRM.org

"Surgery does not deal with the basic molecular foundation of disease. It is a mechanical approach to a biologic problem."
– Dr. Caldwell B. Esselstyn, author of *Prevent and Reverse Heart Disease*; HeartAttackProof.com

People need to reconsider what they consider to be food.
While allopathic doctors release their various reports and announce "recent discoveries" showing "scientific evidence" proving diets low in salt, sugar, oil, and animal products, and high in unrefined plant content

lead to better health and lower cancer risks while improving brain and heart function, the "healthfood fanatics" have always taught that edible plants contain properties that fight and heal diseases, and that a diet free of junk food prevents degenerative diseases while improving the immune system.

> "There is overwhelming evidence that the consumption of a plant-based diet, which is high in fruits, vegetables, grains, and legumes, including soy, and possibly flaxseed, may reduce the risk of breast and other types of cancers."
> – Clare M. Hasler, Ph.D., director, Functional Foods for Health Program, University of Illinois. *Y-Me Hotline* newsletter; March 1996

As the "scientific" studies supporting the role diet plays in the healing process appear more in allopathic medical journals, the U.S. allopathic establishment is taking the results more seriously. Dietary changes are being incorporated into the way doctors treat such conditions as heart disease arthritis, cancer, and diabetes. Nutrition is being used as a way to boost the immune system in cancer patients. Strict vegan diets are being prescribed in combination with exercise and stress reduction to reverse heart disease and diabetes, and to help patients avoid invasive surgery and expensive and risky chemical drugs. But many doctors, nurses, and other healthcare workers themselves are obese, eat unhealthful foods, snack on junk food, drink colas, smoke, don't get enough exercise, and lack an understanding of true high-quality nutrition.

> "Eighty-five percent of common, chronic, killing diseases in Western civilization are diet-related. The single most important thing is what goes through your lips. That determines whether your disease progresses or regresses. If everyone started eating to save their heart, we'd really empty out the hospitals. This same approach doesn't apply only to the heart. It applies to other organs as well."
> – Dr. Caldwell B. Esselstyn, author of *Prevent and Reverse Heart Disease*; HeartAttackProof.com

When one considers that it costs several thousand dollars to send a patient suffering from heart disease to a health retreat, and several times that to perform bypass surgery, it is not too difficult to understand why the health insurance companies are embracing the lower-cost therapies that consist of a vegan diet, daily exercise, yoga, talk therapy, and intellectual stimulation and expression through art, music, and literature.

The "healthfood fanatics" may not have had the so-called "scientific proof" of what a nutritional plant-based diet can do for the human body, but they knew all along of the health and ecological benefits of eating pure unadulterated plant-based foods that are free of animal fats and flesh. The body that is supplied with the proper fuel of a plant-based diet is healthier, feels better, and performs better than a body that has been clogged with the residues of empty calorie, over processed junk foods, and heavy, disease-inducing animal-based foods containing cholesterol, saturated fat, Neu5Gc (N-glycolylneuraminic acid, a problematic sugar molecule in nonhuman mammal meat and milk, and that has been found in human cancer cells), and the hormones of the animals, and saturated with farming chemicals, drugs, and industrial pollutants.

"In the unsanitary conditions typical of confined feedlots, animals are given continual low doses of antibiotics in their feed to prevent sickness, promote faster growth, and boost profits. This contributes to increased antibiotic resistance in the bacteria that infect people – a serious threat to public health. In 2009, 80 percent of all antibiotics used in the U.S. were given to livestock.

Residues of hormones widely used to promote growth in beef cattle, dairy cows, and sheep (especially rBST or rBHG) may increase the risk of breast, prostate, and colorectal cancer. Their use also increases the risk of health problems in animals (especially mastitis), which leads to higher antibiotic use. Hormones are not permitted in pork or poultry products.

According to the FDA, most human exposure to (cancer-causing) dioxins comes from food, almost entirely through animal fats. The best way to reduce health risks associated with dioxins is by limiting dietary exposure to these compounds. Mercury in seafood is also a concern, as this widespread neurotoxin bioaccumulates in large fish. Farmed salmon generally have more dioxin-like PCBs than wild salmon."

– Environmental Working Group, EWG.org

People shouldn't think about following a healthful diet as a restriction. If anything, an unhealthful diet is restrictive. An unhealthful diet restricts you from experiencing the amazing health you can own by following a healthful, low-fat, plant-rich diet. In fact, the more healthful your diet, the better and less restrictive your life can be. The healthful diet opens doors, and eliminates restrictions.

"Food is that material which can be incorporated into and become a part of the cells and fluids of the body. Nonuseful materials, such as chemical additives and drugs, are all poisons. To be a true food, the substance must not contain useless or harmful ingredients."

– Dr. Herbert Shelton, author of *Food Combining Made Easy*

139

It is truly amazing what the body can do if it is provided with the best nutrition. It can rid itself of extra fat. It can eliminate toxic substances from the tissues. It can change its complexion from that of the pallid color of a person who follows an unhealthful diet to the vibrancy of a person who follows a healthful diet. The hair and nails even change on a healthful diet, taking on a more healthful appearance and texture. And these things are reflective of what is going on inside the body when a person switches from a diet that was unhealthful to a diet that is healthful. The pineal gland and the organs, including the brain, become cleaner and function better when a person starts eating healthfully and gets daily exercise.

Changing your diet from horrible, or even from mundane, to that which consists of exceptionally healthful foods can help your body not only to greatly improve in form and function, but can also heal ailments that may have been a problem your entire life.

The human body contains an amazing power to heal. If provided the proper nutrients and exercise, a healthy environment, and positive thoughts, the human body can transform from sickly to healthy in a matter of weeks or months. The longer someone goes about eating a healthful diet; carrying on a daily exercise program to strengthen, stretch, and tone the muscles, tendons, and bones; and works the mind by creating positive thoughts that drives the person to succeed in his or her goals, the more healthful and successful that person will become.

A major part of a successful life is what is put into the mouth. Without a healthful diet, people cannot succeed at experiencing their full potential in life. Anyone who has experienced the sluggishness that is a result of unhealthful food choices, and who has switched to a strictly healthful diet knows of the advantages a healthful diet provides.

The documentary film *May I Be Frank* features a perfect example of what can happen to a human who is on the edge of complete physical collapse, but who then switches to a plant-based diet, a schedule that includes exercise, and a mindset that is fed positive thoughts. The film shows how employees of San Francisco's Café Gratitude focused on the life of one customer, an obese man named Frank Ferrante, who was taking a handful of prescription medications every day, had spent decades abusing himself with drugs, alcohol, and horrible food choices, and held loads of regret, anger, and frustration. For 42 days Frank followed a raw food diet, practiced the philosophy of gratitude, visited with holistic practitioners, faced his frustrations, began yoga, was coached by the three cafe employees, and transformed his life. During those 42 days of filming, and in the months following, Frank dropped the weight that bound him, got off all of the medications he had been taking, began believing in himself, and went back to school. (To see the documentary, Access: MayIBeFrankMovie.com)

> "We must give our bodies the rich nourishment from vegetables, greens, and fruits; and sprouted seeds, beans, and grains. When these foods are combined with proper rest and activity, and a healthy positive attitude, the body and will are strengthened and even the most serious health problems may be overcome."
> – Ann Wigmore, AnnWigmore.Org

When you look around in nature and see what is naturally desirable, which tastes good, which feels right to eat, and is easy to eat, you will most likely be looking at plant structures that we call fruits and vegetables. These are what nature has provided for our sustenance, and are most often naturally created in meal-sized portions. An apple, a tomato, a bunch of lettuce, a head of broccoli, a squash, an orange, a banana, a bunch of grapes, a coconut, a carrot, a stick of celery, an avocado, and many other fruits and vegetables are produced by plants in the perfect size for humans to eat. There are berries that ripen by the handful, and nuts and fruits, such as olives, that are available for harvesting in the amount that is consistent with what is needed to create a satisfying meal. Consider that this is the way nature intended it to be, for plants to provide humans with food.

> "And God said: Behold, I have given you every herb-bearing seed which is upon the face of the earth, and every tree, in which is the fruit of a tree-yielding seed, to be your food."
> – Genesis 1:29

Some of the nutrients that plants have that meat, dairy, and eggs do not are fiber and a broad variety of antioxidants. If we do not get fiber or antioxidants, our health suffers. Plants also contain all of the vitamins, minerals, amino acids, essential fatty acids, enzymes, biophotons, and other nutrients our bodies need to maintain strong immune systems, to form and run our cells, and to experience vibrant health.

It is certainly amazing that plants provide us with the exact nutrients that we need to flourish in health. This is no coincidence. If we simply eat a variety of what nature provides for us through plant matter, our body gets what it needs to grow and carry on in a healthy way. It is only after humans begin to manipulate plant substances by processing them with chemicals and heat that the nutrients in the plants are damaged, and the vibrant energy within the plants is killed.

> "Early human ancestors were not predominantly meat eaters, or even eaters of seeds, shoots, leaves, or grasses. Instead, they appear

to have subsided on a diet of fruit. No exceptions have been found. Every tooth examined from the hominids of the twelve-million-year period leading up to Homo Erectus appeared to be that of a fruit eater."
– Dr. Alan Walker of Johns Hopkins University, in the May 15, 1979, edition of the *New York Times*

Some argue that humans have evolved to the point that they can consume things that their ancestors did not. But just because you can chew something and swallow it without vomiting doesn't mean it is good for you. The same physical structure that humans had thousands of years ago exists today. It is made up of the same design. Only the food has changed. The degenerative diseases caused by the unhealthful foods being consumed by today's humans has resulted in a great diversity of diseases unseen in humans who eat natural diets.

If you were simply created fully grown and were put in a tropical area, alone, with nobody to tell you what to do or what to eat, most likely you would examine what was within your reach. This would include the fruits and berries hanging from the trees and vines. Most likely you would smell and taste them, and you would find that they are good. This would be your natural diet. You would be rained on from the sky, taste the rain, and know that the water is pleasant. This would be your natural source for the fluid you would desire and need.

If, while in this state of innocence, you saw animals, you would likely not taste them. If you did you wouldn't find them to be of a flavor that is desirable. They would also be difficult to eat, especially with the bones, cartilage, tendons, skin, and so forth that would be tough on your teeth and jaw. You would stick to eating the products of the vegetation – fruits, vegetables, herbs, berries, seeds, nuts, and flowers. (Cailiflower and broccoli are flowers. But many common flowers, such as roses and nasturtiums, are also edible – when grown organically.)

Even if, still in your state of innocence, you saw a dead animal, and tasted the flesh, you would still not like the taste of that. It also would not smell good to you. Flesh would not be in your natural diet. This is because it is not natural for you to eat.

If, even still in your state of innocence, by some freak occurrence you came across a dead animal that somehow became burned, such as by a fire caused by a lightning strike, this cooked meat still would be tough on your teeth and jaw, and would likely not taste good to you. It would not be in your natural diet.

Those at the forefront of promoting the plant-based diet understand that all living things are connected, and if we would work with nature, it would provide us with what we need.

A raw or largely raw vegan and organic diet and lifestyle promotes a simplification of living and works toward a balance with nature by adopting activities that contribute to a sound, clean, and natural environment. This can be done by promoting sustainable agriculture, eating only organically grown foods, growing some foods, using only what we need, using only what can be recycled, restoring what we have destroyed, protecting the ecosystems and plant biodiversity of the planet by **not** using toxic chemicals, and by **not** genetically altering plants. When we damage and poison the planet we are doing it to ourselves.

"A vegetarian diet could support a population many times the world's present size."
– *Take a Step Toward Compassionate Living*, 2004; PETA.Org

A vegan diet rich in raw plant matter is a diet most aligned with the natural state of the planet. But it has carried an unfair image problem. Some who hear the word "vegan" turn up their noses. They think vegan means something like limiting the diet to tofu, rice, and carrots. They have not been to a gourmet raw vegan restaurant or to one of these large natural foods stores and sampled the variety of foods, nor have they tasted the wide variety of foods that can be made using simple, raw, unheated ingredients – such as some of those listed in the recipe section of this book.

"As the only black kid in my primary school playground, animals had become my friends. A playground can be the loneliest place in the world when all the kids are playing and nobody will talk to you, so when a cat comes along, you play with the cat, you know? And then the cat comes again the next day and brings a couple of his friends, and you form a community. So that's where my love of animals started, and that was when I went vegetarian and by 15 I was vegan."
– Benjamin Zephaniah

The demand for vegan food is increasing. Restaurants are opening. Chefs are publishing books, maintaining Websites, teaching classes, and being interviewed in the media. Bill Clinton, Mike Tyson, Steve Wynn, Andre 3000, Ben Stiller, Michelle Pfeiffer, Russell Simmons, Casey Affleck, Lea Michele, Jared Leto, Chaka Khan, Paul McCartney, Woody Harrelson, Forest Whitaker, Natalie Portman, Russell Brand, Carrie Underwood, Jessica Chastain, Jane Lynch, Alec Baldwin, Alicia Silverstone, Moby, and others speak of their vegan diet. Tennis stars Venus and Serena Williams, car racer Spencer Pumpelly, boxer Timothy Bradley, running back Montell Owens, tight end Tony Gonzalez, and basketball player Raja Bell are vegan. Brian Greene, author of *The Elegant Universe*, is vegan, as is Twitter founder Biz Stone.

Whether people seek to become healthier by improving the nutritional profile of their diet through eating more plant-based foods, or are ethically driven to eliminate all animal products from their life by becoming vegan, they may find my other book, *Sunfood Traveler: Global Guide to Raw Food Culture*, to be helpful.

> "Veganism has given me a higher level of awareness and spirituality."
> – Dexter Scott King, *Vegetarian Times*, October 1995

Eating in tune with nature is tuning in to the patterns of nature, which is in tune with how cells within your body function.

There are patterns in everything. There are patterns in light, in air, and in water. There are patterns in the seasons and in the day and night. There are patterns in the structures of everything that is living – patterns in the structures of the tissues and other patterns in the microscopic structures of the cells, the walls of the cells, the intercellular structures, and in the nucleus, chromatin, DNA, and in the subatomic electrons and protons. The patterns are created by energy, which is the power of nature, which is of Divinity, which is in us, throughout us, and surrounds us. Every thing is an expression of a pattern of this energy.

> "Every human being has etched in his personality the indelible stamp of the Creator."
> – Martin Luther King, Jr.

When you eat a raw vegan diet you are placing the patterns of nature into your body. The patterns of nature in edible plants are healing, nurturing, uplifting, vibrant, and resonate with a strong energy. These are all things that you should strive for. They are the composers of health.

When you follow a plant-based diet consisting entirely or largely of raw fruits and vegetables, you are eating what is grown in nature and what will complement the patterns of the microscopic structures and energy fields of your body tissues.

Vibrant health cannot exist without the influence of sun. We need to be exposed to the electromagnetic wavelengths of sun through exposure to sun, and by eating foods grown in sun's light. Without regular intake of solar photons to recharge our electrons, our health suffers. Heavily cooked foods not only lack the electrons needed for health, they also clog the system, slowing electrical currents, and certain cooked foods rob the body of health. Raw fruits and vegetables contain the wavelengths of sun energy and help keep our inner fuses charged.

As you sustain a diet consisting of all or mostly raw plant matter, you will be infusing your system with the wavelengths of life that permeate all life forms. When you follow a diet consisting wholly of raw plant substances that have been undiminished by heating, processing, genetic engineering, or artificial chemicals, you will be providing your body with the vital link necessary for your body to experience true health. Let that be your experiment.

"For over forty years, I've been vegetarian. Growing up, my family had little money – I had health problems early in life because of poor nutrition. Eating healthy is a priority for me."
– Rosa Parks, civil rights activist

"Thousands of people who say they 'love' animals sit down once or twice a day to enjoy the flesh of creatures who have been utterly deprived of everything that could make their lives worth living and who endured the awful suffering and the terror of the abattoirs."
–Jane Goodall

"I came home one morning and saw an actress on TV who was talking about how a lot of fast food companies fix chickens, for example. They showed how the chicken would be coming around like an assembly line, and when they get to each place, this thing would cut the heads off and something else would do something else to them. One of my sons who usually cooks for me came over the next morning to make me some bacon and eggs, and I couldn't eat it. And from that time on that's been my protest. I haven't eaten any meat since."
– B.B. King

"In 2010, the U.S. produced a world-leading 696,241,870 pounds of corn. Only 10 percent of that was for human consumption."
– UrbanOrganicGardener.com

A diet relying purely on plants benefits the planet in many different ways. Most significantly, it eliminates the dependence on the wasteful meat, dairy, egg, processed, and corporate food industries. Instead, the sunfood diet consists of edible plant substances, requiring more fruiting trees and culinary plants to be grown. More plants clean the air, provide oxygen, filter water, create homes for wildlife, and manifest a more healthful environment for all forms of life on the planet. Additionally, with fewer people consuming meat, land previously used to raise farm animals – and used to grow tremendous amounts of food for feeding those animals using enormous resources – is turned over to the wilds of nature.

"Chickens raised for food today are covered in excrement, they're diseased, and they're drugged up with all sorts of toxins that you are ingesting if you eat chicken. One recent study found that chicken flesh in this country has four times as much arsenic – yes, arsenic, the poison, which is used in the drugs the chickens are given – as any other meat.
I have been a vegan for many years."
– Russell Simmons

"In our first-ever lab analysis of ground turkey bought at retail stores nationwide, more than half of the packages of raw ground meat and patties tested positive for fecal bacteria. Some samples harbored other germs, including salmonella and staphylococcus aureus, two of the leading causes of foodborne illness in the U.S. Overall, 90 percent of the samples had one or more of the five bacteria for which we tested.
Adding to the concern, almost all of the disease-causing organisms in our 257 samples proved resistant to one or more of the antibiotics commonly used to fight them. Turkeys (and other food animals, including chickens and pigs) are given antibiotics to treat acute illness; but healthy animals may also get drugs daily in their food and water to boost their rate of weight gain and to prevent disease. Many of the drugs are similar to antibiotics important in human medicine."
– *Consumer Reports* investigation: Talking turkey: Our new tests show reason for concern; *Consumer Reports* magazine, June 2013; ConsumerReports.org

"The more we spend on disease care, the sicker and more miserable we seem to become."
– T. Colin Campbell, in his book, *Whole: Rethinking the Science of Nutrition*. Campbell is Professor Emeritus of Nutritonal Biochemistry at Cornell University, and has been involved in the science and research of nutrition for several decades. He advises a low-fat vegan diet with no added (bottled) oils, no salt, no processed sugars, but with whole plant foods. He is also author of *The China Study*; TColinCampbell.org

EATING: IT'S WHAT'S EATING US

"Creatures shall be seen upon the earth who will always be fighting one with another, with very great losses and frequent deaths on either side. These shall set no bounds to their malice; by their fierce limbs a great number of the trees in the immense forests of the world shall be laid level with the ground; and when they have crammed themselves with food it shall gratify their desire to deal out death, affliction, labours, terrors and banishment to every living thing. And by reason of their boundless pride they shall wish to rise towards heaven, but the excessive weight of their limbs shall hold them down. There shall be nothing remaining on earth or under the earth or in the waters that shall not be pursued and molested or destroyed, and that which is in one country taken away to another; and their own bodies shall be made a tomb and the means of transit of all the living bodies which they have slain. O Earth! what delays thee to open and hurl them headlong into the deep fissures of thy huge abyss and caverns, and no longer to display in the sight of heaven so savage and ruthless a monster?"
    – *Of the Cruelty of Man*, Leonardo da Vinci, a vegetarian and outspoken protector of animals and nature

"The beef and meat and sea food industry has contributed to more global deaths than all the wars of this century, all natural disasters, and all automobile accidents, and all AIDS deaths combined. If eating animals is your idea of 'real food for real people,' you'd better live real close to a real good hospital."
    – Dr. Neal Barnard, author of books on diet and health; NealBarnard.org

"Nonviolence leads to the highest ethics which is the goal of all evolution. Until we stop harming all other living beings, we are still savages."
    – Thomas Edison

"We prefer to numb ourselves physically to the fact of the slaughterhouse. We don't like to remember that hamburger is a ground up cow."
    – John Robbins, in his book *Diet for a New America*

"If you have looked at kids in school today, they are more out of shape than any generation in the history of our country. If you could look inside of their arteries, they have the beginnings of artery blockages before they get their high school diploma."
– Dr. Neal Barnard, 2004, NealBarnard.org

"As long as man continues to be the ruthless destroyer of lower living beings, he will never know health or peace. For as long as men massacre animals, they will kill each other. Indeed, he who sows the seed of murder and pain cannot reap the joy of love."
– Pythagoras

"The more red meat and blood we eat, the more bloodthirsty we get, the more violent we get. The more vegetarian food we eat, the more peace is taken into us."
– Ziggy Marley

"As long as people will shed the blood of innocent creatures there can be no peace, no liberty, no harmony between people. Slaughter and justice cannot dwell together."
– Isaac Bashevis Singer, Nobel laureate

"The butcher with his bloody apron incites bloodshed, murder. Why not? From cutting the throat of a young calf to cutting the throat of our brothers and sisters is but a step. While we are ourselves the living graves of murdered animals, how can we expect any ideal conditions on the earth?"
– Isadora Duncan

"Animals do not 'give' their life to us, as the sugar-coated lie would have it. No, we take their lives. They struggle and fight to the last breath, just as we would do if we were in their place."
– John Robbins, author of *The Food Revolution*

"We all love animals. Why do we call some 'pets,' and others 'dinner'?"
– K.D. Lang

"We consume the carcasses of creatures of like appetites, passions, and organs with our own, and fill the slaughterhouses daily with screams of pain and fear."
– Robert Louis Stevenson

"Factory-farm lobbyists are so powerful and so well funded and they do everything in their power to hide the truth about farming. They keep the farms and slaughterhouses in places that most people never visit; they execute huge marketing campaigns in

an effort to make animal production look like a happy, nice, benign institution."
– Moby

"There's no doubt in my mind that going vegetarian has made me feel better not only physically but also because I learned about the suffering of animals who are raised and killed for food. I feel good knowing I'm not contributing to that."
– Sophie Monk

"We will find we can no longer subsidize or ignore the costs of mass-producing cattle, poultry, pigs, sheep, and fish to feed our growing population. These costs include hugely inefficient use of fresh water and land, heavy pollution from livestock feces, rising rates of heart disease and other degenerative illnesses, and spreading destruction of our forests on which much of the planet's life depends"
– *Time* magazine, November 8, 1999

"The raising and eating of animals (livestock [cows, hogs, chickens, turkeys, lamb, and goats] and fish) by our global community ultimately affects food prices, food availability, policy making, and even education to improve agricultural systems in those developing countries. Global factors include control of seed manufacturing and pricing primarily for livestock feed crops by large companies such as Monsanto and Dupont (Pioneer), buying and selling of grain including futures by Archer Daniel Midland, Cargill, and through the processing/slaughterhouses and packaging by Cargill, Swift, Tyson, and JBS. These few but very large and powerful companies control over 65 percent of all seed, grain, and over 80 percent of all final animal products in the world. It is a very monopolized production and economic system manufacturing seeds at one end and spewing out meat at the other. Because of the global demand for meat (all livestock), cultural, social, political, and economic influences remain strongly supportive of the continued dominance of these large companies and the meat, dairy, and fishing industries in general, which then drives how global resources are being used (land, water, rainforests, oceans, atmosphere, biodiversity, etc.), how money is spent, and how policies are determined. The demand for animal products in developed countries drives resource depletion in developing countries as well as exacerbating poverty and hunger."
– Dr. Richard A. Oppenlander, ComfortablyUnaware.com

TUNING IN

"Learn how to see. Realize that everything connects to everything else."
– Leonardo da Vinci

"We are living on this planet as if we had another one to go to."
– Terri Swearingen

"There must have been a moment, at the beginning, where we could have said, 'No!' But, somehow, we missed it."
– Tom Stoppard

AS we are increasingly being bombarded by massive marketing, technomania, economic globalization, industrial agriculture, factory farming, nonstop road building, traffic jams, genetic engineering, threats of nuclear disasters, radioactive waste, perpetual war, environmental damage, and an extinction crisis like no other, it seems that humans have become to Earth as disease is to humans.

"We search for life on other planets and in other regions of our galaxy. Meanwhile, we destroy and ignore other life on this planet."
– A.D. Williams

The human experience has become increasingly distressed because society has disconnected from nature. Business and governments are attempting to control natural systems for shortsighted consumption that favors corporate interests rather than global health. Most often this is done while abusing and misusing all natural resources – and creating extreme amounts of pollution on and in the land and water, and in the air. Much of this is done to feed the people of North America and Western Europe, ranked among the most gluttonous societies of the world.

"When we look back on this time, a couple of hundred years from now, I guarantee you that our diet of today will be considered one of the most radical in history."
– Dr. Sanjay Gupta

As of 2012, on a per-capita basis, the native people of Qatar are considered to be the wealthiest in the world. At the same time, the small country that sits along the Persian Gulf is the fastest growing economy in the world, with its lead export being natural gas. That isn't the only status symbol of Qatar. It is also the fattest country in the world, and one where cigarette smoking is common among males above the age of puberty. Additionally, along with their newly accumulated wealth and girth, their rates of diabetes and cardiovascular disease are skyrocketing, surpassing the U.S. rates of those diseases.

The average diet in Qatar has become rich in animal protein, fat, processed sugar, salt, and mass-marketed foods. While eating high-calorie but poor-quality foods has become common in Qatar, exercise has not. About one-third of the nation's children and one-half of its adults are considered obese.

What their spanking-new wealth has brought Qatar's citizens is a life of luxury, sedentary activities, and degenerative diseases common among the affluent. Air-conditioning services are among the fastest growing industries in the hot, desert nation. To go along with the air conditioning, there is an onslaught of other pampering services catering to the newly wealthy. The fast food industry has quickly grown, as have the posh hotel and luxury automobile industries.

While foreign workers are busy running the restaurants and hotels, the native Qatar people live an increasingly sedate lifestyle, while eating the food prepared for them by their domestic workers, cooks, and other servants.

Along with rising rates of diabetes among the Qatar people, there are increased complications of the disease, including foot ulcers, foot amputations, blindness, diabetic comas, and other unfortunate health events.

Interestingly, genetic and autoimmune disorders have increased in Qatar in alignment with the increase in obesity, diabetes, and cardiovascular disease. In other words, Qatar has become the perfect example of what an unhealthful diet rich in animal protein, fat, salt, and sugar does to humans adapting lifestyles of increasingly reduced physical activity. What is happening to the health of the residents of Qatar helps to reveal that a junk diet plays a lead role in all of the diseases common among the pampered affluent.

In addition to a boom of businesses catering to the wealthy, the medical industry of Qatar is also booming with an increased need for doctors, nurses, and support staff. Hospitals are being built to treat patients suffering from the diseases trailing the increase in a sedentary lifestyle mixed with low-quality foods that some call "comfort foods" or "convenient foods," but which are truly junk foods and sickness-inducing foods. Healthcare in the country is funded by the government, which predicts that, if the decline in health continues among residents, branches of the medical industry treating diseases of affluence will need to double in size in the next couple of decades. At the same time, even with increased medical intervention, the expected lifespan of the average Qatar citizen will decrease.

We may perceive comfort and convenience in our modern and corporate-dominated lifestyle saturated with toxic foods, but the waste and destruction of nature we are creating on Earth degrades the quality of all life and inflicts a great deal of suffering on the other forms of life with which we share Earth.

> "The problem is that humans have victimized animals to such a degree, that they aren't even considered victims. They aren't even considered at all. They're nothing, literally. They don't even count. They don't matter. They're commodities, like TV sets and cell phones."
> – Gary Yourofsky, ADAPTT.org

If people want to protect their health, they can do so by becoming more attuned to their natural surroundings and becoming active in protecting the other beings with whom we share Earth, including animals and plants. When we recognize our kinship with wildlife we rediscover our connection to, and reliance on all life forms.

> "Nearly one-third of the timber cut from national forests is used for paper production. Half of that paper ends up in landfills. Is this making your ears red? Thousand-year-old Doug firs from the Great Bear Rainforest are clearcut to make paper."
> – Malus and John Lorax, Attention Shoppers, Lockdown in Aisle Three!, *Earth First! Journal*, Dec.-Jan. 2002; EarthFirstJournal.Org

> "What we are doing to the forests of the world is but a mirror reflection of what we are doing to ourselves and to one another."
> – Mahatma Gandhi

Currently the way most people are living is not in tune with nature. The way they are leading their lives is in direct opposition to the needs of a healthy planet and contributes to mismanagement of resources, huge amounts of pollution, and the loss and extinction of species. It doesn't help that governments are creating situations of danger, which they then claim they can protect us from, perpetrating the hero syndrome while doing little to nothing about the real problems facing the planet. Often the governments are creating the problems, allowing them to happen, or being the enabler in the most dysfunctional of all relationships, those between corporations and governments, as the neglected and abused citizens and wildlife suffer the consequences.

"All too many politicians are corporate owned and operated, and do whatever their loudest constituents and richest campaign contributors tell them to. All too few show any genuine outrage at the destructive immorality of a small portion of corporate America – the industries that rape and pillage nature, the very lungs of our planet – to make a buck, regardless of what it costs the rest of us.

The honest truth is that humanity needs trees to survive. Trees shade our ground, create topsoil, clean the air and help the land attract, hold, and filter water. The trees and their roots purify the water as the rains fall. Clean streams keep millions of aquatic and other species alive. The cycle is perfect."
– Tim Hermach, President Native Forest Voice; *Forest Voice*, Spring 2006; ForestCouncil.Org

Each day thousands of acres of trees are cut down to make such items as chopsticks, toothpicks, disposable furniture, and paper for junk mail, newspapers, magazines, paper bags, paper plates, take-out food containers, napkins, and tissue. Every year the people of China use about 45 billion pairs of disposable chopsticks, which amounts to about 25 million trees being cut down, killing or displacing huge numbers of wildlife. Around the world there are several hundred billion paper napkins used every year. Hundreds of billions of paper bags, all made from trees, are used every year, and hardly any of the paper is recycled.

"Since 1937, about half the world's forests have been cut down to make paper. If hemp had not been outlawed, most [of those forests] would still be standing, oxygenating the planet."
– Alan Bock, columnist, *Orange County Register*, 1988; as quoted in the documentary *Emperor of Hemp*, EmperorOfHemp.Com

"These mountain lands, which boast some of the most spectacular natural beauty on Earth, are now being devastated to briefly quench the needs of a single generation."
– Al Gore, on the deforestation of the Himalayas

"In a brief moment in the life of our planet, we have destroyed all but a remnant of Earth's ancient forests. The United States has already lost a stunning 97 percent of its native forests. Worldwide, 80 percent of native forests have been cut down, and 25 percent of mammals, 20 percent of reptiles, 25 percent of amphibians, and 34 percent of fish are in danger of extinction. Water around the world is polluted with the soil that washes off bare mountains. The biological inheritance of humanity is being forever diminished, reducing potential sources of medicines, foods, and fibers.

Destruction of forests is a leading cause of global environmental breakdown, including global warming."
– AncientTrees.Org, 2006

Every day thousands of rare trees are being cut down and are sold on the international market for use in furniture, flooring, and construction. At the same time, countries have no laws banning the import of wood from trees that were cut down illegally. Here in North America, where much of that rare tree lumber is used, lumber companies continue to cut down some of the oldest trees on the planet. Meanwhile, law enforcement works to protect the lumber companies while arresting protesters working to block the lumber companies from decimating the ancient trees and the variety of wildlife that exist in them.

Because of both legal and illegal logging in forests around the planet, many species of plants, animals, and other living things are endangered and many have become extinct. That is because each tree and every forest are host to a number of plants, insects, amphibians, reptiles, mammals, birds, fungi, and microscopic organisms that play a role in the network of life on Earth. Because many forests are where the streams and rivers begin, trees and forests support waterlife of all varieties. When a forest is destroyed, so too are the homes to some combination of life, such as butterflies, lichens, amphibians, mushrooms, songbirds, voles, fish, crustaceans, and flowers that may exist only on a small region of the planet.

In Africa, where forests are open to Asian and European logging companies, gorillas are losing their last remaining homes. Because of the logging, eating wild African animal meat of all sorts is more common than ever. Gorillas are still being hunted. Gorillas are also experiencing an Ebola outbreak that scientists estimate has killed about one fourth of the world's gorillas in the last two decades. The hunting, the illness, and the loss of forest habitat are likely to result in the extinction of gorillas in the wild.

On Borneo the logging and farming industries have destroyed 90 percent of the forests. This has placed the orangutans there on the road to extinction that is expected to come to a dead end within decades. As I write this there are more forest fires burning on Borneo. Intentionally set to expand the palm oil plantations, the fires cause orangutans to flee, often to places where humans live. Some of the people torture the orangutans for entertainment. Other people consider the orangutans to be pests and shoot them. Some of the orangutans are captured and sold into the exotic pet, circus, and zoo markets. Some of the orangutans die from burns and injuries suffered in the forest fires, and their babies die of starvation.

"If killing orangutans was the only problem that existed with palm oil, then maybe Earth Balance [a food company that uses palm oil in their product] could get off the hook [Earth Balance claims that their palm oil product is safer as it comes from oil palm plantations in the Peninsular Malaysia]. But, it's simply not. Everywhere that palm oil is grown – very much including Peninsular Malaysia – involves clear cutting rainforest and planning massive monoculture plantations – with serious consequences for both endangered species (the tapir lives in Peninsular Malaysia – does it deserve to go extinct?) and the climate. It also involves displacing communities off their traditionally owned land, which regularly occurs in Peninsular Malaysia. Particularly in Peninsular Malaysia, migrant workers from Indonesia and India are forced into modern-day slavery, forced to work for minuscule wages while paying back the companies for their transportation from their country of origin. It's a wreck."
– Rainforest Action Network, RAN.org

"When I look at animals held captive by circuses, I think of slavery. Animals in circuses represent the domination and oppression we have fought against for so long. They wear the same chains and shackles."
– Dick Gregory

"The Problem with Palm Oil Fact Sheet
Palm oil is a globally traded agricultural commodity that is used in 50 percent of all consumer goods, from lipstick and packaged food to body lotion and biofuels. Used in about half of the products on supermarket shelves, palm oil imports to the U.S. have jumped 485 percent in the last decade, pushing palm oil cultivation into the rainforests and making this crop one of the key causes of rainforest destruction around the globe.

Approximately 85 percent of palm oil is grown in the tropical countries of Indonesia, Malaysia and Papua New Guinea (PNG) on industrial plantations that have severe impacts on the environment, forest peoples and the climate.

Palm oil destroys rainforests. Indonesia's tropical rainforests are among the world's most diverse. They provide critical habitat to species including highly endangered Sumatran tigers, Sumatran elephants and orangutans. The Indonesian government has announced plans to convert approximately 18 million more hectares of rainforests, an area the size of Missouri, into palm oil plantations by 2020.

Palm oil threatens forest peoples. Tens of millions of

155

Indonesians rely directly on rainforests for their livelihoods. A single palm oil plantation can destroy the forests, watersheds, and forest resources of thousands of Indonesians, leaving entire forest communities to face poverty, many for the first time.

Palm oil causes climate change. Rainforests are the earth's largest sinks of carbon, safely storing the greenhouse gases that cause climate change. In Indonesia, rainforests are razed to create industrial palm oil plantations, releasing massive quantities of carbon dioxide into the atmosphere. In fact, deforestation causes eighty percent of Indonesia's CO_2 emissions, making the tropical nation the world's third largest emitter of greenhouse gases.

Who is responsible? North American food and agribusiness companies purchase from, operate, and own many palm oil plantations in Southeast Asia, making our corporations a powerful force in the palm oil market.

The largest privately owned company in the U.S., Cargill dominates the American palm oil market. They own five palm oil plantations in Indonesia and PNG and are the largest importer of palm oil into the U.S., sourcing from at least 26 producers and buying roughly 11 percent of Indonesia's total oil palm output. A large and growing number of investigations have shown that Cargill's palm oil is directly destroying forests, eliminating biodiversity and harming forest peoples.

Rainforest Action Network (RAN) is actively working to stop the destruction of rainforests due to industrial agribusiness expansion. We encourage companies like Cargill to stop producing, trading and purchasing palm oil that destroys rainforests using grassroots pressure, corporate engagement, and nonviolent direct action."
– Rainforest Action Network, RAN.org

Don't use palm oil. Avoid foods containing it. Read labels when shopping at stores, and avoid products that contain "palm fruit oil," "palm margarine," "palm oil margarine," "tropical oils," "red palm oil," and other foods containing palm oil listed in other ways. For more on this issue, access: The ProblemWithPalmOil.org.

What is happening with the destruction of rainforests to expand the oil palm plantations is similar to what is going on with other wildlands as massive monocropping operations spread among every continent and on some islands.

"The single largest contributor to global depletion is the raising, slaughtering, and eating of animals – over 700 billion livestock animals and 1-2 trillion fish (some researchers have estimated as

many as 1.7 trillion chickens are raised and slaughtered in one year).”
– ComfortablyUnaware.com

"Animal agribusiness generates more greenhouse gases than all forms of transportation combined. The livestock sector generates more greenhouse gas emissions than transportation as measured in carbon dioxide equivalent (18 percent vs 13 percent). It is also responsible for 37 percent of all the human-induced methane, which is 23 times more toxic to the ozone layer than carbon dioxide, as well as generating 65 percent of the human-related nitrous oxide, which has 296 times the global warming potential of carbon dioxide. Nitrous oxide and methane mostly come from manure, and 56 billion food animals produce a lot of manure each day.

Livestock use 30 percent of the earth's entire land surface, mostly for permanent pasture but also including 33 percent of global arable land to produce feed for them. As forests are cleared to create new pastures for livestock, it is a major driver of deforestation: some 70 percent of forests in the Amazon have been turned over to grazing.”
– Dr. Dean Ornish, Holy Cow! What's Good For You Is Good For Our Planet: Comment on "Red Meat Consumption and Mortality," *Archives of Internal Medicine*, March 12, 2012. Ornish is the founder of the Preventative Medicine Research Institute, PMRI.org

Every day thousands of trees in the Central and South American forests are cut down to provide grazing land for cattle. Many thousands of other trees are cleared to make room to grow soybeans that are then sold into the world market to feed the billions of massively overbred farm animals. The soybeans grown there are also used to make fried chicken products sold by such tremendously environmentally destructive companies known as *fast food restaurants*.

"Moving away from meat for one day a week is more effective [in terms of energy efficiency and environmental health] than buying everything you eat locally."
– *Harvard Business Review*

Throughout coastal areas of the world the mangrove swampland forests have been and continue to be destroyed to make way for resorts and marinas, and for shrimp and other types of seafood farms. This destruction contributed greatly to the damage done by the tsunami that killed hundreds of thousands of people as it swept away villages and towns throughout the Indian Ocean region in December 2004. Clearing of coastal forests and damage to barrier islands to create fish farms and to drill for oil also contributed to the strength of hurricane Katrina that decimated the New Orleans region in 2005. More of the coastal lands of the Gulf of Mexico are being ruined, and the wildlife in the Gulf and along the coasts are being killed by the massive petroleum tragedy caused by drilling for oil at the bottom of the sea, which should never be done.

"The end of the human race will be that it will eventually die of civilization."
– Ralph Waldo Emerson

"The frogs are sending an alarm call to all concerned about the future of biodiversity and the need to protect the greatest of all open-access resources – the atmosphere."
– Andrew Blaustein, of Oregon State University, and Andy Dobson, of Princeton University, in a commentary in *Nature*, about global warming and the extinction of hundreds of species of amphibians; February 23, 2006. According to the Global Amphibian Assessment, about one-third of the amphibians remaining on the planet are classified as threatened.

Every day thousands of acres of wildlands from the mountains to the coasts and on the islands of the seas are being cleared to make way for roads, stores, restaurants, resorts, amusement parks, golf courses, factories, houses, parking lots, mining operations, office buildings, marinas, airports, military bases, prisons, power plants, fuel processing plants, and animal farming, and also monocropped grain farming to feed billions of farmed animals.

On every continent there are dams built, and more are being built. Dams dramatically alter landscapes that took unknown amounts of time for nature to form, and where varieties of wildlife have lived since the beginning of their species.

Throughout the world large mining operations are altering the landscape. They are digging holes deep into Earth in places like Indonesia, Africa, Canada, and Alaska, and leaving behind toxic heavy metal sediment that poisons water, killing generations of wildlife.

Coal mining companies are cutting down and exploding Appalachian mountaintops in Tennessee, West Virginia, Virginia, and Kentucky. They then fill valleys where rivers and streams ran, killing millions of fish, frogs, toads, snakes, insects, birds and other wildlife. Instead of the ancient mountains and pristine valleys, the people and the remaining wildlife of Appalachia are being left with poisoned rivers that are unfit for swimming, and many water wells that are too poisoned to drink from. The denuded land is subject to mudslides that do more damage to creeks, rivers, and wildlife. To make matters worse, local law enforcement supports the mining companies by arresting those protesting the destruction of the mountains, forests, creeks, and rivers (Access: UnitedMountainDefense.Org and EarthFirstJournal.org).

Those who have protested the works of the coal companies involved with removing mountaintops and destroying river valleys and forests have not only been presented with lawsuits for interfering with business, but have also found themselves to be the focus of the U.S. Department of Homeland Security. Nowadays those involved with protesting huge companies that destroy the planet can find themselves being labeled as "domestic terrorists." Others have been put in prison for years, and even for life because they protested corporate destruction of the environment. This sort of thing is happening in countries around the world. For instance, several years ago when villagers in Sudan gathered to discuss a dam project that would displace farmers and others who lived on the land for generations, police shot at them. This killed three villagers, and others were arrested and charged with waging war against the state (Access: EarthFirstJournal.Org).

As I write this there is a large coal mining operation being set up for the pristine Happy Valley area of New Zealand, home to endangered species and fragile wetlands. The plan is to export coal to China for steel production. Environmental activists are working to stop this mine from opening (SaveHappyValley.Org.NZ), but they are up against corporate giants with deep pockets, and misleading "leaders" who are too eager to please corporations for profit – while Earth and more of her wildlife her suffer.

Meanwhile, instead of providing useful information, the leading news sources are focused on babies being born to selfish movie stars; on which spoiled pop star is dating or divorcing the other; on the most popular fashion styles; and on what company is making the most money.

All of this pop culture news is presented while virtually little information about the state of the planet and what we can do about it is provided by any of the so-called major news sources. Instead we are presented with weak journalism that essentially appeases corporate interests by spreading corporate propaganda that elevates the deity of the dollar bill. Common news sources are all suspect.

Commercial culture is inundating people with ads pushing the coolest things to purchase. Apparently corporations are doing a very good job at convincing children that it is really awesome to become obese while eating toxic junk food and staring at computer games and repetitive television shows, and texting each other about it. In the past 25 years the proportion of overweight adolescents has more than tripled. The obesity of children is part of the result of the $10 billion per year that the junk food industry spends on marketing disease-inducing products to children. The sugary, salty, fatty, fried, and artificially dyed and flavored junk that is marketed as "food" is propagating a lazy generation with high rates of Type-2 diabetes, weak bones, attention problems, and early onset cardiovascular disease. It doesn't help the children when the government keeps reducing funding for sports, music, and arts programs while spending more on jails and prisons. To compensate for these funding cuts, the schools are increasing the number of vending machines on their campuses, and many schools have signed exclusive marketing contracts with soft drink and fastfood companies that pay for access to sell their junk drinks and garbage foods to the students. Meanwhile, every year the government gives billions of dollars in subsidies to corn growers whose crop is turned into disease-inducing corn syrup. Since it was first derived from corn in the 1960s, corn sweetener has become the most popular sweetener in the things children eat. (Because of corn syrup's well-earned association with health problems, in 2010, the Corn Refiners Association sought to change the name to *corn sugar*). The inundation of hydrogenated "transfats" in many of the most commonly consumed foods is also damaging to the health of all those who eat them. Often the children consume this junk while staring at the TV that exposes them to more junk food commercials. The average American child sees 20,000 commercials per year, and the vast majority of those commercials are for processed and fast foods. About half of American children are overweight, and one in four is considered to be obese.

In the adult marketing sector, millions of dollars are spent on ad campaigns to convince people that their lives would be better and they would be much sexier if they drove the right kind of car, if they ate the right kind of artery-clogging dessert, and if their hair coloring looked natural. The lifestyle that mass marketing promotes has helped increase the demand for electricity more than 70 percent in 20 years and has resulted in an adult population that is 65 percent overweight. It is a population that consumes about 100 pounds of sugar additives per year in a diet saturated with hydrogenated fats and farming chemicals that cause a variety of ailments. It is a population that is increasingly obese, and that has made liposuction, stomach stapling, and lap band procedures some of the most popular surgeries.

For the moment, the societal norm is to attempt to look like you belong in a clothing commercial while you create a façade to make it appear as if everything is okay.

But it isn't.

> "Today, the mainstream media is only concerned with profits and ratings, paparazzi, and propaganda. They fail in their responsibility as journalists to report the unbiased truth and present the world as it actually is. For years, most of the scientific

community has believed that we're on the verge of an ecological crisis – the sixth mass extinction. They're predicting that within 100 years HALF of all (nonhuman) species on Earth will be wiped out."
– ZeroImpactProductions.Com

The devastation humans have caused, and are causing, to the planet through their chemically-saturated junk diet, massive packaged and processed food-related pollution, and fossil fuel use is difficult to ignore.

"Americans are producing more and more waste with each passing year. In 1960, the average American threw away 2.7 pounds of trash a day. Today, the average American throws away 4.4 pounds of trash every day."
– Energy Information Administration, EIA, DOE, Gov/Kids/EnergyFacts

Every day millions of fish and other sea creatures are dying from pollution, from fishing, and from damage done by recreational, cruise line, and industrial and military watercraft. In 2010 there were over 24,000 beach closings on U.S. shores triggered by pollution, which was an increase of 5,000 in five years. Throughout the coastal areas of the planet, on beaches in the middle of the oceans, and in areas far from major cities, tons of plastic pollution gather on the sand and rocky shores. Petroleum spills in the oceans remain a serious and growing problem, and are terrible for all life forms; unfortunately petroleum spills are only one part of the many problems humans are causing for wildlife reliant on clean water. (Please see the documentaries *The Big Fix* and The Natural Resources Defense Council's *Acid Trip*.)

"Life is life's greatest gift. Guard the life of another creature as you would your own because it is your own. On life's scale of values, the smallest is no less precious to the creature who owns it than the largest."
– Lloyd Biggle, Jr.

Every day unknown numbers of wild animals are being caught and used for entertainment, for caged hunting, for fur, for zoos, for scientific experimentation, for pet store profits, and for ways to transport drugs.
Every day thousands of animals and millions of plants and other life forms in the mosaic of nature are being killed by human activity in the quest for the suicidal progress we call *global industrialization*.

"The second step toward making America less dependent on foreign oil is to produce and refine more crude oil here at home in environmentally sensitive ways.

By far the most promising site for oil in America is the Arctic National Wildlife Refuge in Alaska."
– George W. Bush, petroleum industry suck-up at the 16th Annual Energy Efficiency Forum; June 15, 2005.

"America is addicted to oil."
– George W. Bush, State of the Union Address; January 31, 2006

The biggest threat to the world is the environmental desecration being carried out by corporate and government interests. One of the most notorious global polluters on the planet is the U.S. military, which is addicted to oil, stuck in perpetual war, overspending and misspending, and regularly abusing power while engaging in flagrant disregard of the most basic human rights.

As of 2011, the U.S. had spent over a trillion dollars on the wars in Iraq and Afghanistan. While this has gone on, the Pentagon keeps up its practice of seeking more money to fund its wars. If less than half of that money had been spent to wean the U.S. off fossil fuels and into a future of plant-based fuels, such as by developing wind energy through household wind turbines; solar electric generating plants on sprawling rooftops; monorail systems in the major cities; localizing the food industry; encouraging home gardening and building school food gardens; and on restarting the industrial hemp farming industry, the nation could have been transformed. Instead, it is in sad shape.

While great destruction is being done, how much are world governments spending to protect the environment? Unfortunately, governments have a history of not protecting the environment. Petroleum is the leading fuel source throughout industrialized society, and despite the knowledge that fossil fuels have caused, and are causing, great damage to Earth, including melting ice caps and ocean acidification, there seems to be no slowing down. Even as the massive oil gusher continues polluting thousands of miles of water in the Gulf of Mexico, there are still oil wells being drilled on land and beneath water, massive numbers of natural gas wells being drilled, the horribly toxic practice of fracking is expanding, and the coal industry continues to expand. Wetlands, grasslands, and what people had thought were protected lands are being "developed," drilled, mined, and clearcut, and this is degrading the terrain of a broad variety of species increasingly at risk of extinction. Ancient forests on every continent and many islands are being cut down. Corporations and government leaders are pushing for more nuclear power plants; cutting deals that favor the fossil fuels industries; allowing corporations to write government policy; shortening science review processes that regulate industrial polluters; and weakening pollution standards.

It does not help that the governments continue to behave as if they are working as concierge services for businesses and industries with horrible environmental records, while helping to propagate the lies spread by the corporations.

The World Meteorological Organization keeps recording each new year as the warmest year since records began in the 1800s. The warmest years on record have occurred in the most recent years, droughts are becoming common, and fire seasons are expanding.

Because of humanities increased use of fossil fuels (coal, petroleum, and natural gas), the polar ice packs are thinning. The far reaches of Earth are under attack by those seeking to exploit resources on land newly exposed by the melting ice. Seemingly unfazed by the threat of global warming, the U.S. is consuming something like 19.6 billion barrels of crude oil every day.

The Bristol Bay, Alaska headwaters region, which is considered one of the most pristine areas on Earth, is under attack of gold and hard rock mining that could end up polluting waters with toxic chemicals. This can kill millions of fish that are also the food for the northern bear and eagle populations, which in turn fertilize the northern forests. These forests provide headwaters for rivers, homes to vast numbers of animals, and the forests produce oxygen for animals throughout Earth.

In the Antarctic waters where the ice is melting, the tiny organisms called phytoplankton are dying, which in turn damages the populations of the tiny marine animals called zooplankton, including the shrimp-like crustaceans called krill, which feed on the phytoplankton. A reduction in both phytoplankton and zooplankton is taking place in many of the world's oceans. This is resulting in a loss of food sources for seabirds, fish, and marine mammals. The resulting loss in food for seabirds has caused a great reduction in the number of nesting birds and an increase in the number of dead seabirds washing up on the coasts. In Antarctica the reduction in food for wild animals has been turning more of them toward cannibalism.

The predator animals living on and near the ice caps are also under threat from a silent danger that is biomagnifying in their food chain. Because the predator animals are at the top of the food chain, they are collecting the industrial pollutants in their bodies that exist in the fatty tissues of the smaller creatures they eat. Although they live far from industrial society, the body tissues of these creatures have been found to contain fire retardants, pesticides, and other industrial chemicals, including perfluorinated compounds used to make Teflon. Seabirds, forest birds, seals, foxes, bears, whales, and fish living in the southern and northern regions of the planet have all been found to contain these chemicals.

"Who has made the decision that sets in motion these chains of poisoning, that ever widening wave of death that spreads out like ripples in a pond. Who has decided – who has the right to decide – for the countless legions of people who were not consulted?"
– Rachel Carson, in her 1962 revolutionary book *Silent Spring*

One of the most common chemicals found in polar bears is a fire retardant used in furniture, carpeting, plastics, and electronics. These chemicals are known to disrupt thyroid and sex hormones, impair mental abilities and motor skills, and to alter brain development. Bears are being found with weak bone structures and weakened immune systems, and the milk of lactating bears has been found to contain enough of these chemicals to jeopardize the health of cubs. These are problems directly attributed to the pollution the bears are accumulating in their body tissues. With only 20,000 to 25,000 polar bears left in the wild, facing problem chemical pollutants and melting ice caps along with the threat of being hunted, their existence on the planet may soon come to an end.

The melting of the ice caps of the planet, which is caused by pollutants, is also one of several factors leading to the warming of the oceans. Ice reflects the heat of sun. Where the ice has melted, the ocean water and the newly bare land are absorbing that heat. Because the polar oceans are becoming far less fresh and more acidic, and the tropical oceans far more salty, the global atmosphere is accumulating more water vapor, which is accelerating the problem.

That is just a small part of the story of what modern human lifestyles are doing to Earth by way of massive use of resources to fuel our environmentally unsustainable choices.

Every minute, enormous amounts of toxic pesticides, fertilizers, fungicides, insecticides, and other agricultural chemicals are being spread over farmland throughout the world. All of these chemicals are known to cause birth defects, hormonal imbalances, learning disabilities, cancers and other disease in both humans and wildlife. Farming and industrial chemicals also accumulate in water and result in large areas of the seas that are void of natural life. Inland, there are people who are told not to drink the tap water because it contains such high levels of chemical fertilizers that drinking the water can cause brain damage. People are left relying on store-bought bottled water, which impacts their income, and leaves billions more plastic bottles polluting the environment for an unknown number of years. What natural gas fracking is doing to the water tables is astoundingly bad. The practice of fracking uses a stew of toxic chemicals that poisons the land and water. (Please watch the documentary, *Gasland*. Learn about the environmental damage being done by natural gas fracking, help to make people aware of this horrible practice, and reduce your use of natural gas.)

"The amount of pesticides and nonorganic fertilizers used in farming today is shocking, and it is being ingested by us and Earth and damaging us both – for example, conventional strawberries use 300 pounds of synthetic pesticides, herbicides, fertilizer, and fungicides per acre."
– Terces Engelhart, co-author with Orchid of *I Am Grateful: Recipes & Lifestyle of Café Gratitude*; CafeGratitude.com

Low-paid farm laborers are exposed to farming chemicals, and often get sick from them. Many of the workers have no idea what the dangers are of the chemicals they are being exposed to. For example, the fumigant chloropicrin that is used on farms contains the same active ingredient as tear gas. A chemical called Nemagon had been used for decades on sugar cane, pineapple, and banana farms. It caused cancers and a variety of terrible ailments in the farm workers. Women repeatedly exposed to it had miscarriages and stillbirths, and their babies that lived often were born with extreme deformities. Today there are similar chemicals being used that are poisoning workers on farms around the planet. These chemicals end up in the food you eat and the water you drink. When farm workers who are exposed to toxic chemicals do get sick they may not know what caused it. If they are able to visit a nurse or doctor they may be misdiagnosed, or their concerns dismissed or lost in translation. Long-term exposure can result in numerous health problems in the workers, and in their children and grandchildren.

"What happens in nature is not allowed to happen in the modern, chemical-drenched world, where spraying destroys not only the insects but also their principal enemy, the birds. When later there is a resurgence of the insect population, as almost always happens, the birds are not there to keep their numbers in check."
– Rachel Carson, *Silent Spring*

Farming chemicals damage soil organisms, such as mycorrhizal soil fungi, that play a large role in soil health and help the plant root systems obtain nutrients and water from the soil. There are many hundreds of billions of chemical reactions that go on in a handful of soil as various forms of microorganisms live and interact through their life processes. If the genetically engineered plants and/or various toxic chemicals produced by industries begin to kill soil organisms or lead to bacteria that largely damages or kills soil organisms, it could stop all plants from growing. If the obscene development of genetically engineered food plants isn't bad enough, there are companies that are developing genetically engineered bacteria. This should be stopped, globally. (Access: OrganicConsumer.org)

Learn about the terrible practices of companies like ADM, Bunge, Monsanto, Cargill, and Bayer CropScience, which are genetically engineering food plants and also producing highly toxic farming chemicals that poison us and the environment. (Access: OccupyMonsanto360.org, LabelGMOs.org, and SayNoToGMOs.org)

There are many people on this planet fighting over land; and the last remaining wildlands are being grabbed up and controlled by governments and corporations that exploit nature's resources. Because of this, many animals and plants have become extinct while others are on the edge of becoming so. The terrible practice of segmenting Earth's rainforests and allowing corporations to control them, giving them invasive permits to alter what grows there, fracturing indigenous cultures, and turning the ancient trees into some sort of tradeoff for carbon exchange, is a big lie that should also stop.

> "There is but one ocean though its coves have many names; a single sea of atmosphere with no coves at all; the miracle of soil, alive and giving life, lying thin on the only Earth, for which there is no spare."
> – David Brower, first executive director of the Sierra Club; founder of Friends of the Earth; founder of Earth Island Institute; father of the modern environmental movement

Wherever a piece of land is changed from its wild state to that of roads, houses, buildings, pavement, timber "management," animal farming, and monocropping, all life on that piece of land is changed – from that of free-living wild animals and plants to that of an unnatural state often unsuitable for most or all of the wildlife that had existed there for many thousands of generations.

> "It has long been apparent that every large, land-based animal on this planet is ultimately fighting a losing battle with humankind."
> – Charles Siebert in his excellent article, Are We Driving Elephants Crazy?: Their behavior in the wild has grown strange and violent in recent years. Researchers say our encroachment on their way of life is to blame; New York Times Magazine, October 8, 2006

Where am I going with all of this information? The point is that everything is interconnected. What you do impacts people and wildlife thousands of miles from you. This is especially true the more you rely on stores and restaurants for food, and the less you rely on self sufficient home gardening or on local organic farmers. As I state elsewhere, the number-one way we interact with Earth is through what we ingest, for instance, our choices of food and water.

Earth is warmer now than it has been in thousands of years. The cause of the warming is human activity, and specifically the burning of fossil fuels. According to studies from various institutions, the meat industry causes more pollution on the planet than any other industry. Intensive livestock farming and the cooking of meat cause more pollution than all cars, trucks, trains, planes, and boats.

> "The livestock sector generates more greenhouse gas emissions as measured in CO_2 equivalent than transport [cars and trucks]."
> – Food and Agriculture Organisation, Rome, Italy; 2006

Meanwhile, vegetation is growing higher on the world's mountains than ever on record. Certain species of insects are appearing in places where they have never been seen, including billions of beetles that are destroying hundreds of millions of trees in the mountain forests of North America. Tropical fish are swimming to parts of the oceans that are closer to the poles. Forms of bacteria and fungi are being found in parts of the world where it was thought they couldn't survive. Tropical diseases are spreading to new regions. Amphibians are increasingly being found with extra legs and other physical deformities caused by industrial pollutants. Algae overgrowth is becoming a problem in the world's largest bodies of fresh water as well as throughout swamplands and saltwater marshes and reefs. Flowers and trees are blooming out of season. Birds are building nests during parts of the year that aren't their traditional breeding season.

What is happening on the land is only a fraction of what is happening to wildlife on the planet.

What is going on in the oceans, which make up the majority of the surface of the planet, is reflective of what is happening on the land.

The oceans continue to show signs that they are dying. Thousands of miles of coral reefs that were filled with life just a decade ago are gone, or sit almost empty of life because of bleaching, dynamite fishing, overfishing, and rising levels of water acidity, or are being strangled by algae overgrowth largely caused by monocropping farm pollution. Kelp and sea grass beds are vanishing, as are the forms of life that depend on them.

Sonar technology being used by the military and fuel industries is killing thousands of sea mammals in excruciating ways by destroying their ears. The Marine Mammal Protection Act continues to be over-ridden by the petroleum companies and U.S. Department of Defense so that the use of sonar equipment can continue to be used by the U.S., by Britain, and by several other nations.

Other sea mammals are absorbing so much pollution that their young suffer and die from the poisons in their mother's milk. Both pollution and industrial sea noise are to blame for the Puget Sound orca whales being declared an endangered species; joining them are their neighbors, dozens of varieties of salmon and steelhead trout, which are on the edge of regional or complete extinction.

The worldwide fishing industry is playing a major role in destroying the oceans. Fish species are becoming rare or extinct in regions where they were common just decades ago, every type of sea turtle is endangered, massive fishing operations are setting billions of hooks every year to capture large fish and are killing sea life of all sorts. It is estimated that 25 percent of the sea life captured is not what the fishing fleets want, so they toss these dead or dying sea creatures back into the water, or they are sold to feed the world's billions of farmed animals – which require massive amounts of land and fossil fuels to breed, raise, slaughter, package, transport, market, and cook.

"The atrocities are no less atrocious when concealed in a convenient package with clever advertising."
– Dr. Holly Wilson

Massive nets are being dragged across the ocean floors at deeper and deeper levels to capture fish that were once abundant, but are becoming sparse or nonexistent in places where they had existed since their species began. This causes a destabilizing of sea life biodiversity, extinguishing populations that rely on others to survive. These deep-sea trawling operations are the equivalent of killing every bird, animal, and bug in a forest during a hunt for several hundred deer. Many of these massively destructive fishing expeditions operate on government subsidies and are protected by laws formed to protect not the oceans or sea life, but the profits of the fishing industry. Because of industrial pollutants the fish that are left are becoming more and more toxic, resulting in fish that can poison predator fish and the wildlife and humans that eat fish.

"No fishing. Because fish have a brain, a central nervous system, and pain receptors. They can feel pain just like cats, dogs, and humans. Just because they can't scream doesn't mean that they are not in pain. Also, other animals, like birds, often strangle or choke to death on lost hooks and lines."
– PETA

"Seafood is simply a socially acceptable form of bush meat. We condemn Africans for hunting monkeys and mammalian and bird species from the jungle, yet the developed world thinks nothing of hauling in magnificent wild creatures like swordfish, tuna, halibut,

shark and salmon for our meals. The fact is that the global slaughter of marine wildlife is simply the largest massacre of wildlife on the planet."
– Captain Paul Watson, SeaShepherd.org

"When we think about animal abuse and environmental destruction on factory farms, we think about cows, pigs, chickens, and turkeys, but we often don't think about fish. However, fish are abused just as awfully as land animals, and fishing is destroying our planet just as quickly as factory farms are. When hauled up from the deep, fish undergo excruciating decompression. Frequently, the intense internal pressure ruptures the swimbladder, pops out the eyes, and pushes the oesophagus and stomach out through the mouth. Most fish are gutted whilst still alive or are left to suffocate."
– Animal Aid

The fishing industry continues to lobby for more protection of their fishing rights, for more government funding for fishing fleets, and spends more and more money to promote the consumption of sea life with no mention of the state of the oceans or the poisons that may exist within the fish. In many parts of the world people can go to their local restaurant or seafood market to get a piece of a sea creature that is a species at risk of extinction.

Additional damage is being caused by the hundreds of millions of pharmaceutical drugs that are being taken every day and that are ending up in the water bodies of the planet. According to the Centers for Disease Control and Prevention, 130 million Americans use prescription drugs every month. The drugs are urinated away, or expired and unwanted prescriptions are flushed down toilets. As the chemical drugs dissolve into the waterways they wreak additional havoc on waterlife.

"Right now is the time to act wisely – by getting wisely informed. The key to saving ourselves (and countless innocent bystanders) from ourselves is education. We must change our ways, or face the collapse of the ocean world… and life on this planet as we know it."
– ZeroImpactProductions.Com

Because of dead zones created by the accumulation of livestock waste, and farming and industrial chemicals flowing into the ocean, and air pollution dropping from the sky, increasingly larger areas of the oceans are devoid of healthy populations of natural sea life. As the dead zones increase, so does the surface temperature of the water, resulting in an increasing number of intense storms.

Because of all this, it is of great importance that we work to preserve and protect what is left of Earth's original beauty, to restore whatever we possibly can, and to start living in ways that are less damaging to the natural cycles of nature: through an organic, plant-based diet, and by greatly reducing fossil fuel use, and eliminating the use of it whenever and wherever possible.

"The Earth has been around for 4.6 billion years. Scaling this time down to 46 years, we have been around for four hours and our Industrial Revolution began just one minute ago. During this short time period we have ransacked the planet for ways to get fuels and raw materials, have been the cause of extinction of an unthinkable amount of plants and animals, and have multiplied our population to that of a plague."
– From Earth Day pamphlet of WorldFestEvents.Com

Without a healthy planet we cannot survive.

We need to stop looking at what is best for the human condition for decades, and start considering what is best for all of Earth's life forms for millennia.

"No one is useless in this world who lightens the burden of it for anyone else."
– Charles Dickens

It is time to realize that each of us can work to make a difference in bringing Earth to a healthier state, for now, and for the future.

"It is no measure of health to be well adjusted to a profoundly sick society."
– Jiddu Krishnamurti

If you are not actively working to make the world a better place, then you are working to make the world a worse place.

"Since becoming a vegan, I have come to realize this. The wider you open your eyes, the darker the world becomes. No matter how hard you try, you can never close them tight enough. The truth sears an everlasting image of the suffering into your retina. From then on, you'll eternally understand that ignoring the pain of others is truly the cruelest action we can do as conscious beings. Inaction is the plague of the world."
– Bianca Nicole Valle

Donate money to or volunteer for an organization that works to protect wild animals, forests, and wildlands, or that aims to improve the condition of Earth. Get involved in other ways to improve the state of the planet. Get closer to nature through your food choices, and through the ways you spend your time, energy, and resources. Clean up your act.

"The only thing necessary for the triumph of evil is for good men to do nothing."
– Edmund Burke

"Every time we witness an injustice and do not act, we train our character to be passive in its presence and thereby eventually lose all ability to defend ourselves and those we love."
– Julian Assange

"Lack of awareness of the basic unity of organism and environment is a serious and dangerous hallucination."
– Alan Watts

"The Earth is not dying, it is being killed. And the people who are killing it have names and addresses."
– Utah Phillips

"Experiencing our own dynamic nature can be the first step towards understanding the dynamic nature of all living systems."
– Adam Wolpert

"We abuse the land because we regard it as a commodity belonging to us. When we see land as a community to which we belong, we may begin to use it with love and respect."
– Aldo Leopold

"There's not a single scientific peer review paper published in the last 25 years that would contradict this scenario: Every living system of Earth is in decline. Every life support system of Earth is in decline. And these together constitute the biosphere. The biosphere that supports and nurtures all of life. Not just our lives, but perhaps 30 million other species that share this planet with us."
– Ray Anderson

"Man's attitude toward nature is today critically important simply because we now have acquired a fateful power to alter and destroy nature. But man is part of nature, and his war is inevitably a war against himself."
– Rachel Carson

"Some day the earth will weep, she will beg for her life, she will cry with tears of blood. You will make a choice, if you will help her or let her die, and when she dies, you will die too."
– John Hollow Horn, Oglala Lakota, 1932

"When we try to pick anything out by itself, we find it hitched to everything else in the universe."
– John Muir

"Humankind has not woven the web of life. We are but one thread within it. Whatever we do to the web, we do to ourselves. All things are bound together. All things are connected."
– Chief Seattle

"You must teach your children that the ground beneath their feet is the ashes of your grandfathers. So that they will respect the land, tell your children that the earth is rich with the lives of our kin. Teach your children what we have taught our children, that the earth is our mother. Whatever befalls the earth befalls the sons of the earth."
– Native American Wisdom

"I tell you truly, you are one with the Earthly Mother; she is in you, and you in her. Of her were you born, in her do you live, and to her shall you return again. It is the blood of our Earthly Mother which falls from the clouds and flows in the rivers; it is the breath of our Earthly Mother, which whispers in the leaves of the forest and blows with a mighty wind from the mountains; sweet and firm is the flesh of our Earthly Mother in the fruits of the trees; strong and unflinching are the bones of our Earthly Mother in the giant rocks and stones which stand as sentinels of the lost times; truly, we are one with our Earthly Mother, and he who clings to the laws of his Mother, to him shall his Mother cling also."
– The Essene Gospel of Peace

"There are two primary choices in life: To accept conditions as they exist, or accept the responsibility for changing them."
– Dr. Denis Waitley

GET INVOLVED in protecting the environment, in protecting animals, in restoring nature.

"Let every individual and institution now think and act as a responsible trustee of Earth, seeking choices in ecology, economics and ethics that will provide a sustainable future, eliminate pollution, poverty, and violence, awaken the wonder of life and foster peaceful progress in the human adventure."
– John McConnell, founder of International Earth Day

We are all part of a bigger picture. We are all connected in one way or another – whether we like it or not. The more the population of the planet explodes, the more this seems to be evident. We can all decide whether we are going to be part of the solution, or part of the problem.

Stop being part of the problem. Stop supporting a system that grows vast quantities of food to feed farmed animals, where most of the farmland on the planet consists of animal farming to supply meat for stores and restaurants in the wealthier countries, while poor people are starving in countries where more than 50 percent of the food grown is fed to farmed animals for exporting meat to wealthy countries.

> "The poverty of our century is unlike that of any other. It is not, as poverty was before, the result of natural scarcity, but of a set of priorities imposed upon the rest of the world by the rich. Consequently, the modern poor are not pitied, but written off as trash."
> – John Berger

Make your daily life part of the solution. Start by eliminating toxic foods from your diet, and tune into a plant-based diet rich in raw fruits and vegetables that are preferably organically grown, including some that are grown by you, and the majority of the rest from organic farms.

> "Certain gardens are described as retreats when they are really attacks."
> – Ian Hamilton Finlay

> "You want to reclaim your mind and get it out of the hands of the cultural engineers who want to turn you into a half-baked moron consuming all the trash that's being manufactured out of the bones of a dying world."
> – Terrance McKenna

Grow and maintain an organic food garden, and compost your food scraps into the soil.

Support organic family farms.

> "We are fellow passengers on the same planet, and we are all equally responsible for the happiness and the well-being of the world in which we happen to live."
> – Hendrick Van Loon

THE MOST NATURAL DIET

HUMANS experience more diseases than their nonhuman counter-
parts. Humans also eat a diet that is much more diverse and far
removed from the natural diets of animals living in the wild. Consider
the connection.

Regionally, humans who follow a certain diet common in their community experience health conditions at rates not seen in regions where
that type of diet is not followed. Those living in areas of the world
where meat, dairy, and egg consumption is highest also have the most elevated rates of heart disease, colorectal cancer, breast cancer, multiple
sclerosis (MS), arthritis, diabetes, certain types of kidney disease, Alzheimer's disease, macular degeneration, and other diseases not experienced among people living in areas of the world where animal protein
consumption is lower.

"To eat is a necessity, but to eat intelligently is an art."
– François de la Rochefoucauld

People in North America who consume the most meat and eggs are
also more likely to consume the most pasteurized dairy, and the most
corn syrup, synthetic food chemicals, and processed foods. These are
the same people who are most likely to be obese, and who experience
maladies common to those who are obese.

"The person who is afraid to alter his living habits, and
especially his eating and drinking habits, because he is afraid that
other persons may regard him as queer, eccentric, or fanatic forgets
that the ownership of his body, the responsibility for its well-being,
belongs to him, not them."
– Dr. Paul Brunton

"Being vegan is easy. Are there social pressures that encourage
you to continue to eat, wear, and use animal products? Of course
there are. But in a patriarchal, racist, homophobic, and ableist
society, there are social pressures to participate and engage in
sexism, racism, homophobia, and ableism. At some point, you have
to decide who you are and what matters morally to you. And once

174

you decide that you regard victimizing vulnerable nonhumans is not morally acceptable, it is easy to go and stay vegan."
– Gary L. Francione

"The fate of animals is of greater importance to me than the fear of appearing ridiculous."
– Emile Zola

Those following a diet that is plant based, low in fat, free of animal protein, and rich in raw fruits and vegetables are less likely to experience a whole list of diseases common among those who follow a diet higher in fat, and contains meat, milk, or eggs, and that is lacking in fresh fruits and vegetables. This book is all about choosing the more healthful foods.

As you change your life and become different from what you used to be, you may find yourself getting attention that you had not been accustomed to receiving — including both compliments and perhaps cynical criticism. When people are accustomed to seeing you maintain a certain lifestyle and appear a certain way, and they then see that you have physically transformed, they also may feel uncomfortable. You will be breaking from the role that you had been playing. People will have to recast you in their minds as no longer being the person they thought you were, and maybe the person they thought you could never be.

Completely changing your diet to the most healthful way available to you will make a huge difference in many areas of your life. When provided with high-quality nutrition, the body will change to a state in tune with those nutrients. Within the body is an amazing power to heal, to detoxify the cells, to reform the tissues, and to reconfigure the shape of the organs. Providing the body with a diet that largely consists of vibrant raw fruits and vegetables can fuel this power.

"You can't turn back the clock. But you can wind it up again."
– Bonnie Prudden

When you become more healthful, people notice. Your skin, shape, and movement change. Your confidence and energy improve. It is then that people may be interested in what you are doing that changed you.

In their excellent book, *Raw Food Revolution Diet*, Cherie Soria, Brenda Davis, and Vesanto Melina offer this advice to those with compromised health and who are switching to a raw vegan diet:
"Find out about your blood cholesterol, triglyceride, and blood sugar levels. Check your blood pressure and body weight. If you are on prescription medications, make sure that your health care

provider knows about your diet plan. You will need to be closely monitored; when people embark on a raw food diet, medications commonly need to be adjusted or stopped completely. This must be done with the approval and assistance of your health care provider. Raw food diets commonly result in weight loss and normalization of blood pressure, blood cholesterol, and blood sugar levels. People who are on medications for high blood pressure, high cholesterol, or Type-2 diabetes may notice rapid changes in their condition and their requirements for these medications. Those on insulin or oral hypoglycemic agents need to monitor their blood sugars closely, as blood sugars may drop too low. In this event, your health care provider may choose to prepare a new medication schedule for you. In any case, regular blood sugar monitoring is essential."

As you follow a fresh foods diet your life will change. This is especially true if you had been eating devitalized, unhealthful, deadened, fried, and otherwise processed commercial foods. Opportunities will arise that you may never have considered. Things will happen that you didn't think were a possibility, or were not even in your conception of how things could happen. You will find yourself feeling and thinking differently from the way you had been. Your perceptions will change. Foods, music, and designs of things may seem different to you. Activities in which you may never have thought about participating may draw your attention. The way you eat, dress, think, and play, and the general way you participate in life may all go through radical changes. The higher frequency that you tune into by eating more vibrant foods can ignite your passions in intense ways you never thought possible.

> "Through our soul is our contact with heaven."
> – Sholem Asch

The power of your soul is what formulated your tissues and it is what is animating you. It is making you think. It is making your heart beat and your lungs breathe. It is making your cells function. It is what is making you seek your desires. It is pushing you to constantly work out your thoughts into actions. You can make it work for you. It is your power source. Honor it with rightful living, self-respect, intentional actions, and vibrant foods that infuse health.

> "The brain gives the heart its sight. The heart gives the brain its vision."
> – Rob Kall

When you follow a plant-based diet that is completely free of animal protein (milk, eggs, and meat), and that is rich in raw vegetables and fruits, and is low in fat, and free of fried oils, sautéed foods, bleached and gluten grains (wheat, rye, barley [See: _The Dark Side of Wheat_ from GreenMedInfo.com]), chemicals (preservatives, flavorings, colors, scents, and sweeteners), refined sugars (white and brown sugar, corn syrup [aka corn sugar], and agave), processed salts, and MSG, the pineal gland, which is located at the center of your brain, functions at a higher level, as does your heart and the brain, muscles, bones, and blood.

Proteins in the pineal gland resemble the photoreceptor proteins in the eyes. It is known that a low-quality diet leads to degeneration of the eyes. Similarly, low-quality foods interfere with the function of the pineal gland. While the cells of the eyes allow you to see and interact with structures, the cells of the pineal gland allow you to interact with spirit, inspiration, and what motivates you in your visualizations. The pineal gland is not walled off behind the blood brain barrier. It receives large amounts of blood, thus it is directly connected to the function and feelings of the heart. For these reasons, the pineal gland is often referred to as _the third eye_. René Descartes called the pineal gland _the seat of the soul_. When your pineal gland is able to function at a high level, you are more likely to receive inspiration that triggers the use of your true talents and intellect emanating from your spirit.

> "When you start using senses you neglected, your reward is to see the world with completely fresh eyes."
> – Barbara Sher

For brain and full body health, follow an organic diet. Foods grown using synthetic chemicals contain weaker energy fields, fewer nutrients, more sugar, and also substances that reduce the release of feel-good chemicals in the brain.

Glyphosate, an herbicide in toxic RoundUp weed killer produced by Monsanto, and used on genetically modified food plants and on cotton, can accumulate in our bodies and interfere with levels of dopamine and serotonin in our brains. Dopamine and serotonin are naturally occurring brain chemicals associated with good mood and health. Low levels of these chemicals are associated with anxiety, depression, bipolar disorder, irritable bowel syndrome, and autoimmune disorders. If you go to an allopathic (typical Western) doctor for these conditions, they will prescribe medications. Instead of relying on chemical drugs and surgery to try to grasp health, it is wise to eliminate from the diet all chemically grown and junk foods, and to get involved with growing your own organic garden, composting your organic food scraps into soil, and supporting local organic farmers. By doing so, you will lower your exposure to toxic chemicals that can cause a variety of health problems, including mood swings, emotional issues, depleted energy, and physical ailments.

A healthful diet rich in raw fruits and vegetables along with daily exercise will get your body, heart, brain, and pineal gland to function at a higher level so that the rest of your life can function at an elevated level.

Do not pollute your body with low-quality foods. Do not allow yourself to eat deadened or otherwise processed foods that lower your frequency and leave residues of toxins in your tissues, clogging and slowing your systems. Follow a diet of high-quality foods that enliven your body, bring about the beauty of health, and improve your level of consciousness. Partake in the living power of nature that is contained in vibrantly alive, organic raw fruits and vegetables, sprouts, and germinates. Let these ignite your health, intellect, passions, talents, craft, confidence, and love.

"And the time came when the risk to remain tight in a bud was more painful than the risk it took to blossom."
– Anais Nin

Start now to eliminate low-quality food, such as foods that are bleached or fried, or that contain clarified sugars, processed salt, or synthetic chemicals. Refrain from eating tissues of animals, and also milk, milk products, or eggs.

"I know in my soul that to eat a creature who is raised to be eaten, and who never has a chance to be a real being, is unhealthy. You're just eating misery."
– Alice Walker

"I learned that you can be a vegetarian and eat food that tastes just as good as if you're not. The foods that we eat right now tend to be foods that come out of the ground looking just the way they look when I eat them. They're unadulterated, they're real foods. I try to eat them raw if I can."
– Dr. Mehmet Oz

"People just don't realize it, that their food choices can have such impact not only on their own health, but now on global health, both environmentally and in terms of public health. But I think slowly but surely these connections are being made from all different directions, and I think it's really an exciting time."
– Dr. Michael Greger, NutritionFacts.org

"Everyone holds the power to save a life or take a life when they choose a meal."
– Ingrid Newkirk

"Vegetarian food leaves a deep impression on our nature. If the whole world adopts vegetarianism, it can change the destiny of mankind."
– Albert Einstein

"Vegan food is soul food in its truest form. Soul food means to feed the soul. And to me, your soul is your intent. If your intent is pure, you are pure."
– Erykah Badu

"After looking at 34 published studies in 16 countries, researchers at Yale University found that countries with the highest rates of osteoporosis, including the United States, Sweden, and Finland, are those in which people consume the most meat, milk, and other animal foods.

Despite the dairy industry funding study after study to try to prove its claims that consuming dairy products will make your bones stronger, the truth is exactly the opposite.

The primary cause of osteoporosis is the high-protein diet most people consume today. Eating a high-protein diet is like pouring acid rain on your bones. (The protein increases productions of acid in the blood, which is then neutralized by calcium taken from our bones). Remarkably enough, if dairy has any effect, both clinical and population evidence strongly implicate dairy in causing, rather than preventing, osteoporosis."
– Dr. John McDougall; DrMcDougall.com

"We cut the throat of a calf and hang it up by the heels to bleed to death so that our veal cutlet may be white; we nail geese to a board and cram them with food because we like the taste of liver disease; we tear birds to pieces to decorate our women's hats; we mutilate domestic animals for no reason at all except to follow an instinctively cruel fashion; and we connive at the most abominable tortures in the hope of discovering some magical cure for our own diseases by them."
– George Bernard Shaw

PROTEIN

"Plant protein can meet requirements when a variety of plant foods is consumed and energy needs are met. Research indicates that an assortment of plant foods eaten over the course of a day can provide all essential amino acids and ensure adequate nitrogen retention and use in healthy adults, thus complementary proteins do not need to be consumed at the same meal."
– American Dietetic Association, 2009

PEOPLE who are vegetarian often get asked if they eat a lot of soy products. The assumption is that because vegetarians don't eat animal tissues they need to have soy protein in their diet. But what many people don't seem to understand is that you don't need to eat protein-dominant plants to get protein into your system.

Some vegetarians and vegans also get caught up in the belief that they need soy in their diet as a sort of replacement for meat. They do this by eating all sorts of soy bean products – soy milk, soy ice cream, soy yogurt, tofu everything, soy burgers, soy powders, soy cheese, and soy custards and puddings.

The structures of our bodies are made of protein. The enzymes, blood, and lymph also consist of protein. People tend to think that we need to eat protein in the form of flesh, eggs, and milk to build our tissues. This is a huge misconception that drives people to focus on eating protein-rich diets, which are rough on the system and trigger degenerative diseases. The misconception helps to fuel the animal farming industry with its slaughterhouses and monocropped GMO grains; the colon, prostate, and breast cancer industries; the diabetes industry; the heart attack industry; the hospital and pharmaceutical industries; the fast food industry; deforestation; and cruelty to animals on a massive scale.

"We've never treated a single patient with protein deficiency; yet the majority of patients we see are suffering from heart disease, diabetes, and other chronic illnesses directly resulting from trying to get enough protein."
– Dr. Alona Pulde and Dr. Matthew Lederman, Forks over Knives

You do not need to eat animal flesh to get protein.

If you don't eat animal flesh, you don't need to eat soy products to get protein.

"A vegetable-based diet for children is generally more healthful than a diet containing the cholesterol, animal fat, and excessive protein found in meat and dairy products. Children and adolescents will get plenty of protein as long as they eat a variety of whole-grains, legumes, vegetables, fruits, and nuts."
– Dr. Benjamin Spock

Your body needs amino acids to build protein. Proteins are made out of chains of amino acids. There is an abundance of amino acids in fresh fruits, vegetables, sprouts, nuts, and seeds. The body makes the protein it needs out of the amino acids obtained through the foods you eat.

There are amino acids in all plants.

"The old ideas about the necessity of carefully combining vegetables at every meal to ensure the supply of essential amino acids has been totally refuted."
– Dr. Charles Attwood

Even when a person eats animal protein, the body does not simply transfer that protein into the tissues of the body. The body takes the individual amino acids from the protein to form the type of amino acid chains it needs.

"You may have heard that vegetable sources of protein are incomplete and become complete only when correctly combined. Research has discredited that notion so you don't have to worry that you won't get enough usable protein if you don't put together some magical combination of foods at each meal."
– Andrew Weil, M.D.

Amino acids that need to be obtained from food:
Isoleucine
Leucine
Lysine
Methionine + Cysteine
Phenylalaline + Tyrosine
Threonine
Tryptophan
Valine
Histidine

Those are the "essential amino acids" – known as such because they need to be obtained from food.

It is essential for children to obtain histidine from food. Adults synthesize it [their systems naturally create it].

In other words, there are nine essential amino acids that children need to obtain from food. But there are eight amino acids that adults need to obtain from food.

There are 22 proteinogenic amino acids in total, which your body uses to create protein. Other than those listed above, the human body synthesizes the others.

The nonessential amino acids are:
Alanine
Arginine
Aspartate
Cyeteine
Glutamate
Glutamine
Glycine
Proline
Serine
Asparagine

These amino acids are unclassified:
Pyrrolysine
Selenocysteine

All fruits and vegetables contain the essential amino acids your body needs to make protein. You will get all of the amino acids you need by eating enough calories of fruits, vegetables, nuts, and seeds.

You don't need to combine fruits and vegetables, or nuts and seeds, or legumes and rice, to get complete protein.

"Complementing proteins is not necessary with vegetable proteins. The myth that vegetable source proteins need to be complemented is similar to the myths that persist about sugar making one's blood glucose go up faster than starch does. These myths have great staying power despite their being no evidence to support them and plenty to refute them."
– Dennis Gordon, M.Ed, R.D.

"It is very easy for a vegan diet to meet the recommendations for protein, as long as calorie intake is adequate. Strict protein combining is not necessary; it is more important to eat a varied diet throughout the day."
– Reed Mangels, Ph.D., R.D.; Vegetarian Resource Group, VRG.org

A balanced live vegan diet provides an abundance of amino acids and other nutrients from a variety of live plant substances.

I use animals as examples of natural vegans. The natural diet of cows, bulls, buffalo, horses, gorillas, giraffes, deer, moose, goats, hippopotamuses, and elephants consists of plants. Their bodies get protein out of the substances within the plants, and their diets chiefly consist of green leaves. Their huge musles are formed on a vegan diet.

When I was in my 20s, I had a lot of kidney problems, to the point that doctors were telling me that I was going to die if I didn't go onto dialysis, and then get a kidney transplant as soon as possible. One of the many doctors told me that I should follow a strictly vegan diet, and I should be okay. Other doctors told me that following a vegan diet would be "difficult." As if having my body cut in half was going to be simple and low risk. Instead of dialysis and undergoing a kidney transplant, I began following a vegan diet. I have since learned very clearly that a high-protein diet is absolutely not good for the kidneys.

"When people eat too much protein, it releases nitrogen into the blood or is digested and metabolized. This places a strain on the kidneys, which must expel the waste through the urine. High-protein diets are associated with reduced kidney function. Over time, individuals who consume very large amounts of protein, particularly animal protein, risk permanent loss of kidney function. Harvard researchers reported recently that high-protein diets were associated with a significant decline in kidney function, based on observations in 1,624 women participating in the Nurses' Health Study. The good news is that the damage was found only in those who already had reduced kidney function at the study's outset. The bad news is that as many as one in four adults in the United States may already have reduced kidney function, suggesting that most people who have renal problems are unaware of that fact and do not realize that high-protein diets may put them at risk for further deterioration. The kidney-damaging effect was seen only with animal protein. Plant protein had no harmful effect.[1]

The American Academy of Family Physicians notes that high animal protein intake is largely responsible for the high prevalence of kidney stones in the United States and other developed countries and recommends protein restriction for the prevention of recurrent kidney stones.[2]"

– Physicians Committee for Responsible Medicine, PCRM.org. Citing
1. Knight EL, Stampfer MJ, Hankinson SE, Spiegelman D, Curhan GC. The Impact of Protein Intake on Renal Function Decline in Women with Normal Renal Function or Mild Renal Insufficiency.

Ann Int Med. 2003;138:460-467; 2. Goldfarb DS, Coe FL. Prevention of Recurrent Nephrolithiasis. *Am Fam Physician.* 1999; 60:2269-2276.

I don't depend on soy, or any one particular plant, for protein in my diet. Soy beans are best consumed raw, such as directly out of the pod, or tossing them into a salad. I eat a variety of fruits, vegetables, herbs, nuts, seeds, and sea vegetables. My body gets more than enough protein-building properties in the form of amino acids from the variety of foods that I eat.

Mushrooms are a protein-dominant food. But they aren't a plant, they are a fungus. They are okay to eat in moderation. They contain the mineral potassium as well as nutritional compounds, including some glyconutrients that improve the immune system and that may help prevent cancer. Mushrooms exposed to sunlight contain vitamin D.

I have reservations about picking my own mushrooms, as I know that certain types of mushrooms can make you very ill, and others can kill you. Of course there are also mushrooms that can open your mind. Mushrooms that fall under the poisonous category make up only a small fraction of the variety of mushroom species. I prefer to purchase mushrooms from people who are educated about mushrooms – such as the family who have a stand at the local farmers' market.

Dietary protein can also be obtained from legumes, which are protein-dominant seeds. These include chickpeas (also known as garbanzo beans), kidney beans, lentils, mung beans, and soy beans. Protein-dominant foods can be harsh on the system. To increase the presence of amino acids and enzymes in legumes, soak them for several hours in water, or germinate them over three to six days by keeping them moist in a clean place (being sure to thoroughly rinse them at least once a day, and preferably two or three times). Soaking, germinating, or sprouting legumes increases their nutritional value, making them less heavy and harsh on the digestive system.

"Modern researchers know that it is virtually impossible to design a calorie-sufficient diet based on unprocessed whole natural plant foods that is deficient in any of the amino acids. The only possible exception could be a diet based solely on fruit."
– Jeff Novick, M.S., R.D.

Don't believe the nonsense put out by the meat, dairy, and egg industries that advise people to consume meat, milk, and eggs to get protein into their diet. Even the United States government programs that supposedly establish nutrition "requirements" – such as the food pyramid – are grandly flawed – in favor of various industries selling food unhealthful food products.

The U.S. Recommended Daily Allowance (USRDA) standards, and the government's food triangle, were largely created using money from trade groups supported by the meat, dairy, and egg industries.

It is no secret that many of the people who work for the FDA and USDA are people who have worked or eventually work for some branch of the meat, dairy, and egg trade groups – often through employment with lobbying groups that work to get laws passed to increase government welfare for the meat, dairy, and egg industries – and usually for large, corporate farming interests.

Much of the nutritional information presented to children in their classrooms is flawed, and is most often provided free to school systems from organizations supported by the meat, dairy, and egg industries. Included in this biased and flawed information is the advice that humans should eat a large amount of animal protein. Again, this information is propaganda financed by the meat, dairy, and egg industries.

What you won't hear in the advertising of meat, dairy, and eggs is that people who consume the largest amounts of animal protein also experience degenerative diseases, such as heart disease, diabetes, arthritis, obesity, macular degeneration, kidney disorders, osteoporosis, cancers, etc., in conjunction with the amount of animal flesh, milk, and eggs they consume.

Some people promote a high-protein diet as a way to become lean. A high-protein diet is clearly not healthful, and can lead to a variety of health problems. Dr. John McDougall, who is one of a group of doctors promoting true health, has some interesting things to say about the high-protein diet. He has written a number of books, including about heart health. He promotes a vegan diet.

"Our Creator designed us to run on carbohydrates. Glucose, one of the simplest, most basic carbohydrates, is our primary fuel. It is more easily converted into energy than fat or protein, and, therefore, our bodies will always burn it first. In addition, it is the cleanest-burning fuel of the body, creating fewer by-products than other nutrients. By our very design, the body needs carbohydrates to operate efficiently and provide ample energy. A testament to their importance is the fact that the brain tissues, red blood cells, and cells of the kidneys will only use glucose as fuel.

When you take the carbohydrates away, your body runs out of glucose and is forced to burn its secondary fuel – fat.

When your cells burn fat instead of glucose, by-products known as ketones are produced. This creates a metabolic state called ketosis, which leads to a loss of appetite and a decrease in food intake, which results in weight loss. Ketosis also has a strong diuretic

effect, resulting in significant water loss, and, again, weight loss. However, ketosis is also associated with fatigue, nausea, and low blood pressure."
– Dr. John McDougall, DrMcDougall.com

To obtain the high-grade protein your body needs to build healthy tissues, stick to eating a variety of edible plants, including fresh fruit, raw green vegetables, some sprouts, and some sea vegetables and soaked raw nuts.

For more information on the topic of nutrients for optimum peformance, read *Thrive Fitness: Mental and Physical Strength for Life*, by Brendan Brazier. Also, *Becoming Raw: The Essential Guide to Raw Vegan Diets*, by Brenda Davis, RD, Vesanto Melina, MS, RD, and Rynn Berry. For prevention of and reversal of common diseases, read Dr. Caldwell Esselstyn's book, *Prevent and Reverse Heart Disease: The Revolutionary, Scientifically-proven, Nutrition-based Cure*. Esselstyn's book also helps kill the myth that we need to consume meat, dairy, and eggs to get protein, and explains how animal protein can degrade health. Read *Whole*, by Dr. T. Colin Campbell.

> "Some Americans are obsessed with protein. Vegans are bombarded with questions about where they get their protein. Athletes used to eat thick steaks before competition because they thought it would improve their performance. Protein supplements are sold at health food stores. This concern about protein is misplaced. Although protein is certainly an essential nutrient which plays many key roles in the way our bodies function, we do not need huge quantities of it. In reality, we need small amounts of protein. Only one calorie out of every ten we take in needs to come from protein. Athletes do not need much more protein than the general public. Protein supplements are expensive, unnecessary, and even harmful for some people."
> – Reed Mangels, Ph.D., R.D., Protein in the Vegan Diet, Vegetarian Resource Group, VRG.org

> "All proteins are made up of the same amino acids. All. No exceptions. The difference between animal and vegetable proteins is in the content of certain amino acids. If vegetable proteins are mixed, the differences get made up. Even if they aren't mixed, all you need to do to get the right amount of low amino acids is to eat more of that food. There is no 'need' for animal proteins at all."
> – Dr. Marion Nestle, Professor, Department of Nutrition, Food Studies, and Public Health, New York University

"If your meals consistently revolve around corpse multiple times daily, you might become one sooner than you planned."
  – Kris Carr, author of *Crazy Sexy Diet*

"Vegetarians and vegans (including athletes) meet and exceed requirements for protein. And, to render the whole we-would-worry-about-getting-enough-protein-and-therefore-eat-meat idea even more useless, other data suggests that excess animal protein intake is linked with osteoporosis, kidney disease, calcium stones in the urinary tract, and some cancers. Despite some persistent confusion, it is clear that vegetarians and vegans tend to have more optimal protein consumption than omnivores."
  – Jonathan Safran Foer, author of *Eating Animals*

"A human body in no way resembles those that were born for ravenousness; it hath no hawk's bill, no sharp talon, no roughness of teeth, no such strength of stomach or heat of digestion, as can be sufficient to convert or alter such heavy and fleshy fare. But if you will contend that you were born to an inclination to such food as you have now a mind to eat, do you then yourself kill what you would eat. But do it yourself, without the help of a chopping-knife, mallet or axe, as wolves, bears, and lions do, who kill and eat at once. Rend an ox with they teeth, worry a hog with thy mouth, tear a lamb or a hare to pieces, and fall on and eat it alive as they do. But if thou had rather stay until what thou eat is to become dead, and if thou art loath to force a soul out of its body, why then dost thou against nature eat an animate thing? There is nobody that is willing to eat even a lifeless and a dead thing even as it is; so they boil it, and roast it, and alter it by fire and medicines, as it were, changing and quenching the slaughtered gore with thousands of sweet sauces, and the palate being thereby deceived may admit of such uncouth fare."
  – Plutarch

"Cruelty to animals is an enormous injustice; so is expecting those on the lowest rung of the economic ladder to do the dangerous, soul-numbing work of slaughtering sentient beings on our behalf."
  – Victoria Moran, author of *Main Street Vegan*

"Personal purity isn't really the issue. Not supporting animal abuse – and persuading others not to support it – is."
  – Peter Singer, author of *The Way We Eat*

The protein per calorie of legumes, vegetables, grains, fruits, and nuts and seeds.

Notice that per calorie, lettuce contains more protein than fruits, nuts, seeds, and some legumes.

Legumes

54%	Soy bean sprouts	29%	Lentils
43%	Mung bean sprouts	28%	Split peas
43%	Soy bean curd (tofu)	26%	Kidney beans
35%	Soy flour2	23%	Garbanzo beans
35%	Soy beans2	6%	Lima beans
33%	Soy sauce	6%	Navy beans
32%	Broad beans		

Grains

31%	Wheat germ	15%	Buckwheat
20%	Rye	12%	Millet
17%	Wheat, hard red	11%	Barley
16%	Wild rice	8%	Brown rice
15%	Oatmeal		

Fruits

16%	Lemons	8%	Watermelon
10%	Honeydew melon	7%	Tangerine
9%	Cantaloupe	6%	Papaya
8%	Strawberry	6%	Peach
8%	Orange	5%	Pear
8%	Blackberry	5%	Banana
8%	Cherry	5%	Grapefruit
8%	Apricot	3%	Pineapple
8%	Grape	1%	Apple

Nuts and Seeds

21%	Pumpkin seeds	12%	Almonds
17%	Sunflower seeds	12%	Cashews
13%	Walnuts, black	8%	Filberts
13%	Sesame seeds		

Vegetables

49%	Spinach	26%	Green beans
47%	New Zealand spinach	24%	Cucumbers
46%	Watercress	24%	Dandelion greens
45%	Kale	26%	Green pepper
45%	Broccoli	22%	Artichokes
44%	Brussels sprouts	22%	Cabbage
43%	Turnip greens	21%	Celery
43%	Collards	21%	Eggplant
40%	Cauliflower	18%	Tomatoes
39%	Mustard greens	16%	Onions
38%	Mushrooms	15%	Beets
34%	Chinese cabbage	12%	Pumpkin

34%	Parsley	11%	Potatoes
34%	Lettuce	8%	Yams
30%	Green peas	6%	Sweet potatoes
28%	Zucchini		

– Nutritive Value of American Foods in Common Units, USDA *Agricultural Handbook No. 456.*

"Human beings have capitalized on the silence of animals, just as certain human beings have historically imposed silence on certain other human beings by denying slaves the right to literacy, denying women the right to own property, and denying both the right to vote."

– Gary Steiner, author of *Animals and the Moral Community*

"Being vegetarian here also means that we do not consume dairy and egg products, because they are products of the meat industry. If we stop consuming, they will stop producing. Only collective awakening can create enough determination for action."

– Thich Nhat Hanh

"I will not eat anything that walks, runs, skips, hops, or crawls. Got knows that I've crawled on occaision, and I'm glad that no one ate me."

– Alex Poulos

"Vegetarian – that's an old Indian word meaning 'lousy hunter.'"

– Andy Rooney

"Men hunt, I think, maybe because they have something wrong with their own equipment and they need something else to shoot."

– Pamela Anderson

"I try to stick to a vegan diet heavy on fruit and vegetables."
– Clint Eastwood

"I'm a big health food freak and a vegetarian devotee."
– Chelsea Clinton

"I sometimes think, would I drink the milk from the breast of a woman I don't know? No. So, I think, why would I drink it from a cow?"

– Devon Aoki

MILK

"The human body has no more need for cows' milk than it does for dogs' milk, horses' milk, or giraffes' milk."
– Dr. Michael Klaper

IF you have been drinking milk and eating cheese, butter, ice cream, creamer, sour cream, yogurt, and kefir, and foods containing milk or milk products, including whey and casein, and other dairy products, there are some things you may like to know.

While the milk industry has a history of promoting milk as if it is a necessary nutrient for humans, the other side of the story about milk and what it does to the human body is one you haven't heard from the dairy industry.

"Scant evidence supports nutrition guidelines that focus specifically on increasing milk or other dairy product intake for promoting child or adolescent bone mineralization."
– *Pediatrics*, March 2005

"Our work showed that casein [the chief protein in milk] is the most relevant cancer promoter ever discovered.

Casein causes a broad spectrum of adverse effects.

Among other fundamental effects, it makes the body more acidic, alters the mix of hormones and modifies important enzyme activities, each of which can cause a broad array of more specific effects. One of these effects is its ability to promote cancer growth (by operating on key enzyme systems, by increasing hormone growth factors and by modifying the tissue acidity). Another is its ability to increase blood cholesterol (by modifying enzyme activities) and to enhance atherogenesis, which is the early stage of cardiovascular disease.

And finally, although these are casein-specific effects, it should be noted that other animal-based proteins are likely to have the same effect as casein.

The biochemical systems which underlie the adverse effects of casein are also common to other animal-based proteins. Also, the amino acid composition of casein, which is the characteristic primarily responsible for its property, is similar to most other animal-based proteins. They all have what we call high 'biological value,' in comparison, for example, with plant-based proteins, which is why animal protein promotes cancer growth and plant protein doesn't."

> – T. Colin Campbell, Ph.D., Cornell University, author of *The China Study* and *Whole*, TColinCampbell.org. Interview conducted by Kathy Freston, author of *Veganist*; KathyFreston.com

"Dairy cows are truly sick, miserable, abused creatures that are fed a high-protein (often animal-based) diet counterproductive to their health. They are then often drugged with bovine growth hormones and antibiotics, and abused to provide more milk than they have been created by nature to give – little or none of which goes to their own young."

> – Howard Lyman, *No More Bull*; MadCowboy.Com

"There's no reason to drink cow's milk at any time in your life. It was designed for calves, not humans, and we should all stop drinking it today."

> – Dr. Frank A. Oski, former Director of Pediatrics, Johns Hopkins University

"Interestingly, many long-term studies have now examined milk consumption in relation to risk of fractures. With remarkable consistency, these studies do not show reduction in fractures with high dairy product consumption. The hype about milk is basically an effective marketing campaign by the American Dairy industry."

> – Walter Willet, M.D., M.P.H., Dr.P.H., Harvard School of Public Health's Nutrition chairman, *Scientific American*, January 2003

"The USDA's food pyramid recommends drinking three glasses of milk a day. What's wrong with that? Well, for one thing, it's a recommendation that's not based on strict science. And some of the 'experts' who helped create the pyramid actually work for the dairy industry, which makes the U.S. Department of Agriculture recommendations reflect industry interests, not science, or our best interests."

> – Dr. Mark Hyman, author of *UltraMetabolism*

"Did you know that 90 percent of hamburger meat in America comes from the dairy industry? When cows no longer give huge amounts of milk after three to seven years, they go to the slaughterhouse. No exceptions. If ever given the chance, cows can live to be eighteen to twenty-five. And dairy cows are like all female mammals. In order for a female mammal to give milk, she has to get pregnant. Every year, every cow on every dairy farm is raped. A long steel device is shoved into their vaginas just to inject them with bull semen. Sometimes they use a bare hand. This forces the milk flow. And after she gives birth, babies are stolen. And why do they take away the babies from their mothers? Well, the dairies can't have little babies sucking up all that milk that was meant for them, when the dairy would rather sell it to you instead. Every time you have a glass of cow milk, some calf does not.

I spent 6 weeks at Thorn Apple Valley pig slaughterhouse in Detroit in 1993. I broke into animal research laboratories. I broke into fur farms. I went behind the scenes of every circus and every rodeo that ever came to Michigan. Worst scream I ever heard? A mother cow on a dairy farm as she screams and bellows her lungs out day after day for her stolen baby to be given back to her."
– Gary Yourofsky, ADAPTT.org

"Of the beasts from whom cheese is made... The milk will be taken from the tiny children."
– Leonardo da Vinci, writing of how taking milk from a cow is stealing from the calf. Da Vinci was a vegetarian and outspoken about his beliefs in protecting the animal kingdom.

I encourage people to eliminate absolutely all dairy from their diet. But if you consume dairy, please avoid dairy from factory farms, pasteurized dairy, dairy containing additives, homogenized dairy, and all heated dairy. If you do consume dairy, which I want to make sure to stress is not something I advise, be sure to stick to raw, organic dairy from cows that graze in open fields, and do only the fermented kefir and yogurt, and no other dairy products. If you consume dairy, or are considering adding any milk product to your diet, please research xanthine oxidase, oxidized cholesterol, and neurotoxic amino acids in dairy, and also the cancer-triggering casein protein that is rich in dairy, and, as mentioned below, the sialic acid sugar protein molecule called Neu5Gc (N-glycolylneuraminic acid).

"Of 14 case studies that have been done on dairy and prostate cancer, 12 have shown a statistically significant relationship – and the other two just aren't strong enough to see anything – and they conclude that all of the predictors of prostate cancer, the consumption of dairy is the best predictor of prostate cancer."
– T. Colin Campbell, Ph.D., Cornell University; author of *The China Study* and *Whole: Rethinking the Science of Nutrition*; TColinCampbell.org

In addition to the cancer-causing casein in milk (including cheese, ice cream, creamer, yogurt, kefir, butter, and whey), consider the sialic acid sugar protein molecule called Neu5Gc (N-glycolylneuraminic acid) in nonhuman mammal milk. Neu5Gc is also in meat. It is produced by nonhuman mammals; can't be synthesized by humans – because they lack the enzymes to produce it; binds to cell surfaces; causes an immune response and inflammation; is often found in human cancers, such as of the breast, colon, and prostate; and can make cancer more aggressive. To avoid Neu5Gc, simply don't consume animal milk or mammal meat. Doing both will also decrease your risk of cardiovascular disease, heart attacks, strokes, diabetes, arthritis, macular degeneration, Alzheimer's, Parkinson's, Crohn's, kidney disease, osteoporosis, and other degenerative and chronic diseases.

In addition to Neu5Gc, if you consume dairy of any kind, you may also like to know about C-reactive protein.

There is a relationship between the consumption of animal protein and C-reactive protein (CRP), which is synthesized in the liver and released into the bloodstream. CRP is also known as *high-sensitive C-reactive protein*, or hs-CRP. A high presence of CRP in the blood is related to conditions of inflammation, tissue necrosis, infection, and inflammatory diseases. CRP binds with phosphocholine on cells that are dead or dying, and also on some varieties of bacteria. Those who consume a diet rich in animal protein are found to have a higher level of CRP. Elevated levels of the protein have been recognized as an indication of rheumatoid arthritis, acute cardiovascular disease, diabetes, renal failure, an increased likelihood of a heart attack, and the presence of cancer. Burn injuries also increase the levels of CRP. In other words, the synthesis of CRP in the liver is part of the body's defense mechanisms – as the body recognizes that something is wrong, or out of place. Nonhuman animal protein is certainly out of place in the human animal, and the body system reacts in relation to that.

Transfats in the diet also raise levels of CRP. Just like meat, milk, and eggs, transfats certainly are also something that should be eliminated from the diet of those wishing to experience the best of health.

The consumption of mammal meat and milk, and foods containing meat and milk derivatives increases the likelihood of Neu5Gc binding to cells and causing inflammation, which increases the production of CRP in the liver and its release into the blood. Additionally, consuming animal protein, including meat, dairy, and eggs, introduces free radicals into the system, and free radicals are damaging to tissues, contributing to heart and kidney disease, vision degeneration, and premature aging. In other words, animal protein consumption plays havoc on the immune system. It is no wonder why people who consume a lot of animal protein have higher rates of a wide variety of diseases.

There is no coincidence that those who consume milk and meat have higher rates of cardiovascular disease, heart attacks, strokes, and a variety of cancers. Certain cancers, especially those of the sex and digestive organs, seem to correspond to higher levels of CRP, and also are known as inflammatory cancers, and have a strong relation to a higher intake of animal protein. However, because CRP is synthesized in the liver, cancer in that organ can interfere with the production of CRP.

In his book about reversing heart disease, Dr. Caldwell Esselstyn tells that patients who switch to following his recommended no-oil vegan diet achieve healthful levels of CRP within about a month after starting the diet. As they continue to follow the diet, cholesterol levels typically drop to a healthful level that is below 150 mg/dl, their blood pressure regulates, their angina disappears, the endothelial layer in their vascular system heals and starts producing healthy levels of nitric oxide, their circulatory system starts to clear away cholesterol plaque, their red blood cells become more permeable and carry more oxygen from the lungs, and their energy increases. Essentially, his patients experience a reversal of cardiovascular disease, and along with it, they experience a wide variety of health benefits.

"My perspective of veganism was most affected by learning that the veal calf is a by-product of dairying, and that in essence there is a slice of veal in every glass of what I had thought was an innocuous white liquid – milk."
– Rynn Berry

Be aware that the dairy industry is the meat industry, as the dairy cows are eventually slaughtered for their meat. To get milk from a cow, the cow needs to become pregnant. Because they can't produce milk and are therefore not needed on a dairy farm, almost all of the baby bulls are killed within days or weeks of their birth. Their bodies are cut up and their muscle tissue is sold as the meat product called "veal."

"On weekends my family, who lived in Chicago, would travel to Wisconsin and stop at this restaurant I didn't like, so I'd wait in the car while everyone else ate. One night, bored, I got out of the car and walked around the parking lot. I noticed this truck full of calves and bonded with one in particular, who kept kissing me. After about an hour the truck driver came out of the restaurant. I asked him what the calf's name was, and he said, 'Veal, tomorrow morning by 7 o'clock.' That was it: I could no longer disassociate the creature from what was on my plate."
– Daryl Hannah

The dairy industry consists of tens of millions of cows the world over, each of them consuming many times the amount of food that would otherwise feed a human following a vegan diet. To produce the feed for those cows, a tremendous amount of land, water, fossil fuels, steel, concrete, and other resources are used. The number-one use of farmland on every continent is to grow food to feed farmed animals.

The dietary requirements for meat, eggs, and dairy for a human body to thrive in health are zero. There is absolutely no nutritional need for humans to consume animal protein, including milk and milk products. The only milk a human needs is that of human breast milk during the initial years of life. Beyond that, once humans enter into the toddler stage, they do not need milk.

Raw, organic milk from animals consuming a natural diet contains beneficial nutrients, such as helpful lactic acid generating bacteria; enzymes, and higher levels of omega-3 and omega-6 essential fatty acids. Pasteurization of milk damages these nutrients. For this reason, even though I do not consume milk, would not advise anyone to consume it, and believe that the milk is best for the animals' young (to turn a small animal into a large animal), as mentioned earlier, I tell people that if they are going to consume dairy products, be sure to consume dairy that is raw, unpasteurized, organic, and from animals spending most of their time outdoors grazing in fields. One example is organic raw goats' milk fermented into kefir rich in probiotics. Find it through local organic family farmers, or natural foods co-ops. Check the Weston A. Price Foundation's Campaign for Real Milk (RealMilk.com). (I also do not endorse the Weston A. Price Foundation, or the meat eating ways they promote and that clearly increase the risk of human diseases.)

Also, if you choose to consume dairy, learn about the difference in the milk of A1 breed cows (Friesians and Holsteins) compared to the milk of A2 breed cows (African, Asian, Guerney, and Jersey). Find an organic farmer who is raising A2 breeds. A1 breeds are common in the U.S., Northern Europe, Australia, and New Zealand. For more information, read *Devil in the Milk: Illness, Health and the Politics of A1 and A2 Milk*, by Keith Woodford.

Milk from animals that are raised eating organic foods where they graze in open fields, and raised in a way that does not expose them to toxic farming chemicals and drugs, is much healthier than milk from factory farms where the animals are fed unnatural diets; exposed to unhealthful conditions that cause stress and disease; treated with growth hormones and other drugs; and exposed to various chemicals.

Because each state seems to have a different law regarding raw milk and raw cheeses, if you are going to consume dairy products, you may need to do some research to know where to get organic, raw dairy products from animals that spend a significant time grazing in meadows. In some states you may have to join a farm co-op or connect directly with organic family farmers to get organic, grass-fed, raw dairy products.

195

Some people join cow- or goat-sharing organizations in which they own a cow or goat with other people. This is based on an old tradition called agistment. The animals are raised on local organic farms, and the milk, butter, cream, kefir, and cheese are made available to the owners of the animals. A sort of "underground" activist movement has formed around this very topic. One book that covers this issue is *The Raw Milk Revolution: Behind America's Emerging Battle Over Food Rights*, by David Gumpert.

I must strongly restate the fact that the dairy industry creates terrible situations for farmed animals, especially the baby bulls, which are killed soon after birth, and, eventually, all of the dairy cows, which are slain for their meat after their milk production has slowed. The environmental impact of raising cows for milk and meat production creates a grotesque amount of damage to Earth, and uses a tremendous amount of resources. Consider all of the information I am providing here about what the consumption of dairy does to the human mechanism. Do yourself a favor: Eliminate milk, butter, cheese, cream, ice cream, and all milk products, and also meat from your diet. Use vegan alternatives.

> "Residues of hormones widely used to promote growth in beef cattle, dairy cows, and sheep (especially rBST or rBGH) may increase the risk of breast, prostate, and colorectal cancer. Their use also increases the risk of health problems in animals (especially mastitis), which leads to higher antibiotic use."
> – Environmental Working Group, July 2011

Recombinant bovine growth hormone (rBGH) is a genetically modified drug given to cows so they produce more milk. It is also known as bovine somatropin (rbST). If you drink milk, please make sure that the cows have not been treated with these terrible drugs.

> "The use of rBGH (rbST) in milk production has been shown to elevate the levels of insulin-like growth factor 1 (IGF-1), a naturally occurring hormone that, in high levels, is linked to several types of cancers, among other things.
>
> rBGH (rbST) use induces an unnatural period of milk production during a cow's 'negative energy phase.' Milk produced during this stage is considered to be low-quality due to its increased fat content and its decreased level of proteins.
>
> Milk from rBGH-injected cows contains higher somatic cell counts, which makes the milk turn sour more quickly, and is another indicator of poor milk quality."
> – Organic Consumers Association

It may surprise those who have lived in a milk-consuming society that people in many parts of the world frown on both drinking milk and eating cheese, and consider it as disgusting to consume milk in any form from another animal.

I used to say that about the only time I could imagine advising anyone to eat dairy products would be if there were no access to raw greens. If that is the case, and they also cannot obtain some quality green powder nutritional supplement, an option would be raw, organic milk that has not been pasteurized, and that is from cows that freely graze in an open field. However, with all I now know about the disease-inducing properties of dairy, I can no longer advise anyone to consume milk, or any milk products or derivatives. They would get much better nutrition by eating edible weeds.

Another issue relating to milk is that of diabetes. This is one topic covered by T. Colin Campbell in his book *The China Study*. He details the situation that may trigger the body to begin attacking the pancreas cells that produce insulin. This immune response situation gone awry is Type-1 diabetes. This may begin to happen after the human consumes milk. It is clear that the countries with the highest consumption of milk and milk products are the very same countries with the highest rates of Type-1 diabetes. Campbell states, "There is strong evidence that this disease is linked to diet and, more specifically, to dairy products. The ability of cow's milk protein to initiate Type-1 diabetes is well documented."

Because of the strong relationship between milk consumption and the development of Type-1 diabetes, I strongly advise parents to refrain from giving milk, or any milk products, including butter, cheese, ice cream, yogurt, or kefir to children of any age. Instead, it is very easy to make alternatives that are vegan, such as by making hemp milk out of hemp seed powder, vanilla, water, and dates. Of course, the best food for babies is human breast milk, and especially during the first few months of life. As soon as the child is weaned, there is no longer any need for a human to consume animal milk.

Most animal milk in industrial society is sold as pasteurized. The pasteurization of milk is a heating process, which damages the fats and creates a product that leads to degenerative conditions in the human body, such as heart disease.

In addition to triggering cancer growth, the casein protein in milk can also cause mood swings, depression, and anxiety. Those who experience depression would be wise to avoid milk and also processed salt, processed sugars (including eliminating all foods containing corn syrup [aka corn sugar], white sugar, brown sugar, agave, and artificial sweeteners), cooked oils, bleached grains, cooked grains, gluten grains, MSG, and synthetic food chemicals, including artificial sweeteners, colors, flavors, scents, and preservatives. They should increase the ratio of organic raw green vegetables and raw fruits in their diet.

"The source of most commercial milk is the 'modern' Holstein, bred to produce huge quantities of milk – three times as much as the old-fashioned cow. She needs special feed and antibiotics to keep her well. Her milk contains high levels of growth hormone from her pituitary gland, even when she is spared the indignities of genetically engineered Bovine Growth Hormone to push her to the udder limits of milk production.

Real feed for cows is green grass in spring, summer and fall; stored dry hay, silage, hay, and root vegetables in winter. It is not soy meal, cottonseed meal or other commercial feeds, nor is it bakery waste, chicken manure or citrus peel cake, laced with pesticides. Vital nutrients like vitamins A and D, and Price's 'Activator X' (a fat-soluble catalyst that promotes optimum mineral assimilation, now believed to be vitamin K2) are greatest in milk from cows eating green grass, especially rapidly growing green grass in the spring and fall. Vitamins A and D are greatly diminished, and Activator X disappears when milk cows are fed commercial feed. Soy meal has the wrong protein profile for the dairy cow, resulting in a short burst of high milk production followed by premature death. Most milk (even most milk labeled "organic") comes from dairy cows that are kept in confinement their entire lives and never see green grass!

Pasteurization destroys enzymes, diminishes vitamin content, denatures fragile milk proteins, destroys vitamins C, B12 and B6, kills beneficial bacteria, promotes pathogens and is associated with allergies, increased tooth decay, colic in infants, growth problems in children, osteoporosis, arthritis, heart disease and cancer. Calves fed pasteurized milk do poorly and many die before maturity. Raw milk sours naturally but pasteurized milk turns putrid; processors must remove slime and pus from pasteurized milk by a process of centrifugal clarification. Inspection of dairy herds for disease is not required for pasteurized milk. Pasteurization was instituted in the 1920s to combat TB, infant diarrhea, undulant fever and other diseases caused by poor animal nutrition and dirty production methods. But times have changed and modern stainless steel tanks, milking machines, refrigerated trucks and inspection methods make pasteurization absolutely unnecessary for public protection. And pasteurization does not always kill the bacteria for Johne's disease suspected of causing Crohn's disease in humans, with which most confinement cows are infected. Much commercial milk is now ultra-pasteurized to get rid of heat-resistant bacteria and give it a longer shelf life. Ultrapasteurization is a violent process that takes milk from a chilled temperature to above the boiling point in less than two seconds. Clean raw milk from certified healthy cows is available commercially in several states and may be bought directly from the farm in many more. (Sources are listed on RealMilk.Com.)

Homogenization is a process that breaks down butterfat globules so they do not rise to the top. Homogenized milk has been linked to heart disease.

Average butterfat content from old-fashioned cows at the turn of the century was over 4 percent (or more than 50 percent of calories). Today butterfat comprises less than 3 percent (or less than 35 percent of calories). Worse, consumers have been duped into believing that low-fat and skim milk products are good for them. Only by marketing low-fat and skim-milk as a health food can the modern dairy industry get rid of its excess poor-quality, low-fat milk from modern high-production herds. Butterfat contains vitamins A and D needed for assimilation of calcium and protein in the water fraction of the milk. Without them protein and calcium are more difficult to utilize and possibly toxic. Butterfat is rich in short- and medium-chain fatty acids which protect against disease and stimulate the immune system. It contains glyco-spingolipids which prevent intestinal distress and conjugated linoleic acid, which has strong anticancer properties."
– RealMilk.Com

"Cows make milk for their babies, and for their babies alone. Case is closed. Forever. Permanently. No debate. No discussion. They don't make milk for baby elephants, baby orangutans, baby hedgehogs, baby rabbits, baby rats, baby humans, adolescent humans, or adult humans. This body of ours has absolutely no need for cow milk, like it has absolutely no need for giraffe milk, and zebra milk, and rhinoceros milk, hippopotamus milk, camel milk, deer milk, antelope milk, horse milk, pig milk, dog milk, or cat milk. The only milk that we ever need is our own mother's breast milk when we are born. And that's it. And when we're done weaning, we never need one drop of milk, ever again. No species on this planet needs milk after they are done weaning."
– Gary Yourofsky, ADAPTT.org.

If you consume cheese made of dairy, you may also be eating the stomach lining of a slaughtered calf. On the label, this ingredient is called "rennet." Some cheese companies will list rennet as an ingredient, and some don't – even when there is rennet in the cheese. Some that don't contain rennet will mention on the label that it is "rennet-less cheese," which means they are being sensitive to the vegetarians that are trying to avoid consuming rennet.

"Different meats affect our health and environment differently. Lamb, beef, cheese, and pork generate the most greenhouse gases. They also tend to be higher in fat and have the worst environmental impacts, because producing them uses the most resources – mainly feed, chemical fertilizer, fuel, pesticides, and water. Lamb has the greatest impact. Beef is second. Cheese is third. Beef has more than twice the emissions of pork, nearly four times more than chicken, and more than 13 times as much as vegetable proteins such as beans, lentils, and tofu. But vegetarians who eat dairy aren't off the hook, because pound for pound, cheese generates the third-highest emissions."
– The Environmental Working Group, July 2011

"Cows' milk is a high-fat food exquisitely designed for turning a 65-pound calf into a 400-pound cow in a year. That is what cows' milk is for."
– Dr. Michael Klaper, author of *Vegan Nutrition*

"According to Dr. Walter Willett (of Harvard School of Public Health), who has done many of the studies and has reviewed the topic extensively, there are many reasons to pass up milk, including: Milk doesn't reduce bone fractures. Contrary to popular belief, eating dairy has never been shown to reduce fracture risk. But dairy may increase the risk of fractures by 50 percent, according to the Nurses' Health Study. Less dairy equals better bones. Countries with the lowest rates of dairy and calcium consumption, like those in Africa and Asia, have the lowest rates of osteoporosis. Next thing is that calcium isn't as bone protective as we thought. Studies of calcium supplementation have showed no benefit in reducing fracture risk. Vitamin D on the other hand, appears to be much more important than calcium in preventing fractures. Also, calcium may raise cancer risk. Research shows that higher intake of both calcium and dairy products may increase a man's risk of prostate cancer by 30 to 50 percent. Plus, dairy consumption increases the body's level of insulin-like growth factor 1, a known cancer promoter.

Calcium has benefits that dairy doesn't. Calcium supplements, but not dairy products, may reduce the chances of colon cancer. And another problem with dairy is that not everyone can stomach dairy. About 75 percent or three-fourths of the world's population is genetically unable to properly digest milk and other dairy products, a problem called *lactose intolerance*. So, based on such findings, Dr. Walter Willett has come to some important conclusions: 1) Everybody needs calcium, but probably not as much as our government's recommended daily allowance of 1,500 mg. 2) Calcium probably doesn't prevent broken bones. Few people in this country are likely to reduce their fracture risk by getting more calcium. 3) Men may not want to take calcium supplements. Supplements of calcium and vitamin D may be reasonable for women. 4) Dairy may be unhealthful; advocating dairy consumption may have negative effects on health.

The Federal Trade Commission recently asked the USDA to look into the scientific bases of claims made in their milk mustache ads. The panel of scientists states the truth clearly. #1) Milk does not benefit sports performance. #2) There's no evidence that dairy is good for your bones or prevents osteoporosis. In fact the animal protein in it may help cause bone loss. #3) dairy is linked to prostate cancer. #4) It's full of saturated fat and is linked to heart disease. #5) Dairy causes digestive problems for 75 percent of people, because of lactose intolerance. And, #6) Dairy aggravates irritable bowl syndrome.

Simply put, the Federal Trade Commission asked the dairy industry, 'Got proof?' and the answer was 'No.' Plus, dairy may contribute to even more health problems, like allergies, sinus issues, ear infections, Type-1 diabetes, chronic constipation, and anemia in children.

'But, what about raw milk?' 'Well, isn't that a healthier form of dairy?' Well, not really. Yes, raw, organic, whole milk eliminates some of the concerns, like pesticides, hormones, antibiotics, and the effects of homogenization and pasteurization. But to me, these benefits don't outweigh dairy's potential risks.

From an evolutionary point of view, milk is a strange food for humans. Until 10,000 years ago, we didn't domesticate animals, and we weren't able to drink milk unless some brave hunter/gatherer milked a wild tiger or buffalo.

Most scientists agree that it is better for us to get calcium, potassium, protein, and fats from other sources, like whole plant foods: vegetables, fruits, beans, whole grains, nuts, seeds, and seaweeds (great source of minerals)."

– Dr. Mark Hyman, author of *UltraMetabolism*

Learn how to make dairy-free, vegan nut and seed milk, yogurt, kefir, and cheeses. There are many recipes for them in the raw vegan recipe books.

"The protein in milk increases growth hormones that promote the development of breast, prostate, colon, brain, and lung cancer."
– Dr. John McDougall, DrMcDougall.com

For more information on milk, see Dr. John McDougall's series of videos on YouTube, titled Marketing Milk and Disease.

Books:
The China Study: Startling Implications for Diet, Weight Loss, and Long-term Health, by T. Colin Campbell, PhD, and Thomas M. Campbell II, MD
Prevent and Reverse Heart Disease: The Revolutionary, Scientifically Proven, Nutrition-based Cure, by Caldwell B. Esselstyn, Jr., MD
Whitewash: The Disturbing Truth About Cow's Milk and Your Health, by Joseph Keon

"Today's dairy cows endure annual cycles of artificial insemination, pregnancy and birth, and mechanized milking for 10 out of 12 months (including 7 months of their 9-month pregnancies). This excessive metabolic drain overburdens the cows, who are considered 'productive' for only two years and are slaughtered for hamburger when their profitability drops, typically around their fourth birthday, a small fraction of their natural lifespan."
– Dr. Michael Greger, *How Much Pus Is There in Milk?*; NutritionFacts.org

"The 9 million cows in America, for the most part, are not healthy. Half the herds in America have cows affected with bovine leukemia virus, half the herds have cows infected with a disease called Crohn's disease, which is caused by a bacterium called mycobacterium paratuberculosis, of which 40 million Americans have been affected with irritable bowel syndrome from this. Every person with Crohn's disease tests positive for mycobacterium paratuberculosis. Every one! One hundred percent! And this was published in 1965 for the Proceedings for the National Academy of Science. So we're talking about real science here, not things I'm making up. You've got thousands of studies published in scientific journals, thousands of converging lines of evidence that tell us that milk does not do the body any good. We drink body fluids from diseased animals."
– Dr. Robert Cohen, author of *Milk: The Deadly Poison*

"To assess the relationship between childhood and adult consumption of milk and breast cancer incidence, Dr. Anette Hjartaker of the University of Oslo, Norway, and colleagues prospectively studied 48,844 premenopausal Norwegian women. The investigators note that 317 incident cases of breast cancer were diagnosed during a mean follow-up of 6.2 years. Dr. Hjartaker's group found that childhood milk consumption was inversely associated with subsequent breast cancer among women between the ages of 34 and 39 years old."

– Hjartåker A, Laake P, Lund E., Institute of Community Medicine, University of Tromsø, Norway

THE FOOD SHORTAGE MYTH

"It takes over 10 times the amount of energy from fossil fuels to produce a calorie of animal-based food than it does to produce a calorie of plant food."
– Forks over Knives, ForksOverKnives.com

"The amount of grain that we grow in the West is mostly used to feed our cattle. Eighty percent of the corn grown in this country is to feed the cattle to make meat. Ninety-five percent of the oats produced in this country is not for us to eat, but for the animals raised for food. According to this recent report that we received of all the agricultural land in the U.S., eighty-seven percent is used to raise animals for food. That is forty-five percent of the total land mass in the U.S."
– John Robbins, author of the books *The Food Revolution*; *May All Be Fed*; *Diet for a New America*; and *Reclaiming Our Health*; FoodRevolution.Org

"ECONOMIC IMPERIALISM
Some 'Third World' countries, where most children are undernourished, are actually exporting their staple crops as animal feed, i.e., to fatten cattle for turning into burgers in the 'First World.' Millions of acres of the best farmland in poor countries are being used for *our* benefit – for tea, coffee, tobacco, etc., while people there are *starving*. McDonald's is directly involved in this economic imperialism, which keeps most black people poor and hungry while many whites grow fat.
GROSS MISUSE OF RESOURCES
GRAIN is fed to cattle in South American countries to produce the meat in McDonald's hamburgers. Cattle consume ten times the amount of grain and soy than humans do: One calorie of beef demands ten calories of grain. Of the 145 million tons of grain and soy fed to livestock, only 21 million tons of meat and by-products are used. *The waste is 124 million tons per year at a value of 20 billion U.S. dollars.* It has been calculated that this sum would feed, clothe and house the world's entire population for one year."
– From the original 1990s *What's Wrong with McDonald's* leaflet distributed by London Greenpeace, which resulted in McDonald's

suing for libel, and the longest court case in England's history; McSpotlight.Org

"A 2010 United Nations study concluded that organic and other sustainable farming methods that come under the umbrella of what the study's authors called 'agroecology' would be necessary to feed the future world. Two years earlier, a U.N. examination of farming in 24 African countries found that organic or near-organic farming resulted in yield increases of more than 100 percent. Another U.N.-supported report entitled *Agriculture at a Crossroads*, compiled by 400 international experts, said that the way the world grows food will have to change radically to meet future demand. It called for governments to pay more attention to small-scale farmers and sustainable practices – shooting down the bigger-is-inevitably-better notion that huge factory farms and their efficiencies of scale are necessary to feed the world."

– Barry Estabrock, Organic Can Feed The World, *The Atlantic*, December 5, 2011. Estabrock is the author of, *Tomatoland*, a book about corporate-produced foods. He blogs at PoliticsOfThePlate.com

"Our food system belongs in the hands of many family farmers, not under the control of a handful of corporations."

– Willie Nelson, founder of Farm Aid, FarmAid.org

"Globalized industrialized food is not cheap. It is too costly for the Earth, for the farmers, for our health. The Earth can no longer carry the burden of groundwater mining, pesticide pollution, disappearance of species, and destabilization of the climate. Farmers can no longer carry the burden of debt, which is inevitable in industrial farming with its high costs of production. It is incapable of producing safe, culturally appropriate, tasty, quality food. And it is incapable of producing enough food for all because it is wasteful of land, water, and energy. Industrial agriculture uses ten times more energy than it produces. It is thus ten times less efficient."

– Vandana Shiva, VandanaShiva.org

"The Pennsylvania-based Rodale Institute is an unequivocal supporter of all things organic. But that's no reason to dismiss its 2008 report 'The Organic Green Revolution,' which provides a concise argument for why a return to organic principles is necessary to stave off world hunger, and which backs the assertion with citations of more than 50 scientific studies.

Rodale concludes that farming must move away from using unsustainable, increasingly unaffordable, petroleum-based [or fossil fuel-based] fertilizers and pesticides and turn to 'organic,

regenerative farming systems that sustain and improve the health of the world population, our soil, and our environment.'"
– Barry Estabrock, Organic Can Feed The World, *The Atlantic,* December 5, 2011.

"GMOs have already clearly shown that they don't produce more than conventional crops, they are hard to market, uninteresting to taste, poorer in terms of nutrition, dangerous for the environment and biodiversity, and are insecure."
– Carlo Petrini, founder, Slow Food International

Water required for producing one pound of food in California, according to soil and water specialists working with the University of California Agricultural Extension:
Water used to produce:

1 pound of lettuce	23 gallons
1 pound of tomatoes	23 gallons
1 pound of potatoes	24 gallons
1 pound of wheat	25 gallons
1 pound of carrots	33 gallons
1 pound of apples	49 gallons
1 pound of chicken	815 gallons
1 pound of pork	1,630 gallons
1 pound of beef	5,214 gallons

"Realize that 82 percent of the world's starving children live in countries where food is fed to animals that are then killed and eaten by more well-off individuals in developed countries like the U.S., U.K., and Europe. One-fourth of all grain produced by third world countries is now given to livestock, in their own country and out.

Globally, even with climate change issues and weather extremes, we are producing enough grain to feed two times as many people as there are in the world. In 2011, there was a record harvest of grain globally, with over 2.5 billion tons, but half of that was fed to animals in the meat and dairy industries. Seventy seven percent of all coarse grains (corn, oats, sorghum, barley, etc.) and over 90 percent of all soy grown in the world was fed to livestock. So clearly the difficulty is not how can we produce enough food to feed the hungry, but where all the food we produce globally is going, in addition to the other factors of pricing, policy making, and education. This will certainly become more of an issue as our planet's human population extends beyond 9 billion before the year 2050."
– Dr. Richard Oppenlander, ComfortablyUnaware.com

CHEMICALS AND DRUGS
IN MILK, MEAT, AND EGGS

M OST farm animals are given drugs by mouth or injection from their first day to nearly their last. These drugs may include hormones, antibiotics, milk stimulants, tranquilizers, and chemicals that influence birth rates. The animals and/or their pens are also sprayed with toxic insecticides, fungicides, miticides, and pesticides.

The insecticides that are used on and around the animals end up in the environment, where they not only kill flies but also kill needed insects such as bees that pollinate plants; praying mantises and ladybugs that help control damaging insects; and other helpful bugs and insects. The chemicals poison the air, water, and land.

The drugs farm animals are given, the pesticides, insecticides and other chemicals used on and around them, and the chemicals used to grow their feed accumulate in the fat cells of the animals. These residues are transferred into the humans that consume the meats, milk products, and eggs.

The fats in farm animals contain residues of all the chemicals used to grow their food. Because the feed given to animals raised in factory farms often contains portions of ground-up farm animals that died prematurely or in accidents, the amount of drug and chemical residue found in meats from these animals contains a larger dose of the residues.

> "Millions upon millions of Americans are merrily eating away, unaware of the pain and disease they are taking into their bodies with every bite. We are ingesting nightmares for breakfast, lunch, and dinner."
> – John Robbins, author of *Diet for a New America* and *The Food Revolution*

As if giving the naturally vegetarian animals a cannibalistic diet were not bad enough, some farm animals are also fed their own excrement. Some pigs are fed their own urine. Poultry waste and feathers are mixed in with feed that is fed to other farm animals. Other farm animal feed contains the leftovers of slaughterhouses, road kill, and the bodies of animals from county and city animal control shelters. Not only does this magnify the amount of chemical and drug residues in the fat of the animals, it also increases the likelihood that the animals are harboring infectious diseases. The farm animals that die are not tested for diseases. Using ground-up animals to increase the protein content of animal feed increases the likelihood that contagious diseases, such as mad cow, are becoming rampant within farm animals.

The consumption of cow milk has been identified as triggering sudden infant death syndrome (SIDS), the condition in which babies simply stop breathing, and which is the leading cause of death among infants considered healthy. As mentioned elsewhere in the book, the consumption of cow milk also increases the likelihood of Type-1 diabetes in children, leading to lifelong health maladies. Pregnant women and nursing mothers may also want to stay away from all dairy products, including foods containing milk and derivatives from milk.

"Penetration of beta-casomorphins (in cow's milk) into the infant's immature central nervous system may inhibit the respiratory center in the brainstem leading to abnormal ventilatory responses, hypercapnia (excess carbon dioxide), hypoxia (lack of oxygen), apnoea, and death."
– Cow's-milk-induced Infancy Apnoea with Increased Serum Content of Bovine Beta-Casomorphin-5; *Journal of Pediatric Gastroenterol Nutrition*, Volume 52, Number 6, June 2011

People, if you want to stay away from not only drugs, but harmful bacteria, in your foods, it is a good idea to stay away from all meat, milk, and eggs – and common commercial and fast foods.

"Consumer Reports recently released a study in which they analyzed U.S. retail pork and found trace levels of an adrenaline-like drug called ractoparmine in about 20 percent of the samples, and a foodborne bacteria that sickens nearly 100,000 Americans ever year called Yersina in two-thirds of the pork samples.

The National Pork Producers Council tried to address concerns about ractoparmine by noting that the levels in meat of this muscle growth promoter, which is fed to pigs in the form of Paylean®, and turkeys in the form of Topmax®, were below the limit set by the U.N. Codex Commission last summer. What they didn't mention was that due to an outstanding safety concern, the Commision's drug residue limit only passed by a single vote out of 143 ballots cast.

The Codex Commission based this drug reside limit in meat on the only human data available, a study of just six people that wasn't designed to establish safety. At highter doses, the study subjects reported their hearts racing and pounding – so much so that one

subject had to be withdrawn from the study. At a lower dose, though, no cardiac changes were noted. So that's the dose the Codex Commission used to calculate the maximum allowable meat residue and acceptable human daily intake levels."
– Dr. Michael Greger, Bugs & Drugs in Pork: Yersinia and Ractopamine. NutritionFacts.org

You can research for yourself, from drugs and farming chemicals used on animal farms and in processed foods, and you will easily find out about a number of drugs and synthetic and natural chemicals that are not good for human health. Dr. Michael Greger often features information about these substances on his Website, NutritionFacts.org.

At every turn, meat, milk, and eggs contain at least several natural or synthetic factors that are deleterious to human health. To avoid any of these substances, simply follow a vegan diet that is all or mostly organic, and that is rich in raw, unheated fruits and vegetables.

Leonardo da Vinci considered the bodies of humans who eat animals to be the tombs of the animals, and he considered taking milk from a cow as stealing from a baby. Leonardo might consider the bodies of modern humans who consume farm animals, eggs, and dairy to be toxic waste dumps of all the farming chemicals and drugs found in the animals raised on today's industrial farms.

"I turned vegetarian after 9/11. A friend of mine came back from New York and said that he couldn't stand the smell of burnt flesh. It immediately reminded me of a barbecue."
– Alyssa Milano

"It is imperative to educate people that there is no moral difference between meat and dairy. There is as much suffering in a glass of milk than in a pound of steak. Indeed, given that animals exploited for dairy live longer, are treated worse, and end up in the same slaughterhouse as do 'meat' animals, we can say with some confidence that there is probably more suffering involved in dairy products."
– Gary L. Francione

"Look, are you a suckling calf? Name one creature on earth that uses milk after it's weaned. Man's the only one. And man's the only one who lives out only half his life span. A cow has four stomachs. You don't. You can't handle whole milk."
– Jack LaLanne

ANIMALS AND FOOD

"The lands of tropical developing countries are made increasingly to produce animal feed and animal products for the rich segment of the world population. Starchy food grains, which double as feed grains, are transformed into costly animal feed products, resulting in less energy and protein than was contained in the original feed. A kilogram of beef provides 1,140 calories of energy and 226 grams of protein, but the feed grain required for producing that kilogram of beef, if directly consumed as food grain (instead of being transformed into beef), provides as much as 24,150 calories and 700 grams of protein."
– Utsa Patnalk, Origins of the Food Crisis in India and Developing Countries, *Monthly Review*, July-August 2009

"New research suggests at least 51 percent of carbon emissions are from animal-farming industries but no-one in the mainstream media wants to mention that. We can't wait for those in power to do something about it – politicians are followers, not leaders. People can buy a Prius or put solar panels on their roof but those things cost money. Going vegan is cheap and the best single thing you can do for the planet."
– Sienna Blake, *Vegan Voice* magazine

"More animals are being subjected to more torturous conditions in the United States today than has ever occurred anywhere in world history…
Today, because of the way animals are raised for market, the question of whether or not it's ethical to eat meat has a whole new meaning and a whole new urgency. Never before have animals been treated like this. Never before has such deep, unrelenting, and systematic cruelty been mass produced."
– John Robbins, author of *The Food Revolution*

"One kg of chicken eggs requires 2 kg of grain and gives 1,090 calories and 259 grams of protein.
The grain used to produce that kg of eggs would have provided 200 grams of protein and 6,900 calories to a human.

One kg of pork requires 3 kg of grain and gives 1,180 calories and 187 grams of protein.

The grain used to produce that kg of pork would have provided 300 grams of protein and 10,350 calories to a human.

One kg of beef requires 7 kg of grain and gives 1,140 calories and 226 grams of protein.

The grain used to produce that kg of beef would have provided 700 grams of protein and 24,150 calories to a human."

– *Monthly Review*, Origins of the Food Crisis in India and Developing Countries, by Utsa Patnaik, professor of economics, Centre for Economic Studies and Planning at Jawaharlal Nehru University, New Delhi. Author of *The Republic of Hunger and Other Essays*.

"The greatness of a nation and its moral progress can be judged by the way its animals are treated."
– Mahatma Gandhi

ALL plant structures grown in nature consist of soil nutrients, water, gasses, and sun energy transformed into a plant. When you are eating plants you are eating these substances as they have been transformed. When you eat living plants, you are transferring that energy into your system.

Spiritual leaders throughout history have advised a plant-based diet as a way to connect with the spiritual, cleanse the body of unhealthful energies, and to be more in tune with the powers of nature.

All food carries energy.

Meat, especially from the modern-day factory farming industry, carries the energy of suppression and confinement, and the fear, violence, illness, and horror of the slaughterhouse.

"Ever seen them butcher a cow for hamburger? It's incredibly brutal and violent."
– Brad Pitt

Dairy, especially from the modern-day factory farming industry, carries the energy of animals that are incarcerated.

Plants contain the energy of sun and nature.

Relatively few dairy cows in North America are allowed to graze in open fields, where they would feel the sun and energy of nature. Instead, they spend nearly their entire lives indoors, eating unnatural diets that are so problematic for their systems that they are regularly treated with pharmaceutical drugs.

"Deliberate cruelty to our defenseless and beautiful little cousins is surely one of the meanest and most detestable vices of which a human being can be guilty."
– William Randolph Inge

Other farm animals are also treated in lousy, horrible, and heinous ways, never seeing the light of day, and being denied their natural diet.

"The broiler chicken industry produces 6 billion chickens a year for slaughter. This industry is ruled by only 60 companies, which have created an oligopoly. Broiler chickens are selectively bred and genetically altered to produce bigger thighs and breasts, the parts in most demand. This breeding creates birds so heavy that their bones cannot support their weight, making it difficult for them to stand. The birds are bred to grow at an astonishing rate, reaching their market weight of 3 1/2 pounds in seven weeks. Broilers are raised in overcrowded broiler houses instead of cages to prevent the occurrence of bruised flesh, which would make their meat undesirable. Their beaks and toes are cut off and the broiler houses are usually unlit to prevent fighting among the birds."
– In Defense of Animals, IDAUSA.org

Meat holds the energy of fright chemicals. These stress hormones are created by and rush through the body tissues of the animals as they are aware that they are about to be slaughtered – often hearing and seeing other animals being killed right before them. According to many people that work or have worked in the animal slaughter industry, many cows, pigs, chickens, turkeys, and other animals are sliced to pieces while they are still alive (Access: VeganOutreach.org, IDAUSA.org, Meat.org, FarmSanctuary.org, FarmUSA.org, PETA.org, and Earthlings.com).

"Our awareness has to be applied to understanding that slaughtering is killing. To achieve inner harmony and world peace, we must eradicate the mentality of violence, and therefore, there goes the slaughter."
– Sri Swamini "Mother Maya" Mayatitananda

"If slaughterhouses had glass walls, everyone would be a vegetarian."
– Paul McCartney

When the human body is put into a stressful situation the body cells respond by releasing stress hormones into the tissues. The hypothalamus sends signals through the sympathetic nerves near the spinal cord and triggers the adrenal glands to release epinephrine and norepinephrine. The pituitary gland releases a chemical signal into the blood that triggers the adrenal glands to release other hormones, including cortisol. The body under stress also produces higher levels of hormones labeled inflammatory cytokines, which cause inflammation, pain, and swelling. A similar scenario happens within the bodies of nonhuman animals when they are exposed to stressful situations.

"My life experience has given me a better understanding of what is happening, and what a mistake it is to believe there is anything called humane slaughter. Animals have families and feelings, and to think that kindness before killing them is an answer is totally wrong. Humans have no need for animal products. And when we consume animal products, we're not just killing the animals. In the long run, we're killing the planet, and ourselves."
– Howard Lyman, author of *No More Bull*, MadCowboy.com

Animals raised in the loud, stressful, unhealthful, and unnatural situations of today's factory "confinement" farms are filled with illness. Stress, drugs, and bad diet destroy the health of farmed animals in the same way that drugs, stress, and bad diet destroy the health of humans.

"The question is not, 'Can they reason?' nor, 'Can they talk?' but, 'Can they suffer?'"
– Jeremy Bentham

"We cannot have peace among men whose hearts find delight in killing any living creature."
– Rachel Carson

"Recognize meat for what it really is: the antibiotic- and pesticide-laden corpse of a tortured animal."
– Ingrid Newkirk

"Modern meat production, modern dairy production, treat the animals with a level of cruelty, brutality, that if you saw how severe it is – you wouldn't have to be a vegetarian, you wouldn't have to be an animal rights activist – to be appalled. I'm not talking about the fact that the animals are killed. I don't want to deny that, but what I'm talking about is how they live, how they are treated in a factory farm by corporate agribusiness, and it is really ugly. And you don't have to support it."
– John Robbins

"As soon as I realized that I didn't need meat to survive or to be in good health, I began to see how forlorn it all is. If only we had a different mentality about the drama of the cowboy and the range and all the rest of it. It's a very romantic notion, an

213

entrenched part of American culture, but I've seen, for example, pigs waiting to be slaughtered, and their hysteria and panic was something I shall never forget."
– Cloris Leachman

Stress hormones damage brain cells and impair memory. They also raise the blood pressure and trigger the endocrine system to produce and release inflammatory hormones, which helps lead to damaging plaque buildup in the arteries. The hormones thicken the blood, increasing the likelihood of stroke and heart attack, and of irregular heartbeat. The hormones also cause fat to build up in the abdominal area, which is a risk factor in a slew of health conditions, such as heart disease, hypertension, and diabetes. In fact, there is no part of the body that is not damaged by long-term stress, from the skin, hair, and nails, to the lungs and stomach, to the intestines, bones, joints, and nerves. Mental function is altered, as stress ages the brain and brings about depression, psychosis, and other types of mental derangement. The immune system is degraded by stress and this sets the stage for bacteria, viruses, inflammation, and cancers to gain hold within the tissues. When a person is under heavy stress while also consuming low-quality foods, their health can quickly degrade in all areas.

"I think of veganism humbly and holistically. It's about taking personal responsibility in a world so full of needless suffering. It's challenging one's self to open one's eyes and question society's assumptions and habits. It's about critical thinking and compassion and how we would like to see the world evolve."
– Michael Greger, VeganMD.org

When people consume animals raised in an unhealthful atmosphere, animals that are unhealthy because of the way they are treated, and the bad food and toxic drugs and poisonous farming chemicals the animals are exposed to, the people are eating animal tissues that contain all of the unhealthful substances these animals have in their systems. The animal meat people are eating contains residues of all of the poisonous farming chemicals the animal has been exposed to, and all of the toxic drugs it was given, which cause disease. They are eating the fright chemicals that are released into the animal's body tissues when the animal knows it is about to be slaughtered, and the hormones that alter their blood flow and breathing patterns, and that surge their senses with alarm.

When a person eats meat from factory confinement farms, they are eating the energy of illness, abuse, incarceration, suppression, violence, fear, and slaughter. They are putting sickness into their body.

"If one person is unkind to an animal it is considered to be cruelty, but where a lot of people are unkind to animals, especially in the name of commerce, the cruelty is condoned and, once large sums of money are at stake, will be defended to the last by otherwise intelligent people."
    – Ruth Harrison

"The thinking man must oppose all cruelties, no matter how deeply rooted in tradition or surrounded by a halo."
    – Albert Schweitzer

The modern meat diet is extremely wasteful of resources. It takes three-quarters of a gallon of petroleum oil and 2,500 gallons of water to produce one pound of beef. Raising one steer to market weight takes 283 gallons of petroleum oil, including for producing the food to feed the steer, farming chemicals, and fuel for the engines on the farms.

"The love for all living creatures is the most noble attribute of man."
    – Charles Darwin

You can decide what sort of energy you will allow into your body simply by selecting the types of foods you eat. You can either bring into your system the destructive energy that exists in the tissues of slaughtered animals, which is the product of sickly and incarcerated farm animals, or you can bring in the good energy of nature through following a diet that consists of nutrient-rich plant matter.

"The consumption of animals causes more harm to the environment than all the forms of transportation put together. That's one thing. And, of course, I don't think when they said dominion over the animals they meant the abuse of 10 billion farm animals every year, which is what we do here in America."
    – Russell Simmons

When people or other animals are mistreated, the pain they feel in their mind creates energy waves and molecules of emotion that saturate their body tissues. The molecules leave the body, traveling into the surrounding atmosphere and substances. This creates a ripple effect that impacts humanity. It is part of the horror spread through war, animal farming, animal slaughter, child abuse, the destruction of and misuse of nature, and all of the other ugly, unkind, and cruel behaviors of humans. Ending factory farming would be a big step in the right direction.

"We must fight against the spirit of unconscious cruelty with which we treat the animals. Animals suffer as much as we do. True

humanity does not allow us to impose such sufferings on them. It is our duty to make the whole world recognize it. Until we extend our circle of compassion to all living things, humanity will not find peace."
– Albert Schweitzer

If a person disrespects other life forms and nature, they are unlikely to tune in to the life-affirming power to be gained by respecting life. Truths of the unity with animals are more likely to be closed off to them. The abuse of farm animals, the mass breeding of them into the tens of billions, the vile factory farming of them, the slaughter and consumption of them, and the destruction of nature in relation to raising billions of farm animals are damaging to the collective health of all life.

"Humanity's true moral test, its fundamental test, consists of its attitude towards those who are at its mercy: animals. And in this respect humankind has suffered a fundamental debacle, a debacle so fundamental that all others stem from it."
– Milan Kundera

Imagine being kept in a box your entire life, indoors, fed an unnatural diet, and surrounded by and slathered with your own and others' excrement that is always present. This is how factory farmed animals live out their entire lives, in torturous total confinement with the constant smell of urine and shit, and the continual sound of clanging cages, while never smelling fresh air; never feeling sun on their skin; never having a sip of water from a river, pond, or lake; never knowing what it is like to walk in open fields; and never knowing what it is like to graze on fresh plants, which is their natural diet.

Then their flesh, milk, and eggs are sold in packaging that feature drawings of happy animals living in pleasant, pristine country farm settings. The marketing of these products is a lie, and the belief that people cannot survive without eating animal products is not true.

"The animals of the world exist for their own reasons. They were not made for humans any more than black people were made for white, or women created for men."
– Alice Walker

The publicity and advertising campaigns of the animal farming industries present the image that Americans are not eating enough animal products and that eating more of those products rather than less promotes better health. The truth is that the amount of animal products Americans already eat is unhealthful, and increasing the amount of the products would be even more unhealthful.

"If you allow the media to guide your food choices, the next step will be to ask *your* doctor is if *this drug* is right for you."
– Brigitte Mars, *The Sexual Herbal: Prescriptions for Enhancing Love and Passion*; BrigitteMars.com

What the commercials and promotional materials do not tell you is that the more meat, dairy products, and eggs a person consumes, the more likely he is to get cancer and experience other degenerative diseases, like colitis, arthritis, and muscular sclerosis. Studies have shown over and over that the less meat people consume and the more their diets are based on fruits, vegetables, raw nuts, seeds, and seaweeds, with a tilt toward a low-fat diet, the less likely they are of experiencing heart disease and a variety of other ailments.

"If we – that is, society – switched to a vegetarian diet, atherosclerotic coronary artery disease, which accounts for most heart disease, would vanish."
– Dr. William C. Roberts, editor of the *American Journal of Cardiology*

In addition to heart attacks, a person's risk of experiencing strokes, kidney disease, diabetes, arthritis, obesity, and various types of cancer corresponds with the amount of meat, eggs, and milk products that person consumes. Degenerative diseases are also related to the consumption of processed salts and sugars, fried oils, and synthetic food additives.

The foods that contain heart-choking cholesterol – meats, dairy, and eggs – also contain harmful fat: saturated fat. Cholesterol and saturated fat clog the blood systems in the body and this causes heart disease and strokes. This is especially true if a person is consuming foods rich with fried oils, and processed salts and sugars.

In a study involving 27,000 men over 14 years, scientists at the University of California, San Francisco, found that men who consumed 2.5 or more eggs per week had an 81 percent higher risk of developing lethal prostate cancer compared to men who consumed fewer than half an egg per week on average. The study was published in the September 19, 2011 edition of the journal *Cancer Prevention Research*, and considered the possibility that the cholesterol and choline in eggs, which are also "highly concentrated in prostate cancer cells," played major roles in the incidence of the disease. The study also identified the consumption of meat, processed meat, and chicken as risk factors in the development of prostate cancer. The study recognized that the men who consumed the most eggs also were more likely to smoke, to be overweight, to lack adequate exercise to keep fit, and to follow a poor diet, which all increase the risk of experiencing prostate cancer.

"Regarding cancer mortality, red meat intake has been associated with increased risks of colorectal cancer and several other cancers. Several compounds in red meat or created by high-temperature cooking, including N-nitroso compounds (nitrosamines or nitrosamides) converted from nitrites, polycyclic aromatic hydrocarbons, and heterocyclic amines, are potential carcinogens. Heme iron and iron overload might also be associated with increased cancer risk through promotion of N-nitroso compound formation, increased colonic cytotoxicity and epithelial proliferation, increased oxidative stress, and iron-induced hypoxia signaling."
– Red Meat Consumption and Mortality, An Pan, PhD, Frank B Hu, MD, et al; Harvard Health Professionals Follow-Up Study; Harvard School of Public Health; *Archives of Internal Medicine*, March, 12, 2012. Study tracked 37,698 men from the Harvard Health Professionals Follow-Up Study and 83,644 women from the Harvard Nurses Health Study for more than 20 years.

"Cancer of the prostate is strongly linked to what men eat. Again, animal products are consistently indicted: Milk, meat, eggs, cheese, cream, butter, and fats are found, in one research study after another, to be linked to prostate cancer. And it is not just dairy products and meats. Some studies have also pointed a finger at vegetable oils. Most recently, milk consumption has been linked to prostate cancer due to high levels of the compound insulin-like growth factor (IGF-1), both present in dairy products and in increased levels in the bodies of those who consume dairy on a regular basis. A recent study showed that men who had the highest levels of IGF-1 had more than four times the risk of prostate cancer compared with those who had the lowest levels."
– Dr. Neal Barnard, Prostate Cancer: Prevention and Survival, The Cancer Project; CancerProject.org; Physicians Committee for Responsible Medicine, PCRM.org

For men, the consumption of meat, dairy, and eggs and the cholesterol imbalances these substances cause increases the incidence of both prostate cancer and erectile dysfunction.

"Because arteries in the penis are smaller, atherosclerosis shows up there sooner, perhaps three to four years before the onset of cardiovascular disease."
– Dr. Robert Kloner, cardiologist, Keck School of Medicine, University of Southern California

Numerous studies have concluded that men who are overweight are more likely to experience prostate cancer, and that men and women who are overweight are more likely to experience cancers of the colon, kidney, liver, and pancreas. People who are vegetarian or vegan are less likely to be overweight, especially if they refrain from fried and sautéed foods, and if their diet consists largely of raw fruits and vegetables.

Some of the carcinogens that meat eaters are exposed to are the residues of the toxic pesticides, insecticides, and other chemicals that are used on and around the livestock, and on the grains and other things fed to the farm animals. Additionally, the antibiotics, breeding drugs, and other drugs fed to and injected into farm animals, as well as the fertilizers in the feed, often are present in the meat, dairy, and eggs consumed by humans. The large majority of the antibiotics used in North America are given to livestock.

> "Autopsies of soldiers during the Korean and Vietnam wars showed the effects of America's artery-clogging diet even on the very young. The arteries of Asian soldiers were largely clean, free of fatty deposits. But almost 80 percent of American battlefield casualties showed gross evidence of coronary artery disease – clogging and damage that, had the soldiers lived, would have grown worse with every passing decade. What's more, in recent years, researchers have observed that as residents of areas with a low incidence of cardiovascular disease begin to adopt a more Western style of life and diet, the incidence of disease – especially coronary artery disease – rises dramatically."
> – Dr. Caldwell B. Esselstyn, author of *Prevent and Reverse Heart Disease*; HeartAttackProof.com

Besides being major risk factors in the most common types of heart diseases and strokes, meats are a major source of destructive free radicals that damage body tissues. Eating meat products introduces prostaglandin-2 into the body and increases the uric acid level, and these both induce arthritic conditions.

In the U.S., osteoporosis causes more deaths than cancers of the breast and cervix combined. Americans have the highest rate of osteoporosis in the world. Americans are always listed in the top ten in consumption of meat and dairy products in the world. Osteoporosis is most common in exactly those countries where dairy products are consumed in the largest quantities.

After heart disease, the second-leading cause of death in the U.S. is cancer. The second-leading cause of cancer-related death in the U.S. is colorectal cancer. This type of cancer is most common in people who eat an abundance of meat, dairy, and egg products.

For these and other reasons, the last thing people need to do is eat more animal-based foods. It would be more healthful to eliminate all meat, dairy, eggs, and animal protein and animal fats from the diet – and instead, eat a low-fat, plant-based diet rich in unheated fruits and vegetables.

"After years of increasing consumption, Americans began cutting back on beef in the 1970s as health and cost concerns about red meat pushed people toward poultry. Falling from the 1976 peak of 91 pounds, beef eating per person is projected to sink to 52 pounds in 2012, a 43 percent drop off the high. The national beef cattle herd is now smaller than it has been in any year since 1962. The record heat and drought that desiccated grazing lands and curtailed hay production in the Southern Plains in 2011 has led to further culling of herds as well as a mass movement of cattle from drought-ridden Texas to Nebraska."
– Janet Larsen, Peak Meat: U.S. Consumption Falling; Earth Policy Institute; March 7, 2012; Earth-Policy.org

"Having a bad diet right now is a better predictor of future violence than past violent behavior."
– Stephen Schoenthalerf

"It is very significant that some of the most thoughtful and cultured men are partisans of a pure vegetable diet."
– Mahatma Ghandi

"True benevolence, or compassion, extends itself through the whole of existence and sympathises with the distress of every creature capable of sensation."
– Joseph Addison

"My doctrine is this, that if we see cruelty or wrong that we have the power to stop, and do nothing, we make ourselves sharers in the quilt."
– Anna Sewell, author of *Black Beauty*

"Because one species is more clever than another, does it give it the right to imprison or torture the less clever species? Does one exceptionally clever individual have a right to exploit the less clever individuals of his own species? To say that he does is to say with the fascists that the strong have a right to abuse and exploit the weak – might is right, and the strong and ruthless shall inherit the earth."
– Richard Ryder

THE MEAT INDUSTRY: RAPE, INCARCERATE, MURDER, DISMEMBERMENT FOR PROFIT

"Animals have done us no harm and they have no power of resistance. There is something so very dreadful in tormenting those who have never harmed us, who cannot defend themselves, who are utterly in our power."
– Cardinal John Henry Newman

"Although other animals may be different from us, this does not make them less than us."
– Marc Bekoff

"Every living thing feels pain and should be protected from cruelty. Farm animals are no different."
– Kim Basinger

"Cows are amongst the gentlest of breathing creatures; none show more passionate tenderness to their young when deprived of them; and, in short, I am not ashamed to profess a deep love for these quiet creatures."
– Thomas de Quincey

"As infuriating and disheartening it is to have your pleas for compassion fall upon deaf ears, never give up. Animals don't have a voice, so make sure people never stop hearing yours."
– Felix Sampson

"A pound of conventional grain-fed beef requires a gallon of fuel and 5,169 gallons of water."
– Paul Roberts, *Mother Jones Magazine*, April 2009

"Would Nature have placed our very means of survival – food – in mobile animals, another mammal's skin, and under a hen, or in 260,000 varieties of plants spread over Earth?"
– Rex Bowlby, author of *Plant Roots: 101 reasons why the human diet is rooted exclusively in plants*

"The meat industry is one of the most destructive ecological industries on the planet. The raising and slaughtering of pigs, cows, sheep, turkeys and chickens not only utilizes vast areas of land and

vast quantities of water, but it is a greater contributor to greenhouse gas emissions than the automobile industry."
  – Paul Watson, SeaShepherd.org

Meat wasn't so common in the human diet at large until the invention of modern refrigeration. Now, it is common for many people to consume a variety of animal proteins, including meat, dairy, and eggs, at every meal.

From the Centers for Disease Control and Prevention:
- Heart disease is the leading cause of death in the U.S.
- In recent years, heart disease played a role in one in every four deaths.
- In 2008, 405,309 people died from coronary heart disease.
- Every year about 785,000 Americans have a first heart attack.
- Another 470,000 who have already had one or more heart attacks have another attack.
- In 2010, coronary heart disease alone cost the United States $108.9 billion. This total includes the cost of health care services, medications, and lost productivity.
- Heart disease is the leading cause of death for people of most ethnicities in the United States, including African Americans, Hispanics, and Caucasians.
- For American Indians or Alaska Natives and Asians or Pacific Islanders, heart disease is second only to cancer.

MORE land on this planet is used to support the animal farming industry than any other human land use. Most of the farmland on the planet is used to grow food for farm animals. That translates to most of the water used for farming, and most of the fuel used for farming, and most of the toxic chemicals used for farming. That is just the start of the damage done to the planet by the animal farming industries.

> "I challenge the idea that anyone can eat meat 'in peace.' It's a contradiction in terms. How can you talk about peace if your plate is swimming in blood? America raises and kills about 10 billion animals for food every year. The overwhelming majority of those animals – cows, pigs, chickens, turkeys, lambs – are raised in hideous, overcrowded factory conditions. Ever wonder why we're experiencing all those salmonella and swine flu outbreaks? A peek inside these factory farms would give you food for thought."
>   – Jane Velez-Mitchell

"The livestock sector generates more greenhouse gas emissions as measured in CO_2 equivalent than transport [pollution from all cars and trucks combined]."
– Food and Agriculture Organisation, Rome, Italy; 2006

"The less animal-based food you eat, and the more you replace those calories with plant-based food, the better off you are, in terms of your health as well as your contributions to the health of the planet."
– Gidon Eshel, assistant professor of geophysics, University of Chicago. Co-author of study concluding that becoming a vegan does more to reduce greenhouse gasses than reducing car use.

"The crowded, often unsanitary conditions promote disease, which has led to the overuse of antibiotics and to a class of superbugs that are resistant to those same antibiotics. Even the modern corn-based livestock diet causes problems. It makes meat fattier and may have helped some strains of the *E. coli* bacteria evolve from benign microbe to one of the deadliest pathogens in the food supply. And, of course, to grow all the grain we now feed our livestock, we've converted much of the Midwest into a huge corn and soybean plantation."
– Paul Roberts, *Los Angeles Times*, Aug. 23, 2008. Author of *The End of Food*.

"One day the absurdity of the almost universal human belief in the slavery of other animals will be palpable. We shall then have discovered our souls and become worthier of sharing this planet with them."
– Dr. Martin Luther King, Jr.

Please read Howard Lyman's books, *Mad Cowboy* and *No More Bull*, and John Robbin's book, *The Food Revolution*.

"In recent years, nearly a billion pounds of this ammonia-laced burger filler have been mixed annually into the ground beef sold in the U.S. As a result, more than two-thirds of the nation's pre-made burger patties have contained pink slime.

The name 'pink slime' sounds, well, slimy, but what exactly is it? The answer isn't reassuring. In fact, it's as gross as it seems. Just 10 years ago, according to Mary Jane's Farm, 'the rejected fat, sinew, bloody effluvia, and occasional bits of meat cut from carcasses in the slaughterhouse were a low-value waste product called 'trimmings' that were sold primarily as pet food.' But then Beef Products, Inc., began converting the stuff into a mash and treating it with ammonium hydroxide to kill bacteria. The resulting product was given the name pink slime by Gerald Zirnstein, a microbiologist working for the USDA Food Safety and Inspection Service. He said it was 'not meat,' but 'salvage.' Zirnstein added: 'I consider allowing it in ground beef to be a form of fraudulent labeling.'

Does such fraudulent labeling still take place? In March, ABC World News with Diane Sawyer reported that 70 percent of U.S. supermarket ground beef contained pink slime, and that it is often labeled '100 percent ground beef.'"
– John Robbins, Pink Slime and Mad Cow Disease: Coming to a Burger Near You, *Huffington Post*, April 26, 2012

"Poultry, once a rarity on American dinner tables, made a meteoric rise after World War II as industrial production systems took over from small farm flocks. Until 1940, Americans consumed less than a pound of poultry per person each month. By 1990, they were eating more than a pound each week. Intake of poultry first surpassed beef in the mid-1990s and then surged ahead, only recently beginning to falter. If 2012 forecasts play out, consumption will be down to 70 pounds per person, more than 5 percent below the 2006 peak."
– Janet Larsen, Peak Meat: U.S. Consumption Falling; Earth Policy Institute; March 7, 2012; Earth-Policy.org

Unfortunate facts about the animal farming and meat industry:
• The number-one reason why tropical rainforests are cut down is to provide land to grow corn, soy, and other food for farmed animals. The forests are clearcut and/or burned, releasing the greenhouse gas, carbon dioxide, into the atmosphere.
• The destruction of the Brazilian rainforests to make way for cattle grazing and grain fields has turned Brazil into the world's leading exporter of beef and soy.
• According to the 2007 report, *Livestock's Long Shadow*, produced by the United Nations Food and Agriculture Organization, the animal farming industry produces more pollution than all cars, trucks, ships, trains, and airplanes combined. It is responsible for 65 percent of nitrous oxide emissions and 37 percent of methane emissions. Transportation causes 13.5 percent of the worlds global greenhouse gasses, and the livestock industry produced 18 percent. According to the report, 265 gallons of fossil fuels are used to produce the meat consumed annually by the typical American family of four.
• The number-one use of synthetic chemical fertilizers on the planet is to grow food for farmed animals. The fertilizers are made using fossil fuels, are spread on the land using petroleum burning engines, and

release tremendous amounts of CO_2 into the atmosphere. The nitrogen-based fertilizers release nitrous oxide, which is nearly 300 times more damaging than CO_2.

• Produces the greenhouse gasses carbon dioxide, methane, and nitrous oxide as a result of the manure and gasses from tens of billions of farm animals. Methane is emitted from the mouths of cattle and sheep and is 23 times stronger than CO_2. One cow can produce as much as 130 gallons of methane per day.

• In the 30 years starting in 1975 the global production of farmed meat from cows, chickens, turkeys, hogs, and lambs rose from 130 million tons to 230 million tons.

• In 2007, meat consumption in the U.S. was 55 billion pounds.

• Nearly 1/3 of Earth's fertile land is used to grow livestock feed.

"Migrant laborers are being employed by huge international enterprises on soya bean farms. Can you imagine they are cutting down the old growth forests of the Amazon and replacing it with soya bean farms to feed cattle to give us hamburgers? And after ten years those farms are useless because the soil only supports rainforest. It was never intended to grow soya beans. What an incredible mistake we are making. If the root cause of this problem is poverty, then let us solve that problem. The entire problem of the Amazon can be solved with six months' spending in Iraq. We could have the Amazon secure forever with just six months' spending in Iraq. All that is really needed is to pay the people of the Amazon to look after it, to protect this precious treasure for the world. Instead, because of short-sighted, ignorant, greedy thinking we are allowing this incredible resource to be destroyed. We are literally burning the lifeboat in which we all live. It is madness."
– Graham Hancock

"It is only by softening and disguising dead flesh by culinary preparation that it is rendered susceptible of mastication or digestion, and that the sight of its bloody juices and raw horror does not excite intolerable loathing and disgust."
– Percy Bysshe Shelley, _Queen Mob Notes_

"I actually get quite sad when I smell bacon. Factory farming has made life an unimaginable hell for the billions of pigs raised and killed for food. Sows are kept in gestation crates the size of their bodies and never able to turn around or even scratch themselves. These pigs, which have an I.Q. comparable to dogs, routinely become psychotic.

Stacked by the thousands in dark warehouses, these sentient beings live out their miserable lives never seeing the sky or taking in a single breath of fresh air. Americans are decent people and the only consumers who still enjoy bacon are those from whom the pork industry has managed to hide the truth. I defy anybody to look at those pig gestation crates and walk away with a hankering for a slice of bacon."
– Jane Velez-Mitchell

"Anyone who isn't vegan simply doesn't comprehend what we've done to nonhumans – sentient beings just like us. They don't get the language, the sentiment, the horror. And it is a horror. For we have taken everything from them: their homes, their children, their land, their families, their dignity, their joy, their sanity, their liberty, and their lives. Try telling that to your average meat eater, and watch them glaze over."
– Sienna Blake

"While inefficiently producing unhealthful food, and contributing to heart disease and cancer, factory farms leave a wake of toxic waste, disease, declining aquifers, global warming, obesity for the affluent and malnutrition for the excluded."
– Christopher Cook

"We eat animals for four reasons: habit, tradition, convenience, and taste. Not because we need to. Not for our health. These animals are trapped, imprisoned, and bred to be raped, tortured, and killed so we can satisfy our taste buds. It's an industry of murder. We are all animals and deserve equal rights to pursue our lives freely. It's not cool, it's not necessary, and it's time to wake up and stop supporting murder."
– Markus Rafael Nylund

"Animals pay a dear price, simply for being born into a world where humans see them as 'property.' These beings are not 'resources.' They are living, breathing, hurting members of our global family."
– Anthony Damiano

"We cannot have two hearts, one for the animals and one for men. In cruelty towards the former and cruelty to the latter there is no difference but in the victim."
– Alphonse Marie-Louis d'Lamartine

Animals Australia, AnimalsAustralia.org
Farm Animal Reform Movement, FARMUSA.org

Farm Sanctuary, FarmSanctuary.org
Howard Lyman, MadCowboy.Com
Humane Myth, HumaneMyth.org
Mercy for Animals, MercyForAnimals.org
No Veal, NoVeal.org
People for the Ethical Treatment of Animals, PETA.org
John Robbins, FoodRevolution.org
SAFE, New Zealand, SAFE.org.NZ
Woodstock Farm Animal Sanctuary, WoodstockFAS.org
Vegetarian Society, VegSoc.org/environment

"It should not be believed that all beings exist for the sake of the existence of man. On the contrary, all the other beings too have been intended for their own sakes and not for the sake of something else."
– Maimonides

"A man can live and be healthy without killing animals for food; therefore, if he eats meat, he participates in taking animal life for the sake of his appetite. And to act so is immoral."
– Leo Tolstoy

"Many years ago, I was fishing, and as I was reeling in the poor fish, I realized, 'I am killing him – all for the passing pleasure it brings me.' And something inside me clicked. I realized, as I was watching him fight for breath, that his life was as important to him as mine is to me."
– Paul McCartney

"I became a vegetarian because I was persuaded that Life is as valid for other creatures as it is for humans. I do not need dead animal bodies to keep me alive, strong and healthy. Therefore, I will not kill for food."
– Scott Nearing

"When I was old enough to realize all meat was killed, I saw it as an irrational way of using our power, to take a weaker thing and mutilate it. It was like the way bullies would take control of younger kids in the schoolyard."
– River Phoenix

"We universally condemn supremacism, elitism, and exclusivism for destroying peace and social justice, yet we unquestionably and even proudly adopt precisely these attitudes when it comes to animals."
– Dr. Will Tuttle, author of *The World Peace Diet*, WorldPeaceDiet.org

"Don't talk to me about peace and nonviolence when there's a dead animal on your dinner plate."
– Colleen Polito

"We manage to swallow flesh, only because we do not think of the cruel and sinful things we do."
– Rabinadranath Tagor, *Glimpses of Bengel Letters*

"We consume the carcasses of creatures of like appetites, passions, and organs with our own, and fill the slaughterhouses daily with screams of fear and pain."
– Robert Louis Stevenson

"Thus far, our responsibility for how we treat chickens and allow them to be treated in our culture is dismissed with blistering rhetoric designed to silence objections: 'How the hell can you compare the feelings of a hen with those of a human being?' One answer is, by looking at her. It does not take special insight or credentials to see that a hen confined in a battery cage is suffering, or to imagine what her feelings must be compared with those of a hen ranging outside in the grass and sunlight. We are told that we humans are capable of knowing just about anything that we want to know – except, ironically, what it feels like to be one of our victims."
– Karen Davis, United Poultry Concerns; UPC-Online.org

"In all the round world of Utopia there is no meat. There used to be. But now we cannot stand the thought of slaughterhouses. And it is impossible to find anyone who will hew a dead ox or pig. I can still remember as a boy the rejoicing over the closing of the last slaughterhouse."
– Herbert G. Wells, *A Modern Utopia*

"Love animals. God has given them the rudiments of thought and joy untroubled. Do not trouble their joy, don't harass them, don't deprive them of their happiness, don't work against God's intent. Man, do not pride yourself on superiority to animals; they are without sin, and you, with your greatness, defile the Earth by your appearance on it, and leave the traces of your foulness after you – alas, it is true of almost every one of us!"
– Fyodor Dostoyevsky

LIVESTOCK BY THE BILLIONS:
A GLOBAL ENVIRONMENTAL DISASTER

"The fact is that there is enough food in the world for everyone. But tragically, much of the world's food and land resources are tied up in producing beef and other livestock – food for the well off – while millions of children and adults suffer from malnutrition and starvation."
– Dr. Walden Bello

"Ask the questions, 'Who produced my food?' 'What did they use on it?' 'What's it doing to me, the environment, and the animals?' I want you to think about this. Is it right? Is it right that we should end up with more cancer? Should it be right that we end up with less top soil? It is right that we end up with fewer trees? When are we as the American people going to stand up and say, 'Enough is enough!' When in God's world are we going to wake up to the fact that we are destroying the planet?"
– Howard Lyman, MadCowboy.com

In addition to the incapacitating degenerative diseases, the fueling of the pharmaceutical and hospital industries, the food poisoning, and the suffering issues of raising, killing, and eating billions of animals, there are also the issues of the ecological damage to the planet caused by the livestock industry.

"Of all agricultural land in the United States, 87 percent is used to raise animals for food. Twenty thousand pounds of potatoes can be grown on one acre of land, but only 165 pounds of beef can be produced in the same space.

[South and Central American] Rainforests are being destroyed at a rate of 125,000 square miles per year to create space to raise animals for food. Fifty-five square feet of land are consumed for every quarter-pound fast food burger made of rainforest beef."
– PETA, VegNow.Com

"Nationwide, factory-farmed animals produce 130 times more manure than the human population – the equivalent of five tons of

manure for every U.S. citizen. U.S. factory farms generate more than 350 million tons of manure each year."
– Farm Sanctuary, VegForLife.Org

"Cattle and sheep grazing is ecologically destructive and an abomination against our national park system in areas as pristine as the Grand Canyon Park.

Grazing causes rapid depletion of wooded areas by clearing, cultivating and eroding the soil. Soil losses are as high as 44 tons per acre annually on steep slopes. Woodlands, waterways and wildlife habitats have been significantly reduced or eradicated entirely due to overgrazing."
– FarmSanctuary.Org

"Most wars are fought over control of natural resources: land, water, oil, and minerals. Yet, animal agriculture is by far the largest user and despoiler of natural resources."
– Citizens for Healthy Options in Children's Education, CHOICE.USA

The livestock industry and companies that exist to service it, including the petroleum industry, chemical companies, and the grain industry, collectively use up more land and resources and create more pollution and ecological damage on the planet than any industry. There are tens of billions of chickens and turkeys, billions of pigs, over a billion cattle, and hundreds of millions of lambs and other farm animals being raised on millions of acres of land all over the world and this is ravaging the biodiversity (the full spectrum of living things including plants, insects, birds, and other land and water life) of the planet.

"Cattle are a chief source of organic pollution; cow dung is poisoning the freshwater lakes, rivers, and streams of the world. Growing herds of cattle are exerting unprecedented pressure on the carrying capacity of natural ecosystems, edging entire species of wildlife to the brink of extinction. Cattle are a growing source of global warming, and their increasing numbers now threaten the very dynamic of the biosphere."
– Jeremy Rifkin, in his book *Beyond Beef: The Rise and Fall of the Cattle Culture*

"Livestock (like automobiles) are a human invention and convenience, not part of pre-human times, and a molecule of CO_2 exhaled by livestock is no more natural than one from an auto tailpipe. Moreover, while over time an equilibrium of CO_2 may exist between the amount respired by animals and the amount photosynthesized by plants, that equilibrium has never been static. Today, tens of billions more livestock are exhaling CO_2 than in preindustrial days, while Earth's photosynthetic capacity (its capacity to keep carbon out of the atmosphere by absorbing it in plant mass) has declined sharply as forest has been cleared. (Meanwhile, of course, we add more carbon to the air by burning fossil fuels, further overwhelming the carbon-absorption system.)"

> – Robert Goodland, a former World Bank Group environmental advisor, and Jeff Anhang, an environmental specialist at the World Bank Group's International Finance Corporation. They concluded that, of the world emissions of global greenhouse gasses related to human activity, 51 percent could be attributed to the meat diet. That is a huge jump from the 18 percent figure devised in 2006. *World Watch* magazine, April 2012

Raising of livestock for human consumption and all of the ecologically destructive chemicals used by the animal-farming industry cause massive damage to the delicate ecosystems throughout the world. Livestock in the U.S. produces more than 130 times the amount of bodily waste of the nation's human population. As more people around the world are converting to an American diet style of meat and junk food, expansive stretches of virgin land and land that had been used to grow food for human consumption are being converted to provide space for cattle grazing and for growing feed for livestock.

"The less animal-based food you eat, and the more you replace those calories with plant-based food, the better off you are, in terms of your health as well as your contributions to the health of the planet."

> – Gidon Eshel, assistant professor of geophysics at the University of Chicago, co-author of a study concluding that becoming a vegan does more to reduce greenhouse gasses than the type of car you drive. (*Earth Interactions* journal, April 2006; It's better to green your diet than your car, *New Scientist Magazine*, Dec. 17, 2005)

"Rainforests cover less than two percent of the Earth's surface, yet they are home to nearly half of our planet's living creatures. Butterflies and birds fill the air, their colors are so intense, no artist could ever match them. Noble jaguars, howler monkeys, vines, fish, gorillas, orchids, lizards, and orangutans flourish there – and nowhere else on Earth.

A four-square-mile area of rainforest teems with colorful variety: 750 types of trees, 1,500 different flowers, 125 mammal species, and 400 kinds of birds.

But rainforests are disappearing at the rate of a football field every second. The destruction of the Earth's most ancient complex ecosystem threatens the very survival of the human species.

Over 99 percent of the rainforest species has not yet been studied for possible medical use. A plant that holds the cure for AIDS – or a future epidemic – may be growing somewhere in the rainforest. Or a bulldozer may be crushing the last one right now as you read this.

Rice, potatoes, bananas, chocolate, coffee, oranges, tomatoes, yams, and dozens of other food crops originated in the rainforests. The wild strains still found there provide genetic material necessary to keep world agriculture stocks hardy and healthy. Undiscovered rainforest species could provide new sources of food in the future.

Once the rainforest is gone, the vanished species won't return. And once the proud, ancient indigenous cultures are destroyed, the knowledge they possess – knowledge that could benefit all of humanity – will be lost forever."
– The Rainforest Action Network, RAN.Org

Anyone who considers the story of a Brazilian rubber tapper named Chico Mendez will begin to get an idea of how much corruption and damage the cattle industry has caused to the life-sustaining rainforests.

The main reason millions of acres of rainforests in South and Central America continue to be destroyed by cutting and burning is to clear new land for cattle grazing and feed crops. This kills off many kinds of plants, insects, animals, amphibians, and birds, and also destroys natural water filtration systems within the rainforests that have existed for an unknown number of years. The cattle that are raised on the defiled rainforest land are used to supply beef to the Orient, to the Middle East, to North America, and to Europe – where millions of acres of land are already being ruined to raise, feed, and grow feed for hundreds of millions of cattle and billions of other farm animals.

"The livestock population of the United States today consumes enough grain and soybeans to feed over five times the entire human population of the country. We feed these animals over 80 percent of the corn we grow, and over 95 percent of the oats… Less than half the harvested agricultural acreage in the United States is used to grow food for people. Most of it is used to grow livestock feed. This is a drastically inefficient use of our acreage. For every sixteen pounds of grain and soybeans fed to beef cattle, we get back only one pound as meat on our plates. The other fifteen are inaccessible to us. Most of it is turned into manure."
– John Robbins, in his book *Diet for a New America*

In 1994 the U.S. Fish and Wildlife Service announced that California's state fish, the golden trout found in the waters of the High Sierras of California, was a candidate for the endangered species list. The declining population of the fish was blamed on cattle grazing in the U.S. government-owned Golden Trout Wilderness land adjacent to the streams where the fish spawn. The cattle the U.S. government allows ranchers to graze there have eroded the land and widened the river banks. As the cattle trample the soil it becomes compacted, making it unsuitable for new plant growth and prevents rainwater from being absorbed. Instead, the rainwater runoff carries soil into rivers and streams and the plants that do take up root are often invasive weeds. The vegetation degradation, soil erosion, and the manure from the cattle have affected the water temperature and clarity, smothered fish eggs, and have had a negative impact on the population of insects, on which the fish and birds survive.

"In California, the number of gallons of water needed to produce one edible pound of wheat: 25 gallons; beef: 5,214 gallons.

Energy expended to produce one pound of grain-fed beef: equivalent to one gallon of gasoline."
– EarthSave.Org

"McDonald's equals slavery and starvation."
– Graffiti on a wall in Quito, Ecuador

"More than half of all the water and 33 percent of all the raw materials used for all purposes in the United States are used in meat production… the average chicken-processing plant may use 100 million gallons of water daily. More than 260 million acres of U.S. forest have been cleared to grow crops to feed to cattle. Cattle grazing in the western United States has led to soil erosion and desertification."
– *Take a Step Toward Compassionate Living*, by the People for the Ethical Treatment of Animals, PETA-Online.Org; 2004

Raising livestock and growing grains to feed livestock is not energy efficient. It takes significantly larger amounts of land, water, and other resources to produce cattle, poultry, and hog meat than it does to produce fruits, vegetables, herbs, legumes, and grains for human consumption. More than half of the water used in the U.S. goes to grow feed crops and to provide water for livestock. Those uses of water have been blamed for the droughts in California, where water consumption by the livestock industry exceeds that of the state's human population. The beef industry in California is the state's third-largest agricultural sector. The number-one reason California has had periods in droughts when people were told not to use water and some people were fined for using more of their share is that so much water goes for raising grains for feed and water for the livestock herds that it depletes the water supplies during the times there is no rain. Water for farm animals, and to grow their food, is pumped out of the ground, draining aquifers; or is taken from streams, lakes, and rivers, damaging wildlife populations, including fish, amphibians, land mammals, and birds, that depend on that water and the life in and around it.

"More than half of U.S. grain and almost 40 percent of world grain is being fed to livestock rather than being consumed directly by humans. In the United States, more than 8 billion livestock are maintained, which eat about 7 times as much grain as is consumed directly by the entire U.S. population.

Producing 1 kg of fresh beef requires about 13 kg of grain and 30 kg of forage. This much grain and forage requires a total of 43 000 liters of water.

A quarter-pound burger with cheese takes 26 oz of petroleum and leaves a 13-lbs carbon footprint. This is equivalent to burning 7 lbs. of coal.

At a time when 20 percent of people in the U.S. go to bed hungry each night and almost 50 percent of the world's population is malnourished, choosing to eat more plant-based foods and less red meat is better for all of us – ourselves, our loved ones, and our planet."

– Dr. Dean Ornish, Holy Cow! What's Good for You Is Good for Our Planet: Comment on "Red Meat Consumption and Mortality," *Archives of Internal Medicine*, March 12, 2012. Ornish is the founder of the Preventative Medicine Research Institute, PMRI.org

Enormous amounts of government money in the U.S. and other countries is spent to help irrigate livestock grain fields, and to build and manage water systems for the cattle industry. This water is then polluted by the chemicals used to grow the feed for the farm animals and by the farm animals themselves, and the drugs used on them. The pollution and the soil erosion caused by livestock poison streams, rivers, ponds, lakes, and oceans. Farming chemicals and genetically modified crops grown to feed farm animals can alter the organisms in soil, in water, in the intestines of the animals, and the microflora in our intestines.

"Livestock grazing on public lands accounts for less than one-tenth of one percent of employment in the eleven western states, including in Colorado (according to a study by Thomas Powers, chairman of the University of Montana's Department of Economics). However, this activity costs taxpayers anywhere from three to five hundred million dollars per year (according to the Cato Institute). More significantly, cows and sheep on public lands pollute streams and rivers, and jeopardize the continued survival of

many rare wildlife species (according to the Congressional General Accounting Office)."
– *Colorado Wolf Tracks*; 1996; WildEarthGuardians.org

"Last April (2011), Congress eliminated federal protection for wolves in the Northern Rocky Mountains. Hunting in Idaho and Montana has resulted in 410 wolves killed this winter alone – yet, less than 1,300 wolves live in those two states."
– WildEarthGuardians.org

"The U.S. government spent $22 billion to build 133 water projects in the West. Every year the government spends $7 billion on these water projects. Farmers pay less than $1 billion per year to the government for water."
– *NPR*, 1997

The farming of all the grains that are grown to feed farm animals takes up the majority of farmland on the planet, and has been and is causing a huge amount of damage and erosion to the land, streams, rivers, lakes, and oceans, as well as to underground water tables. Growing food for farm animals is a tremendous waste of fuel, water, equipment, and all those used to manufacture and maintain the farm equipment needed to grow all that food for all the billions of animals grown on this planet to feed the humans who choose to eat dead animals – the very same humans who would be a lot healthier if they did not eat animals and dairy products, but instead subsisted on a vegan diet.

"You can use your food choices, your daily habit of eating, to say yes to life in a very profound way, and to say no to the corporate culture that is destroying the planet, and our communities. You can use your food choices, every meal, every bite, as an opportunity to take a stand for life, to take a stand for compassion."
– John Robbins, *The Food Revolution*; TheFoodRevolution.Org

The California dairy industry is a billion-dollar industry that relies on the milk from of a population of 1.7 million dairy cows. These cattle create 65 billion pounds of manure each year, and this results in ammonia emissions that add significant amounts of pollution. Much of the manure is spread on farmland in the surrounding regions. Many dairies produce so much manure that it can't be used and it ends up poisoning the land, rivers, lakes, and ocean. A small fraction of California's 2,100 dairies have their manure carried away by companies that bring it to "methane digester" plants that heat the slurry so that bacteria break it down to release methane gas to generate electricity.

Scientists at UC Davis have discovered that cows also emit a significant amount of gasses from their chewing and regurgitating. Combined with the nitrogen oxide emissions from vehicles and factories, the ammonia and methane from millions of cattle create particulate-laden smog. This pollution is damaging to human lung tissue, and is especially a risk to babies, children, pregnant women, the elderly, people with weakened immune systems, and really everyone who breathes it. Smog also affects plant life in that it reduces growth and photosynthesis, and speeds aging within the leaves. This has an impact on crop farming as well as on forests, wildlands, and on wildlife of all varieties. Smog is the main reason that the dairy farming regions of California often have some of the worst air quality on the continent.

"When emissions from land-use and land use change are included, the livestock sector accounts for nine percent of CO_2 deriving from human-related activities, but produces a much larger share of even more harmful greenhouse gases."
– Food and Agriculture Organisation, Rome, Italy; in a report on worldwide pollution caused by the cattle industry; 2006

According to a 1995 estimate by the San Joaquin Valley Air Pollution Control District, the average dairy cow releases 19.3 pounds of volatile organic compounds every year. California's vast San Joaquin Valley contains the most dairy cows of any region of the continent, and it also has the smoggiest air in North America. If you've bought California milk or cheese, you've supported that industry and have also played a part in that pollution. Got pollution?

The world would be a more healthful place if people would stop eating animals as well as milk and eggs and foods made with them.

"Raising animals for food causes more water pollution than any other industry in the U.S. because animals raised for food produce one hundred thirty times the excrement of the entire human population. It means 87,000 pounds per second. Much of the waste from factory farms and slaughterhouses flows into streams and rivers, contaminating water sources.

Each vegetarian can save one acre of trees per year. More than 260 million acres of U.S. forests have been cleared to grow crops to feed animals raised for meat. And another acre of trees disappears every eight seconds. The tropical rainforests are also being destroyed to create grazing land for cattle."
– Eating for Peace, by Buddhist teacher Thich Naht Hanh, on mindful consumption. From the FoodRevolution.Org Website of John Robbins.

According to the United Nations, global meat production in 2001 was 229 million tons. It is expected to double by the year 2050. The milk industry produced an estimated 580 million tons of milk in 2001. It is expected to nearly double by 2050.

"The animals you eat are not those who devour others; you do not eat the carnivorous beasts, you take them as your pattern. You only hunger after sweet and gentle creatures who harm no one, which follow you, serve you, and are devoured by you as the reward of their service."

– John Jacques Rousseau

"Raising animals for food consumes more than half of all the water used in the United States. It takes 2,500 gallons of water to produce a pound of meat, but only 25 gallons to produce a pound of wheat. The amount of water used in the production of the meat from an average steer could float a destroyer."

– People for the Ethical Treatment of Animals, VegNow.Com

"I think there will come a time when civilized people will look back in horror on our generation and the ones that have preceded it; the idea that we should eat other living things running around on four legs, that we should raise them just for the purpose of killing them! The people of the future will say 'meat eaters' in disgust and regard us in the same way that we regard cannibals and cannibalism."

– Dennis Weaver

"Remote from universal nature and living by complicated artiface, man in civilization surveys the creature through the glass of his knowledge and sees thereby a feather magnified and the whole image in distortion. We patronize them for their incompleteness, for their tragic fate of having taken form so far below ourselves. And therein do we err. For the animal shall not be measured by man. They move finished and complete, given with the extension of the senses we have lost or never attained, living by voices we shall never hear. They are not brethren, they are not underlings: they are other nations, caught with ourselves in the net of life and time, fellow prisoners of the splendour and travel of earth."

– Henry Beston, *The Outermost House*

WAR ON WILDLIFE: HOW THE MEAT INDUSTRY CAUSES EXTINCTION OF SPECIES

"But it [cattle ranching] is anything but benign. It is the number-one source of water pollution in the West. It's the number-one source of soil erosion in the West. It's the number-one cause of species endangerment in the West. It's the reason we don't have wolves throughout the West. It's one of the major reasons that more than four-fifths of all native fish west of the Continental Divide are endangered or threatened."
— George Wuerthner of Eugene, Oregon. From *Dispelling the Cowboy Myth*, by Tim Lenerich, Earthsave.org/News/03Summer/Cowboy_Myth.htm; 2004

"Every year, tens of thousands of bison, coyotes, wolves, and other wildlife are maimed, shot, poisoned, and even burned alive because the meat industry claims these animals interfere with raising animals for food. This war on wildlife is carried out with the full support of state and federal agencies, which fund so-called predator control programs."
— FarmSancturary.org

"Animal agriculture directly kills annually nearly 50 billion animals worldwide, after subjecting them to the cruelties of factory farming. It also kills uncounted numbers of wildlife on land and in the seas."
— Citizens for Healthy Options in Children's Education, CHOICE.usa

"In reality, ranchers are the most pervasively destructive force on our public land, with logging as a distant second. Via outlandish subsidies, you, I, and Uncle Sam support the cattle industry with drought and fire relief, fencing, water tanks, windmills, and bargain-basement grazing fees. Our government kills hundreds of thousands of wild creatures each year to protect ranchers' herds against predators such as wolves, mountain lions, and coyotes.

In return we get erosion, endangered species, habitat destruction, flash floods, exotic weeds, desertification, and some of the most degraded landscape on Earth."
— Tim Lenerich, *Dispelling the Cowboy Myth*

"Nearly 20 million taxpayer dollars fund the trapping, poisoning, and shooting of native predators deemed a threat to agriculture by the USDA Wildlife Services agency, which each year kills approximately 100,000 coyotes, bobcats, foxes, bears, wolves, and other predators. In 2001 the program also killed 1.6 million other 'nuisance' animals.

Almost two-thirds of all large mammal species are threatened or endangered in the lower 48 states. Less than 10 percent of all endangered and threatened species in the U.S. is improving.

About 20 percent of all endangered and threatened species are harmed by grazing."
– A Voice for Animals, VoiceForAnimals.net; 2004

"In response to ranchers' complaints of coyotes attacking cattle in southern Arizona, the federal government took to the air this past January, killing 200 coyotes. The hunt was conducted by Wildlife Services, a division of the U.S. Department of Agriculture, and took place on both public and private land."
– *Earth First! Journal*, May-June 2006; EarthFirstJournal.org

SOME people would like the public to believe that pollution is the only and worst offender to wildlife in the U.S. While pollution does take an enormous toll, the reason populations of native animals in the U.S. have dwindled is that the animals have been killed to provide grazing land for livestock, and to protect farm animals and grazing livestock.

To make it possible for cattle and other livestock to graze in open fields there has to be a safe haven created for them. This means that native animals have to be killed off. These animals include wolves, coyotes, foxes, lynx, mountain lions, bobcats, bears, elk, bighorn sheep, deer, porcupines, beavers, badgers, skunks, possums, prairie dogs, and antelopes, and many types of birds.

"In 1914, Congress first appropriated money for the U.S. Biological Survey (now known as Animal Damage Control) to exterminate wolves from the face of the continent. Though the agency failed to eradicate the species entirely, by 1945 it had killed every wolf in Colorado."
– *Colorado Wolf Tracks*; 1996; WildEarthGuardians.org

Eliminating the native animals is done with poisons, with steel jaw leghold traps, with flame torches, by shooting them from helicopters, and by damaging their food supplies. The government offices involved in these activities include the Bureau of Land Management (BLM) and the Animal Damage Control (ADC) program of the Department of

Agriculture. According to *Wildlife Damage Review*, in 1994 the government spent over $56 million of federal, state, and cooperative funds to kill 783,585 wild animals.

The land that has been cleared of native wildlife is then used as pasture for grazing livestock such as cattle, sheep, and goats. The ranchers lease the land from the government, and they do so at very low rates that do not make up for the money spent by the government to manage the land for the ranchers. The balance is made up from tax dollars – thus providing government welfare programs for ranchers.

In addition to killing wild animals for pastureland, the U.S. Department of Agriculture also is involved in killing millions of birds. They regularly use poisoned rice laced with DRC-1339 to kill grain-eating birds, such as grackles, red-winged blackbirds, ravens, magpies, vultures, and yellow-headed blackbirds. The killing doesn't stop there. That's because predator birds, such as Cooper's hawks and prairie falcons that eat the poisoned birds, also die.

Killing predator animals damages the natural cycle of native animal life. When the predator animals are killed off, the animals they feed on are able to reproduce in massive numbers. This has resulted in large populations of animals such as mice, rats, gophers, squirrels, badgers, prairie dogs, skunks, possum, rabbits, chipmunks, deer, and raccoons.

The ADC programs attempt to control the populations of the smaller animals by sending out trappers to eliminate them. They eliminate the smaller animals by burning them, by bludgeoning them, and by poisoning their young. Many smaller native animals are also killed to prevent them from eating the crops that are being grown to feed livestock, and to prevent them from creating nesting and dwelling holes in the ground, which may result in livestock injuring their legs.

To help control the population of some animals, such as deer, hunters are allowed to enter into controlled areas to kill a certain number of animals every year. When bows are used to hunt deer, about half of the deer escape with the bow stuck in them, and then the deer suffer slow, agonizing deaths.

The techniques used to kill off smaller animals, and to eliminate brush and other native plants used by larger animals, also harm the bird populations. Not only do birds die when they get caught in traps and when they eat poison meant for other animals, large birds die after eating animals that have been poisoned. A decrease in the bird population allows more insects to populate the land. To kill off the insects, the government and farmers use more chemical poisons. The pesticides then do even more damage to the bird population, create insects that are resistant to pesticides, destroy beneficial insects, and pollute the land and water, and so forth, in a cycle that would naturally take care of itself if man would not interfere.

"The ADC program, created by the Animal Damage Control Act of 1931, is greatly responsible for the virtual extinction of the grizzly and wolf in the lower 48 states as well as for putting the black-footed ferret, jaguar, black-tailed prairie dog, bald eagle, and other wild animals in, or close to, the endangered category. ADC reported it poisoned 1.8 million animals in 1991 and distributed thousands of pounds of restricted-use pesticides to private individuals who poisoned untold numbers more. The U.S. Agency for International Development works with ADC to export ADC pest control practices and chemicals, including those banned in the U.S., to developing countries."
 – *Wildlife Damage Review*, 1997; WildEarthGuardians.org

"Trapping and/or hunting are allowed on more than half of the 540 U.S. National Wildlife Refuges.
 According to the U.S. Fish & Wildlife Service, of 27 million people who visited refuges, 22 million came for wildlife observation, while only 1.2 million visited to hunt or trap animals."
 – A Voice for Animals, VoiceForAnimals.net, 2005

Ranchers and BLM workers eliminate shrubs that are used for food and shelter by native animals, and then plant grasses to feed grazing cattle. By eliminating native plants that provide food and shelter for wild animals, by eliminating small animals that provide food for predator animals, and by killing all kinds of native animals, the government has had an enormous negative impact on the populations, life cycles, migrating patterns, and social structures of native animals of North and Central America. This is done at great cost to taxpayers to provide grazing land for livestock ranchers. It is welfare farming and it is destroying the biodiversity and ecosystems of the continent. Sadly, because more and more cattle are being raised on other continents, these practices are becoming the standard in other countries.

Predator animals not only manage populations of large animals in the natural circle of life, they also improve conditions for small animals, fish, insects, and plants.

When wolves were reintroduced to Yellowstone National Park, willow trees, cottonwoods, and aspen trees began to grow more abundantly there. This was the result of elk seeking the safety of higher ground away from the wolves. The new vegetation has attracted other wildlife. The banks of the rivers and creeks, which had been damaged by elk, began to show more vegetation growth, which in turn improved the health of the rivers and creeks. This improved conditions for fish populations. And the new trees have also attracted native birds to nest there and provide shade for certain varieties of plants to grow.

"Next to an all-out nuclear war, today's intensive animal agriculture represents the greatest threat to human welfare in the history of mankind."
– Farm Animal Reform Movement, FarmUSA.org; 2005

"The love for all living creatures is the most noble attribute of man."
– Charles Darwin

"The fact is, in our country, meat is not a necessity in order to preserve life. It is simply a profit-driven industry and an extravagance that humans are unwilling to live without, regardless of its effects on health, environment, and the livelihood of conscious creatures.

Moral principles must be considered when any thought is given to the process of bringing meat to your plate. By simply researching the subject, it is easy to realize that the meat and dairy production industries are cruel. One could research veal production, foie gras, humane-slaughter regulations for poultry (nonexistent), the de-horning process for cows, gestation crates for pigs, the cruel confinement of battery hens, and countless more subpar standards that are a sad reflection of man's superiority. If evolution or man's ascribed status in the food chain is the culprit behind these acts, then perhaps it is prudent to consider that something may have gone awry in nature.

Arguments made for the necessity of meat in our culture are ill founded. Converting to a vegetarian-based diet has proven again and again to improve general health, reduce risks of disease, improve symptoms of existing ailments, and with an appropriately balanced plan, lead to a healthier community. The *China Study* provides a strong correlation between diet and disease by documenting the relationship between a vegetation-based diet and lower rates of various cancers and degenerative heart disease.

In addition to health issues, meat consumption affects many global, social, and economical factions as well. Between the methane gas output assisting in the destruction of the ozone layer, the rainforests that are being torn down to provide land for grazing cows abroad and the large amounts of grain fed to cows to produce small amounts of meat, animal agribusiness proves time and again that the driving force is in the almighty dollar."
– Joanna Strittmatter

POLLUTION CAUSED BY FARMING ANIMALS

MOST pollution on this planet is caused by the meat, dairy, and egg industries – including the meat and dairy packaging, distribution, marketing, cooking, and consumption process. This is because of the misuse and abuse of resources such as fuel, metal, plastics, paper, electricity, and other items used to get meat on the plates of humans who choose to eat meat, dairy, and eggs. Consider the following:

1. The supplies and fuel used to manufacture the equipment that is used to farm the food for billions of farm animals.

2. The supplies and fuel used to run and maintain the equipment that grows the food for billions of farm animals.

3. The supplies and fuel used to transfer the food to feed billions of farm animals.

4. The supplies and fuel used to manufacture the equipment that is used to raise billions of farm animals.

5. The supplies and fuel used to run and maintain the equipment that is used to raise billions of farm animals.

6. The supplies and fuel used to transfer billions of farm animals to the slaughterhouses.

7. The supplies and fuel used to create and maintain the trucks and other equipment used to transport billions of farm animals to slaughterhouses.

8. The supplies and fuel used to manufacture the equipment that runs the slaughterhouses where billions of farm animals are killed.

9. The supplies and fuel used to run and maintain the slaughterhouses.

10. The supplies and fuel used to manufacture the equipment that transfers the dairy products to processing and storage facilities.

11. The supplies and fuel used to run and maintain those processing and storage facilities.

12. The supplies and fuel used to manufacture the equipment that transfers the meat and dairy products to the markets.

13. The supplies and fuel used to run and maintain the equipment that transfers trillions of pounds of meat and dairy products to the markets.

14. The supplies and fuel used to manufacture the equipment that is used in the markets — from the buildings to the shelving to the heating and air conditioning and refrigeration units.

15. The supplies and fuel used to run the markets that sell the meat and dairy products.

16. The supplies and fuel used to manufacture all the equipment used to advertise the meat and dairy products.

17. The supplies and fuel used to advertise the meat and dairy products — which take up millions of pages of newspaper and magazine pages, all sorts of outdoor advertising, and hordes of radio and TV commercial time.

18. The supplies and fuel used to keep and display the meat and dairy products in stores.

19. The supplies and fuel used to manufacture and maintain all the hundreds of millions of refrigerators, stoves, and microwaves used in the stores, restaurants, hotels, homes, cruise ships, schools, hospitals, prisons, military bases, and other places where meat and dairy products are kept and prepared for consumption.

20. The supplies and fuel used to fuel all the hundreds of millions of refrigerators, stoves, and microwaves.

21. The massive amounts of water, soaps, and other cleansers used to clean the farms, slaughterhouses, equipment, markets, and kitchens of all sorts where all of that meat and dairy are produced, killed, sold, prepared, cooked, and eaten.

22. All the pollution left from the manufacture, marketing, packaging, and shipping of the meat and dairy products.

23. All the supplies and fuel used to deal with all of that pollution.

When a considering the environmental destruction caused by the meat, dairy, and egg industries, people should take into account the litter from fast-food and junk food that is strewn among the roads and highways of the cities, towns, and country. These are the main sources of litter. The other two main sources of litter are products that also lead to health problems: cigarettes and unhealthful drinks. Beer, soda, energy drinks, coffee, and sweetened-juice bottles, cans, and cups, along with cigarette butts, are tossed around by the billions — every day. If the North American diet were factored based on the litter found around towns and cities, and along country roads, one might conclude that we are eating the worst foods ever, topped off by beer, booze, cola, coffee, and candy. In reality, that is what a large number of people are putting into their bodies on a daily basis. The environment pays the price for our low-quality food choices and sugar, caffeine, tobacco, and alcohol addictions. And the medical, surgery, and pharmaceutical industries cash in on the ignorance, neglect, addictions, and abuse that nurture polluted land, toxic bodies, illness, and degenerative diseases.

Then there are all the resources used to run the allopathic medical industry, which largely exists to treat the results of unhealthful living. It does this by utilizing toxic drugs and risky, invasive surgery.

The entire obesity industry – from liposuction to stomach stapling and intestinal bypass to "diet" pills and programs – is the result of unhealthful living. The large majority of heart surgery is the result of people eating unhealthful food (especially dairy, meat, eggs, and processed, chemically-saturated foods), and not exercising.

All of this pollution, the animal farming, and the products associated with it, are not good for human health, or the health of Earth.

Humans do not need to drink soda or eat meat or dairy, fried foods, grilled or barbecued foods, or anything containing artificial dyes, preservatives, flavors, scents, emulsifiers, or sweeteners. The world would be a much healthier place without any of these toxic concoctions.

Again I ask, which industries use up the most amount of petroleum in North America?

> "This is a global business, and it's not only that we need to add to supply, but we need to reduce demand... In the United States alone, we have about two percent of world oil reserves, five percent of the population and yet we use about 25 percent of the world's consumption of oil."
> – James J. Mulva, chairman of ConocoPhillips Co., speaking on NBC TV's *Meet the Press*, June 18, 2006. On the same show, Shell Oil Co. President John Hofmeister explained that oil companies are holding "discussions with the White House quite frequently" with the goal of gaining greater access to U.S. federal lands (such as nature preserves and national parks), as well as local waters to explore and drill for oil and natural gas. That is truly deplorable.

The large majority of the food we grow on the continent is fed to farm animals. Raising, slaughtering, packaging, marketing, refrigerating, and cooking billions of farm animals every year uses tremendous amounts of fuel.

If you want to help save the world, stop eating meat, dairy, eggs, and processed foods.

> "The typical U.S. diet, about 28 per cent of which comes from animal sources, generates the equivalent of nearly 1.5 tons more carbon dioxide per person per year than a vegan diet with the same number of calories... By comparison, the difference in annual emissions between driving a typical saloon [sedan] car and a hybrid

car, which runs off a rechargeable battery and gasoline, is just over one ton."
> – According to study done at the University of Chicago: It's better to green your diet than your car, *New Scientist* magazine, Dec. 17, 2005

"Raising animals for food requires more than one-third of all raw materials and fossil fuels used in the United States. Producing a single hamburger patty uses enough fossil fuel to drive a small car 20 miles and enough water for 17 showers."
> – PETA, VegNow.Com, 2004

"If anyone wants to save the planet, all they have to do is just stop eating meat. That's the single most important thing you could do. It's staggering when you think about it. Vegetarianism takes care of so many things in one shot: ecology, famine, cruelty."
> – Paul McCartney

Following a vegan diet is the single most effective way you can improve the environment and the health of the world.

If you are a meat eater and think that eating meat, dairy, and eggs is your business, and none of mine, think again. Similarly to how Howard Lyman and others have stated it, I repeat the defense of the stance of vegans: If your diet style is relying on the mass breeding of animals, then it is my business, and it is the business of everyone on the planet. It impacts us environmentally, socially, physically, and financially. Your diet style pollutes the air I breathe, the water I drink, and the food I eat. It has led to, and is leading to the extinction of species, and the entire animal farming industry, including the resources needed to support it, is the main cause of global warming.

A vegetarian diet uses substantially fewer resources than the wasteful and unhealthful meat-based diet. A plant-based diet is not only healthier for humans, but also for farm workers, for the land, for plant life, for the water, for the air, for the animals, and for Earth.

"It makes me sad to be in a world where innocent animals are literally turned into products and ingredients that people can, without even the slightest thought of the suffering and cruelty that went into the making of that 'product,' simply toss into their shopping carts at the grocery stores. Worse yet are those who see the suffering and cruelty and are made aware and do nothing about it, say nothing about it, or even go as far as to defend it."
> – Sarah Kiser

HOG FARM POLLUTION

"Factory farms pose a serious public health hazard, so why are they subsidized by public money? These facilities pump out high-fat, high-cholesterol meat products and often pollute waterways – yet they also receive generous subsidies under the Farm Bill. We want Congress to stop rewarding facilities that endanger public health.

Animal waste runoff from factory farms, where chickens, pigs, and cows raised for food are confined in small spaces, has in the past contaminated waterways and even drinking water supplies and has led to disease outbreaks among humans and aquatic life. Waste from hog farms, for example, has been implicated in the contamination of North Carolina waters with the microorganism pfiesteria, killing more than 1 billion fish. The widespread use of antibiotics on factory farms has led to a proliferation of antibiotic-resistant bacteria, making it harder to treat infections among humans.

Sixty-three percent of the government's agricultural subsidies for domestic food products in recent history have directly and indirectly supported meat and dairy production. Less than 1 percent of these subsidies have gone to fruits and vegetables."
– Physicians Committee for Responsible Medicine, 2012; PCRM.org

"In our everyday lives, it may be difficult for us to relate to pigs or any farmed animal for that matter. Most of us have never met a pig in person or had the opportunity to discover that these highly social animals possess an amazing capacity for love, joy, and sorrow."
– Erica Meier

WHEN pigs live in a natural, wild environment they walk and explore many miles a day, and sleep with other pigs in a bed of twigs and/or grass. They are clean, smart, and social animals.

"Pigs are smart individuals fully aware of their own existence, and enjoy their lives when given the chance. They can spend hours playing, rooting in the ground, lying in the sun and exploring their surroundings with their keen sense of smell. They take pleasure in doing these things and like us, want to continue experiencing and enjoying their lives. Possibly those who suffer most in this industry are the 'sows' used for breeding. They are repeatedly forcibly impregnated throughout their lives, often severely confined, and then separated from their babies soon after giving birth. They suffer both physically and mentally. The lives of these pigs, and their capacity to reproduce, are seen as no more than a way of creating more units of production. Mothers unable to give birth to the required number of piglets are sent to the slaughterhouse."

    – Animal Equality

Today most pigs that are grown for human consumption are raised indoors in smelly, filthy, noisy conditions with cement floors that deform their feet. They are kept in cramped pens and fed horrible diets that are a far cry from what they would naturally eat. Pregnant pigs are kept in narrow cages that restrict their movement to the point that they can't turn or lie or stretch. Often the pregnant pigs are kept with a chain or leash around their neck that is tied to the floor or pen.

When the babies are born, the piglet's teeth are cut, their tails are sliced off, and their ears are clipped off. Then they are placed in a pen where they will spend their entire lives with hundreds and often thousands of pigs living a similar grim fate of confinement. They are limited to eating a poisonous diet that will make them as fat as possible as fast as possible. Most U.S. pigs have respiratory infections at time of slaughter. Several hundred thousand of them are slaughtered every day in the U.S., and more than that are being born.

"Basically, pork producers figured out some years ago that if they packed the maximum number of pigs into the minimum amount of space, if they pinned the creatures down into fit-to-size iron crates above slatted floors and carved out giant 'lagoons' to contain the manure – if they turned the 'farm,' in short, into a sunless hell of metal and concrete – it made everything so much more efficient. An obvious cost-saver, and from the industry's standpoint, that should settle the matter.

… It turns out that when you trap intelligent, 400- to 500-pound mammals in gestation crates 22 inches wide and seven feet long, when their limbs are broken from trying to turn or escape and they are covered in sores, blood, tumors, 'pus pockets,' and their own urine and excrement, they tend to act up a bit.

Indeed, the most notable thing is how the appearance of any human being causes a violent panic. A mere opening of the door brings on a horrific wave of roars, squeals and cage-rattling from the sows. Another memorable sight is the 'cull pen,' wherein each and

every day, the dead or dying bodies of the weak are placed, the ones who expired from the sheer, unrelenting agony of it.
– Matthew Scully, author of *Dominion: The Power of Man, the Suffering of Animals, and the Call to Mercy*; in an article published in the *Arizona Republic*, February 9, 2006

"A typical pig factory farm generates raw waste equivalent to that of a city of 12,000 people."
– PETA, VegNow.Com, 2004

Raleigh, North Carolina, *News and Observer* newspaper reporters Joby Warrick and Pat Stith, along with editor Melanie Sill, worked for several months on a series of articles that exposed the environmental disasters and health risks of hog farming in factory farms in North Carolina. In April 1996 the newspaper won the Pulitzer Prize gold medal for meritorious public service.

The articles, known as the *Boss Hog Series*, told how politicians involved in hog farming helped pave the way for a billion-dollar hog farming expansion where corporations are taking over the industry and elbowing out the small farmers. The politicians did so by influencing state agencies, introducing bills, helping to pass laws, and forming policies that provide weaker environmental regulations and zoning protection for corporate hog farming. Many legislatures in North Carolina have a history of receiving money from the hog industry, and some are investors in hog farming.

The expansion of big business hog farming in North Carolina was done in spite of complaints and concerns voiced by long-time residents, local leaders, and environmental groups. But key to the rapid expansion is the way self-serving politicians, along with contributors to political campaigns, make millions from the hog industry. The issues detailed in the *News and Observer* are not confined to North Carolina; they are issues being faced by farming and business communities all over the world. Corporate pig farm interests spent $1 million in 1998 to defeat legislators who were working to clean up the environmental hazards of factory hog farm cesspools.

The massive amounts of pollution from the hog farms in eastern North Carolina come from housing several million hogs in large steel barns (factory farms). The combination of the hogs, barns, flies, and pollution has changed the landscape, real estate value, smell, and water quality of the region. The odors from the hog farms have invaded the homes, schools, churches, and businesses of residents angered that their communities are being spoiled by the rapidly expanding hog industry.

The hog population in North Carolina resulted in the state jumping from the seventh to the second largest hog-farming state in the U.S.

Since the 1990s there are more hogs than humans in North Carolina. Each hog produces two to four times as much waste as the average human.

By the year 2000 it was estimated that hog farms in North Carolina were producing more than ten million tons of waste every year. With millions of hogs in such a small area producing that much waste, North Carolina hog farms are turning out more raw sewage than both New York City *and* the suburbs surrounding it.

The pollution produced by the hog farms in North Carolina is overwhelming the land and the people who live there. By 2005 the state had over 16 million hogs producing raw waste equal to at least 32 million people. The situation has been able to magnify so fast because North Carolina has weaker and imposes fewer environmental regulations for hog farms than any major hog-producing state.

> "Animals raised for human consumption in the U.S. generate 2.2 trillion pounds of waste each year."
> – A Voice for Animals, VoiceForAnimals.Net; 2002

The putrid waste from the hog farms is stored in thousands of cesspools that the hog industry likes to charmingly refer to as "lagoons." Those in the hog industry say the hog waste safely decomposes in the cesspools before it is sprayed onto cropland. The problem is that the land cannot absorb that much waste. The waste stored in the cesspools also leaks into ground water.

The *60 Minutes* TV show reported in December 1996 that over 30 percent of water wells near hog farms were contaminated by hog waste. The cesspools also overflow into streams and rivers during heavy rains. Millions of gallons of hog farm sludge, hog feces, hog afterbirths and blood, as well as cropland fertilizer have leaked into surrounding waterways where it has been killing aquatic life and causing algae overgrowth that chokes waterways. In one incident an estimated 25 million tons of hog waste flowed out of an eight-acre cesspool when a levee broke. Many farms have been caught dumping hog waste directly into surrounding streams, rivers, and lakes. The pollution has killed millions of fish and many other types of waterlife and caused rivers and lakes to be closed off to swimming and water sports.

In 1995 a 120,000-square-foot hog cesspool lagoon released over 25 million gallons of crap into the headwaters of North Carolina's New River. It took months to reach the ocean and killed millions of fish and unknown numbers of water mammals unfortunate enough to be in the contaminated river. In 1999 Hurricane Floyd caused so much flooding in Eastern North Carolina that it is estimated that well over 120 million gallons of hog waste made its way into the rivers and out to the sea. It carried with it tens of thousands of drowned pigs, and killed unknown millions of fish. There were too many dead fish for birds to eat, and too many pigs in the ocean for sharks to feast on.

Nitrate-nitrogen from the hog cesspools continues to leak into ground water. This is a major problem because the chemical causes methemoglobinemia, a disease that hampers the ability of the blood to absorb oxygen. It can be particularly lethal to infants who drink contaminated water.

Other ingredients of hog waste that may threaten human and animal health include bacteria, viruses, and parasites. Pfiesteria piscicidia is one of the microbes. It results in massive fish kills. When humans are exposed to this microbe they can experience skin sores, nausea, vomiting, headache, blurred vision, breathing difficulties, liver and kidney problems, memory loss, and cognitive impairment. The putrid smell from the hog farms can saturate everything in the community, including well water, food, laundry, and the structures of the homes.

In addition to the hog waste that is polluting the air, water, and land of North Carolina, the people regularly find dead hogs dumped in the countryside. The corporation may own the pigs, but the farmers who are under contract with the corporation are supposed to take care of the pigs that die and the hog waste. When the farmers under contract raise thousands of pigs they can quickly get overwhelmed with the waste and carcasses.

What is a growing problem in North Carolina is not limited to that state. The corporate players in the hog industry have expanded in several states as well as to other countries, including Eastern Europe. The type of hog farm pollution happening in North Carolina and Iowa is now a growing problem in other countries, including Poland and Brazil.

Some factory hog farm facilities are designed to hold several hundred thousand hogs with adjoining cesspools holding millions of gallons of urine mixed with feces containing all the drugs the animals were given, all of the toxic sprays they were treated with, all of the farming chemicals used on the foods the pigs ate, and a wide variety of bacteria. In addition, the lagoons contain the afterbirth of hogs, as well as stillborn pigs and piglets that died soon after birth.

One hog factory in Utah has about 500,000 pigs. Since hogs produce about three times as much excrement as humans, those 500,000 hogs produce more waste than 1.5 million people. It is a subsidiary of Smithfield Foods, a company responsible for the slaughter of about 27 million hogs in 2005. An article that appeared in *Rolling Stone* compared this Smithfield Foods slaughter in body weight to killing all of the human population of America's 32 largest cities (*Boss Hog*, by Jeff Tietz, *Rolling Stone*, Dec. 14, 2006). That same article estimated that the

251

excrement from Smithfield Foods hog farms for one year would fill four Yankee Stadiums. The article tells of factory hog farm workers who have died in these cesspools of waste, including five members of one family.

> "We've thumped as many as 120 pigs in one day. We just swing them, thump them (smashing their heads onto concrete), then toss them aside. After you've thumped then, twelve, fourteen of them, you stack them up. If some are still alive, you do this all over again. There've been times I've walked in and pigs would be running around with an eyeball hanging down the side of their face, just bleeding like crazy, or their jaw would be broken. I've seen them with broken backs still trying to get up. Some of these guys thump them, then just stand on top of their throat, smashing their jaw and everything, until they die. If you get a pig that can't move you take a meat hook, stick it into his anus and drag him backwards. A lot of times the meat hook rips out of the bunghole. I've seen hams – thighs and even intestines spill out. If the pig collapses near the front, you shove a meat hook into his cheek and drag him forward. I've seen sows being beaten with gate rods, stomped on, and dragged having their throats slowly cut with a tiny scalpel while they were still fully conscious and moaning. One day there were twenty little hogs out there and these two guys were having themselves a good old time, beating them to death with metal pipes."
> – *Slaughterhouse: The Shocking Story of Greed, Neglect, and Inhumane Treatment inside the U.S. Meat Industry*, by Gail A. Eisnitz

Heart attacks, strokes, and bypass surgery are too kind for people who support factory hog farming.

> "The animal-rights people want to impose a vegetarian's society on the U.S. Most vegetarians I know are neurotic."
> – Joseph Luter III, Chairman of Smithfield Foods, the world's largest pig farming company. It produces several billion pounds of hog meat every year, as quoted in *Boss Hog*, by Jeff Tietz, *Rolling Stone*, Dec. 14, 2006. The Environmental Protection Agency has cited Smithfield Foods for thousands of violations of the Clean Water Act.

> "When nonvegetarians say that 'human problems come first' I cannot help wondering what exactly it is that they are doing for human beings that compels them to continue to support the wasteful, ruthless exploitation of farm animals."
> – Peter Singer, *Animal Liberation*, 1990

SLAUGHTERHOUSE WORKERS: A MOST DANGEROUS JOB

"I have unfortunately been inside slaughterhouses and can tell you that the animals are not willingly walking up to the end of the kill line and sticking their necks out. These animals fight with every bit of strength they have left at the end of that kill line. They fight to get out of that kill line. They don't want to die, and they know it's coming. They see, and they know exactly what's going to happen to them. There is absolutely no truth that any process of slaughtering is humane. From the moment those animals are taken from those trucks and forced through the slaughtering process, it is the most inhumane treatment that I have ever witnessed."
– Cayce Mell

"Think occasionally of the suffering of which you spare yourself the sight."
– Albert Schweitzer

"Cowardice and selfishness among many other reasons. Hired hitmen, your money funds their knives. Paying someone else to do your dirty work doesn't make the blood any less on your hands."
– Felix Sampson

THE injury rate of slaughterhouse workers is among the highest of any industry. In 1995, according to the U.S. Occupational Safety and Health Administration, 36 percent of meatpacking plant workers sustained serious injuries. Poultry slaughterhouse workers had a 22.7 percent injury rate.

"According to the Bureau of Labor Statistics, meatpacking is the nation's most dangerous occupation. In 1999, more than one-quarter of America's nearly 150,000 meatpacking workers suffered a job-related injury or illness. The meatpacking industry not only has the highest injury rate, but also has by far the highest rate of serious injury – more than five times the national average, as measured in lost workdays. If you accept the official figures, about 40,000 meatpacking workers are injured on the job every year. But the actual number is most likely higher. The meatpacking industry has a well-documented history of discouraging injury reports, falsifying injury data, and putting injured workers back on the job quickly to minimize the reporting of lost workdays."

    — *The Chain Never Stops*, by Eric Schlosser, *Mother Jones* magazine, July/Aug. 2001

"There are no magical slaughterhouses where animals are fed their favorite meal, make a last phone call to a loved one, and voluntarily hold their breath until they die. The act of slaughter is violent, vicious, bloody, and hellish. The animals do not sacrifice themselves for your pleasure, tradition, or greed. They are dragged in kicking and screaming until their last breath. Don't fool yourself into thinking that you can eat meat, dairy, and eggs and remain disconnected from this violence. The only way out is vegan."

    — Gary Smith

"Slaughterhouses are nothing less than hells on earth. Animals are stunned, bled, hung upside down, skinned, disemboweled, and chopped into pieces that will be wrapped in cellophane... The whole process is unspeakably filthy, as agricultural science, despite its best efforts, has yet to breed a cow or pig or chicken that can be chopped up without its blood, urine, feces and vomit inconsiderately spilling out all over and mucking up the whole proceedings...

Only a single industry in America has been cited by the group Human Rights Watch for violating human rights: the nation's meatpackers and slaughterhouses. In January 2005, the group issued a detailed, 175-page report calling meatpacking 'the most dangerous factory job in America.' "

    — Former Montana cattle rancher Howard Lyman, in his book *No More Bull: The Mad Cowboy Targets America's Worst Enemy: Our Diet*, MadCowboy.Com

"In 1998, nearly 30 percent of U.S. meatpacking plant workers sustained a work-related injury or illness, making meatpacking the most dangerous job in the country in terms of nonfatal injuries. Data from the Bureau of Labor Statistics shows (from 2003-2007) the rate of illnesses and injuries for workers in 'animal slaughtering and processing' was over twice as high as the national average, and the rate of illnesses alone was over ten times the national average. Common ailments among slaughterhouse workers include back problems, torn muscles and pinched nerves, as well as more dramatic injuries such as broken bones, deep cuts and amputated fingers and limbs."

    — Slaughterhouses and Processing, SustainableTable.org

A man I knew grew up in Mexico where he began working in a slaughterhouse at the age of 13. He eventually moved to the United States, where, as an undocumented worker, he continued to work in slaughterhouses. He spent a total of 14 years in that line of work. He often began his day by slitting the throat of a cow and drinking the fresh blood as it poured out of the wound. At the last slaughterhouse he worked in there would be about five additional workers kept on hand every day, in addition to the 30 who were scheduled to work. The extra five were there to take over for the workers who got injured that day. Every day there would be injuries that required a worker to take the rest of the day off, or to be taken to a hospital for stitches, or worse. He saw workers lose fingers, break bones, and get kicked in the face by cows, sometimes breaking facial bones. And he often saw cows being cut up before they were fully dead. He finally left the business after he suffered a stab wound on his arm that cut through tendons and nerves that controlled half of his left hand.

"Improperly stunned hogs kick and scream as they are drowned in tanks of scalding-hot water, used to soften their skin. Cows struggle as the skin is ripped from their bodies. Chickens, who aren't even included in the only federal law designed to protect animals killed for food, have their throats slit while they're still conscious and are scalded to death in tanks of hot water by the millions."
– *Slaughterhouse Workers: Dying for a Job*, by Lindsay Rajt, OpEdNews.com

The injuries combined with the hellish visions the slaughterhouse workers are exposed to take a toll. Apparently killing and cutting up farm animals all day is not a very enjoyable job, and most workers do not hold onto their jobs for very long. Some animal-killing and meatpacking companies experience more than an 80 percent annual employee turnover rate. The low wages slaughterhouse workers are paid become even lower as companies may deduct charges for lunch meals, work clothes, and, when living on company property, rent.

"No one knows more about the suffering farmed animals endure than the workers in slaughterhouses and on factory farms, many of whom are desperate for employment and working for low wages in horrific conditions.

Although it seems easy to think of these workers as cold and uncaring individuals who abuse and torture animals for a living, there are many who took these jobs out of desperation – or were simply unaware of the conditions inside. In many ways they too are victims of a brutal industry."

> – Behind Closed Doors: Former Factory Farm & Slaughterhouse Workers Speak Out; *Outrage: The Magazine of Mercy for Animals*, Summer/Fall 2006; MercyForAnimals.Org

The high turnover rate among workers in the $100-billion animal-killing and meatpacking industry has caused many U.S. slaughterhouses to rely on the cheapest and most uneducated labor they can find – often those labeled as "illegal immigrants," who may have been recruited by the meatpacking companies from their native towns in Mexico and Central America, from U.S. towns on the Mexican border, or from the Asian immigrant populations of larger U.S. cities.

During 2006, agents of the U.S. Immigration and Customs Enforcement office conducted a series of raids on slaughterhouses and meatpacking plants. In this raid that took place in December of that year, there were 1,282 "legal" and "illegal" immigrants arrested at Swift & Co. meatpacking plants in six states. The raids were part of a ten-month investigation into allegations that the immigrants were using fake or stolen identities of U.S. citizens. Swift & Co. executives say they relied on the government's own Basic Pilot system to check the identities of the employees, but that the system is flawed. The company operated nine plants in eight states, turning a profit of about $10 billion a year, and was the third largest beef and pork processor in the country. About 10 percent of its employees were taken away in the raids.

Many of the immigrants were transfered to a detention center in Atlanta, while others were taken to Camp Dodge, a National Guard base in Johnston, Iowa, where they faced deportation hearings.

Random raids on slaughterhouses continue. Even though many slaughterhouse workers are married to U.S. citizens and have children in the U.S., they are deported and face a future far away from their families. Many other workers who do not get arrested in the raids go into hiding so they avoid deportation. Often the households with children that are suddenly single-parent households rely on government assistance and charities to make up for lost income.

Hiring recent immigrants to work in the U.S. meatpacking plants is something that has been going on for decades. It has been mentioned in many books, and it was the subject of a special investigation, The New Jungle, that appeared in the September 23, 1996, edition of *U.S. News & World Report* magazine. That investigative report told of how meatpacking giant IBP regularly advertised for workers on Spanish-language radio stations in southern Texas.

A report in the *Los Angeles Times* told of chicken slaughterhouses in Missouri, Mississippi, North Carolina, Arkansas, and Georgia recruiting workers from the Rio Grande Valley in southern Texas where unemployment is high and cheap laborers are easy to find. The recruiting was often done by placing English and Spanish help-wanted newspaper ads saying that no experience is necessary, transportation to Missouri is provided, and housing is available for those who want to work in the slaughterhouses (1,000 Miles of Hope, and Heartache, by Jesse Katz, *Los Angeles Times*, November 10, 1996). While the events of 2001 changed some things for people immigrating illegally to the U.S., the hiring of undocumented workers by slaughterhouses continues.

Some slaughterhouses and meatpacking plants also use connections in Mexico to find workers to come to America. When officials working for the Immigration and Naturalization Service raided the Swift & Company meatpacking plant in Marshalltown, Iowa, in the mid-1990s they detained at least 125 suspected illegal workers out of the approximately 900 workers at the site. The raid took place after it was discovered that many of the employees had submitted false information to the company. This kind of raid where "illegal immigrants" are found working in U.S. meatpacking plants is not unusual. The New Jungle article told of a 1,000-an-hour hog-processing plant in Storm Lake, Iowa, owned by meatpacking industry giant IBP Inc, where 78 "illegal immigrants" were detained and sent back to Mexico.

Three companies have a history of controlling a majority of the beef and pork industry in America: Cargill's Excel Corp., Con-Agra's Monfort, Inc., and Tyson.

The pay at the meatpacking plants is what entices the workers to come from Mexico and Central America. While workers in Mexico may make a few dollars a day, and unemployment is high, they can work for $6 to $10 or more per hour in the U.S. meatpacking plants. Towns in Mexico have maintained long-term relations with certain meatpacking plants in the Midwest.

With more and more meatpacking plants being located in rural areas away from big cities, living quarters can be relatively cheap compared to city housing prices. The number of recent immigrants working at large meatpacking plants can transform surrounding towns into Spanish-speaking communities. It strains the towns to have to provide schooling for the large number of foreign-speaking immigrant children. It allows the meatpacking companies to keep expenses low by employing recent immigrants who work for the low pay without medical or other benefits. While there may be more employment in the town, that doesn't mean it is necessarily a good thing for the town or for the workers. It may mean that the workers end up living in rural slums.

> "There are 220 packing plants in Iowa and Nebraska. Our estimate is that 25 percent of the workers in those plants are illegal."
> – Jerry Heinauer, district director of the INS, quoted in The New Jungle, by Stephen J. Hedges, Dana Hawkins, and Penny Loeb, *U.S. News & World Report*, Sept. 23, 1996

Being an undocumented worker in America means that you do not get unemployment benefits if you lose your job, may not get proper medical care if you are injured on the job, and at any moment you can be deported if you are caught by agents working for the U.S. Federal Immigration and Naturalization Service, who may raid your place of work. If you do receive health insurance, you may not be able to afford the premium, and you may avoid going to the doctor altogether because you fear authority figures who may report you and have you deported. If you get deported before you get your weekly pay there is a strong likelihood that you will never receive it.

Finding work in a meatpacking plant is relatively easy for workers carrying fake immigration papers. While you may be able to get the papers, your employer doesn't have to prove the documents are legitimate; that is the job of the immigration agents who may show up at your workplace. It is also easy to find work in the meatpacking plants because many of them are no longer unionized. That presents another combination of problems because, as a nonunion worker and nonresident, if you have a grievance about your work conditions you have nobody to turn to, and little if any legal recourse.

> "Workers on the killing floor are in constant contact with feces, vomit and diseased animals, so it's no surprise that they often fall ill themselves. One study of slaughterhouse workers by the Johns Hopkins Bloomberg School of Public Health found that half tested positive for campylobacter bacteria, which can cause diarrhea, stomach cramps and fever."
> – Slaughterhouse Workers: Dying for a Job, by Lindsay Rajt, OpEdNews.com

> "As long as there are slaughterhouses, there will be battlefields."
> – Leo Tolstoy

For more information on this topic, read Eric Schlosser's book *Fast Food Nation*. It is also a theatrical film directed by Richard Linklater and featuring an excellent cast of actors, including Greg Kinnear. Parts of the film take place in a real slaughterhouse, and are very gruesome as they show the real process of killing and chopping apart animals.

> "Although slaughterhouses account for a small portion of most meats' overall carbon footprint, they dump millions of pounds of

toxic pollutants into America's waterways (nitrogen, phosphorus, ammonia, etc.). Eight slaughterhouses consistently rank among the nation's top 20 industrial polluters, responsible for discharging 30 million pounds of contamination in 2009."
 – Environmental Working Group, July 2011

"As I cannot kill, I cannot authorize others to kill. Do you see? If you are buying from a butcher you are authorizing him to kill – to kill helpless, dumb creatures which neither you nor I could kill ourselves."
 – Paul Troubetzkoy

"I was the merchant banker whose favorite meal was filet mignon and lobster. Around twelve years ago I was mandated to act for a large corporate client and visited one of their main subsidiaries. It turned out to be a slaughterhouse. And I had never seen a slaughterhouse before. My blood ran cold. This didn't just turn me into a vegetarian. It turned me into a genuinely compassionate human being. Anybody who eats the murdered carcass of an innocent animal cannot claim to be compassionate – not with a straight face anyway.

The slaughterhouse turned my life around. I ultimately became vegan eight years ago when I saw what happens to millions of chickens – their beaks burned off, millions of tiny male chicks being hurled to their death into grinders, premature calves being deliberately induced and being killed by crushing to death. It is a crime of unimaginable proportions. It is so tiresome to still hear the hideous lies and self-delusion from those who profit from this ghastly trade.

I am a vegan because I love life in all its forms. The life of a human necrovore is not a life. It is a life sentence. Short, nasty, and brutish."
 – Philip Wollen

"May our daily choices be a reflection of our deepest values, and may we use our voices to speak for those who need us most, those who have no voice, those who have no choice."
 – Colleen Patrick-Goudreau

"The problem is that humans have victimized animals to such a degree that they aren't even considered victims. They aren't even considered at all. They're nothing, literally, they don't count, they don't matter, they're commodities, like TV sets and cell phones."
 – Gary Yourofsky, ADAPTT.org

"It's not a requirement to eat animals, we just chose to do it, so it

becomes a moral choice and one that is having a huge impact on the planet, using up resources and destroying the biosphere."
– James Cameron

"Until we have the courage to recognize cruelty for what it is – whether its victim is human or animal – we cannot expect things to be much better in this world. We cannot have peace among men whose hearts delight in killing any living creature. By every act that glorifies or even tolerates such moronic delight in killing we set back the progress of humanity."
– Rachel Carson

"Whereas predators kill to survive, sport hunters and fishers wound and kill for fun. Whereas nonhumans rarely prolong the act of killing, bullfighters, vivisectors, and other humans routinely torture to death. Each day, fish purveyors kill millions of birds, mammals, and fishes for profit. For mere convenience and taste, consumers eat the remains. Directly or indirectly, most humans routinely, knowingly participate in the needless infliction of suffering and death. While boasting of 'human kindness,' our species treats nonhumans – and often humans – with extreme injustice and cruelty."
– Karen Davis, United Poultry Concerns

"Egg-laying hens don't just appear out of thin air. They are bred in an industrial system where 250 million male chicks are either ground up alive or suffocated [because the male chicks are of no use since they can't grow up and lay eggs]. This is the same whether that hen finds herself on a factory farm or a small family farm. And when her body is broken down from years of abuse, she is murdered for chicken sandwiches or nuggets. So yes, there is violence and murder in your eggs."
– Gary Smith

VEAL: A SPECIAL SORT OF CRUELTY

"Endless multitudes will have their little children taken from them, ripped open and flayed and most cruelly cut in pieces."
– Leonardo da Vinci, who was outspoken against the killing and consumption of animals

"Think of me tonight. For that which you savor. Did it give you something real, or could you taste the pain of my death in its flavor?"
– Wayne K. Tolson

"We manage to swallow flesh only because we do not think of the cruel and sinful thing that we do."
– Rabindranath Tagore

"A dead cow or sheep lying in the pasture is recognized as carrion. The same sort of carcass dressed and hung up on a butcher's stall passes as food."
– J.H. Kellogg

"A newborn baby is taken from his mother and placed in a 'crate' so narrow he can't turn around or even lie down comfortably. Instead of nourishing mother's milk, he is fed a substitute liquid that is purposely deficient in iron and fiber – the better to keep his flesh pale. And since he can hardly move in his confined space, his muscles won't develop and he will stay soft and tender. He will endure this for four months… and then he'll be slaughtered and eaten.

Male calves are an unwanted 'by-product' of the dairy industry, as they cannot produce milk. They are trucked to livestock auctions within hours or days of being born and sold for just a few dollars to veal producers. If the calves are too weak or ill to sell after the grueling truck ride, they may be left to die in pens or back alleyways at the auction yards.

At the veal factories, each calf is chained at the neck in a crate only 22 inches wide, so he can't walk or turn around. Because the iron-deficient diet makes him anemic and sickly, his formula routinely contains drugs… that can get passed on to the unsuspecting consumer. The calf suffers from chronic diarrhea, and he is not even allowed to have water to drink – just the liquid diet that produces what is misleadingly labeled 'milk-fed' – and also 'fancy' or 'white' – veal.

Because this is considered a 'common agribusiness practice' it is typically exempt from animal-cruelty laws. As a matter of fact, the production of veal is specifically excluded from anticruelty laws in the majority of U.S. states. In Europe, several nations have banned the inhumane, severe confinement producer for calves that is standard operating procedure in the U.S. But, the meat and dairy industries are a wealthy, powerful lobbying and advertising force… and they have been defeating farm animal protection efforts for decades."
– Farm Sanctuary No Veal Campaign; FarmSantuary.Org

"I observe the spirit of Mother's Day every day by not eating anyone's children."
– Victor Sjodin

"If you had to kill your own calf before you ate him, most likely you would not be able to do it. To hear the calf scream, to see the blood spill, to see the baby being taken away from his momma, and to see the look of death in the animal's eye would turn your stomach. So you get the man at the packing house to do the killing for you."
– Dick Gregory

"I became a vegan the day I watched a video of a calf being born on a factory farm. The baby was dragged away from his mother before he hit the ground. The helpless calf strained its head backwards to find his mother. The mother bolted after her son and exploded into a rage when the rancher slammed the gate on her. She wailed the saddest noise I'd ever heard an animal make, and then thrashed and dug into the ground, burying her face in the muddy placenta. I had no idea what was happening respecting brain chemistry, animal instinct, or whatever. I just knew that this was deeply wrong. I just knew that such suffering could never be worth the taste of milk and veal. I empathized with the cow and the calf and, in so doing, my life changed.
– James McWilliams

"Let no one regard as light the burden of his responsibility. While so much ill treatment of animals goes on, while the moans of thirsty animals in railway trucks sound unheard, while so much brutality prevails in our slaughterhouses, we all bear guilt. Everything that lives has value as a living thing, as one of the

manifestations of the mystery that is life."
– Albert Schweitzer

"Your ability to confine, mutilate, and destroy does not place you at the 'top of the food chain.' Your inability to comprehend their language does not by default make them 'stupid.' Your use of written language, organized religion, and adhering to societal norms do not obviate personal responsibility. Today is a great day to go vegan."
– Dr. Holly Wilson

"'But… What about cheese?' Spare me your hysteria and emotional attachment to this food. What about the enslaved cows and their stolen babies? What about the pure absurdity in consuming another mammal's milk? What about the rape rack and the veal crate? Before you ask, answer these questions."
– Dr. Holly Wilson

"What are we to think of people who, despite knowing about the animal abuse they are contributing to, continue to buy animal products? To me, this is the most difficult aspect of being vegan: trying to understand why otherwise 'good people' continue to cling to products of horrific cruelty, when none of it is necessary."
– Jo Tyler

"As infuriating and disheartening it is to have your pleas for compassion fall upon deaf ears, never give up. Animals don't have a voice, so make sure people never stop hearing yours."
– Felix Sampson

"All nature protests against the barbarity of man, who misapprehends, who humiliates, and tortures his inferior brethren."
– Jules Michelet

"All beings tremble before violence. All fear death. All love life. See yourself in others. Then whom can you hurt? What harm can you do?"
– Buddha

Compassion Action Institute, PleaseBeKind.Com
Farm Sanctuary East, POB 150, Watkins Glen, NY 14891; 607-583-2225; FarmSanctuary.Org; FactoryFarming.Com; NoVeal.Org
Farm Sanctuary West, POB 1065, Orland, CA 95963; 530-865-4617; FarmSanctuary.Org; FactoryFarming.Com; NoVeal.Org
Humane Society of the United States, HSUS.Org

Vivisection: Animal torture

"Atrocities are not less atrocities when they occur in laboratories and are called medical research."
– George Bernard Shaw

"They laugh, like us. They are devoted to their families, like us. They show compassion, like us. They have unique personalities, like us. When they are confined, hurt, or experimented on, they get depressed, they get angry, they cry, and they grieve. Like us."
– ReleaseChimps.Org

"Vivisection is the blackest of all the black crimes that a man is at present committing against God and his fair creation."
– Mahatma Gandhi

"Each year an estimated 28 million animals in the U.S. are used in research, testing, and education, including:
• 70,000 dogs
• 23,00 cats
• 54,000 nonhuman primates
• 266,000 guinea pigs
• 201,000 hamsters
• 280,000 rabbits
• 155,000 farm animals, including cattle, sheep, and pigs
• 165,000 others, such as gerbils, ferrets, and minks
• Approximately 20–25 million rats and mice."
– A Voice for Animals, VoiceForAnimals.Net; 2006

ANIMALS kept in "science labs" are often purposefully injured, such as by burning them, breaking their bones, cutting off their limbs or facial parts, and having drills and surgical tools put into their brains and other parts of their body. Some have their eyes sewn shut. Others have harsh chemicals put into their eyes, on their skin, or into their mouths. Some have electrodes implanted into their skin, muscles, and brain. Some are exposed to extreme noise, nonstop wind, heat, cold, and other experiments. When they are of no more use to the lab workers these horribly abused animals are left to die, or are killed.

"The relationship of homo sapiens to the other animals is one of unremitting exploitation. We must employ their work; we eat and wear them. We exploit them to serve our superstitions: Whereas we

used to sacrifice them to our gods and tear out their entrails in order to foresee the future, we now sacrifice them to science, and experiment on their entrails in the hope – or on the mere off chance – that we might thereby see a little more clearly into the present. To us it seems incredible that the Greek philosophers should have scanned so deeply into right and wrong and yet never noticed the immorality of slavery. Perhaps 3,000 years from now it will seem equally incredible that we do not notice the immorality of our own oppression of animals."
– Brigid Brophy

Who funds these laboratory experiments? Many of them are paid for by grants from the National Institutes of Health, which is funded by tax dollars. Another tax-supported agency involved with animal experimentation is the U.S. Department of Agriculture. Other labs are supported by businesses, such as those that manufacture various products. Some animal farming businesses use animals to experiment on to develop new ways of slaughtering farm animals. It is all horrible.

"But aren't these experiments necessary to save human lives?
No, absolutely not. There are better ways to study human physiology, disease, and injury than inducing disease and injury in a different species.   – –
Clinical human studies, autopsies, epidemiology, human tissue studies, and imaging technologies are only some of the better ways to study human health and disease."
– New England Anti-Vivisection Society, NEAVS.Org

Many cosmetics companies have been involved in animal experimentation. Federally funded agencies that have been involved in vivisection include the National Institute of Neurological Disorders and Stroke; the National Center for Research Resources; the National Institute of Diabetes & Digestive & Kidney Diseases; and the National Heart, Lung and Blood Institute. Many universities also run labs where animals are tortured. These include Boston University, Harvard University, the University of Massachusetts Medical School, and UCLA. But that is a very short list. For more information on companies, government agencies, schools and others conducting animal experimentation, contact the organizations listed in this section.

"In the past three years, approximately $15 million taxpayer dollars went into federally funded cat experiments in the state of Massachusetts alone."
– New England Anti-Vivisection Society, NEAVS.Org; 2002

265

"If you agree with vivisection, go and be vivisected upon yourself."
– Morrissey, during concert in London, May 2006. Commenting about a new £20 million animal testing lab at Oxford University. The week before, Oxford University won a legal appeal to keep demonstrators away from the "biomedical" animal torture facility.

"What do they know – all these scholars, all these philosophers, all the leaders of the world? They have convinced themselves that man, the worst transgressor of all the species, is the crown of creation. All other creatures were created merely to provide him with food, pelts, to be tormented, exterminated. In relation to them, all people are Nazis; for the animals it is an eternal Treblinka."
– Isaac Bashevis Singer, 1978 Nobel Prize winner

"That vivisectors can look them in the eyes while perpetrating one atrocity after another on them is testament to the amorality that science permits itself. The poor, orphans, criminals, the mentally ill, Jews, and African-Americans were all at some time within the vivisector's reach. Equally disturbing is that chimpanzees still are."
– Theodora Capaldo, EdD, President of the New England Anti-Vivisection Society, NEAVS.Org

"It is easy for me to see the connection between the entertainment industry and biomedical research for chimpanzees because I face it every day. I see their faces, and I think about what their lives were like before [arriving at The Fauna Foundation]. Half of my chimpanzee family began their lives in entertainment only to end up being used for biomedical research. I am ashamed by the lack of respect they were shown by humans. They deserve so much more."
– Gloria Grow, The Fauna Foundation; FaunaFoundation.Org

"There are many reasons why the rat is an unsound model for toxicity testing and other experiments. Rat anatomy and physiology differ enormously from that of humans, and the dissimilarities render research invalid and harmful when extrapolated to humans. For example, rats rarely vomit; do not have a gall bladder; do not have sweat glands; cannot pant; are poor regulators of body temperature; have twice the concentrating ability for urine; and, have a heart rate four times that of a human.
Many drug studies on rats were inaccurate and dangerous when extrapolated to humans, including Flosint, an arthritis medication, which proved fatal to humans; Zelmid, an antidepressant, which caused neurological damage in humans; and Clioquinal, an

antidiarrheal, which caused blindness and paralysis in humans – all despite animal testing."
– New England Anti-Vivisection Society, NEAVS.Org; 2002

"Let me say it openly: we are surrounded by an enterprise of degradation, cruelty, and killing which rivals anything the Third Reich was capable of, indeed dwarfs it, in that ours is an enterprise without end, self-regenerating, bringing rabbits, rats, poultry, livestock ceaselessly into the world for the purpose of killing them."
– John Maxwell, South African author

"If you don't like my opinions leave. But just remember, the animals can't leave the cages that hold them. They are captive and suffering. As you cozy into your bed tonight, try to imagine the pain and the suffering that they endure day after day and night after night. Next time you get some soap in your eyes, try to imagine that pain for 3 or 4 days at a time. Next time you have a stomachache, try to imagine liquid plumber being poured down your throat till you puke so much blood that you bleed to death. Next time you bump your head, try to imagine being a monkey and getting a steel plate smashed into your skull at 50 miles per hour. Then, only then should you feel compelled to tell me that I'm wrong about my opinions. For all these things have happened in the name of science. They continue in abundance till this day."
– Rikki Rocket

"If a man aspires towards a righteous life, his first act of abstinence is from injury to animals."
– Leo Tolstoy

"Every year tens of thousands of animals suffer and die in laboratory tests of cosmetics and household products – despite the fact that the test results do not help prevent or treat accidental or purposeful misuse of the products. Please, join me in using your voice for those whose cries are forever sealed behind the laboratory doors."
– Woody Harrelson

American Anti-Vivisection Society, AAVS.Org
AnimalAid.Org.UK
Animal Protection Institute, API4Animals.Org
AnimalsNeedRights.Net
AnimalSuffering.Com
British Anti-Vivisection Society, BAVA.PWP.BlueYonder.CO.UK
British Union for the Abolition of Vivisection, BUAV.Org
Coalition to Abolish Animal Testing, OHSUKillsPrimates.Com
Dawn Watch, DawnWatch.Com/Animal_Testing.htm

FreeAnimals.Org
The Humane Society of the United States, HSUS.Org
In Defense of Animals, IDAUSA.Org; VivisectionInfo.Org
Irish Anti-Vivisection Society, IrishAntiVivisection.Org
Italian Anti-Vivisection Scientific Committee, AntiVivisezione.IT
Last Chance for Animals, LCAnimal.Org
National Anti-Vivisection Society, NAVS.Org
New England Anti-Vivisection Society, NEAVS.Org
New Zealand Anti-Vivisection Society, NZAVS.Org.NZ
People for the Ethical Treatment of Animals, PETA.Org;
   StopAnimalTests.Com
Physicians Committee for Responsible Medicine, PCRM.Org
Stop Animal Exploitation Now, All-Creatures.Org
Uncaged.CO.UK
Vivisection-Absurd.Org.UK

"I am not interested to know whether vivisection produces results that are profitable to the human race. The pain which it inflicts upon unconsenting animals is the basis of my enmity toward it, and it is to me sufficient justification of the enmity without looking further."
– Mark Twain

"There's really no such thing as the 'voiceless.' There are the deliberately silenced, or the preferably unheard."
– Arundhati Roy

"While the experience of each individual and each group that has endured oppression and injustice is unique and must be recognized and respected as such, the mindset of those benefiting from the exploitation of others remains remarkably consistent across culture and context, and across centuries. Pro-slavery advocates systematically worked to manipulate the public into focusing on the manner of treatment, rather than the injustice of the enslavement itself. The parallels with today's struggle for justice for other-than-human animals are stunning, with industry lies and manipulations shifting the emphasis towards 'humane' treatment rather than questioning the privilege of domination itself."
– James LaVeck

"Around the time I got beaten up for being gay, gasping for breath, surrounded by people looking down at me laughing, I caught a very big fish. When I pulled him on the boat, it was just an ugly flounder, and he was gasping for breath, too, and in that instance, the flounder was the only creature I could relate to. I had turned into the bully."
– Dan Mathews

FUR INDUSTRY: CRUELTY, PAIN, SUFFERING, KILLING, AND MINK COATS

"Not to hurt our humble brethren in fur, feather or fin, is our first duty to them, but to stop there is not enough. We have a higher mission: to be of service to them whenever they require it."
– Francis of Assisi

"Where we find wrongs done to animals, it is no excuse to say that more important wrongs are done to human beings, and let us concentrate on those. A wrong is a wrong, and often the little ones, when they are shrugged off as nothing, spread and do the gravest harm to ourselves and others."
– Matthew Scully

"When I was a little girl, I rescued hurt animals, always had pets, rats, mice, dogs, etc. And I helped my neighbor with her farm. I've always loved animals immensely. I have been known to tell people with fur on how disgusting they look. I'm pretty vocal. I have had plenty of bad reactions, but it doesn't stop me. At the end of the day, I will always side with the animals. Cruelty is cruelty, plain and simple."
– Pink

"Fur used to turn heads, now it turns stomachs."
– Rue McClanahan

"Dog and cat fur is often falsely labeled to obscure the true source of the fur. Dog fur products have been sold as Gae-wolf, Asian wolf, Asiatic raccoon, China wolf, Corsac fox, Goupee, Pommern wolf, Loup d'Asie, Asian jackal, Dogue de Chine, Sobakigae-wolf, Mongolian dog fur, and Asiatic raccoon, Mountain Goat skin, Sakon Makhon lamb, Kou pi, Dog skin plasters (sold in Chinatowns as a cure for rheumatism). Cat fur has been sold as Housecat, Wildcat, Katzenfelle, Goyangi, Mountain cat, rabbit, maopee, gatto cinesi, natuerliches mittel, and chat de Chine. Fur manufacturers in China told (Humane Society of The U.S. (HSUS) investigators they could sew any label they asked for onto dog and cat fur products to make them more marketable.

Since 1997, HSUS has investigated and documented the international trade in dog and cat fur and skins. This undercover

269

investigation has spanned the globe from source countries in China, the Philippines, and Thailand to retailers and wholesalers in the U.S., Russia, and the European Union.

Over two million dogs and cats are slaughtered each year for their furs and skins, mostly in China and other Asian countries. Investigators documented 50,000 to 100,000 cat pelts stockpiled at animal byproduct factories in China. At least ten dogs are slaughtered to make a single coat, more if puppies are used. Up to 24 cats are slaughtered to make one fur coat. Dog and cat fur is used in trims, linings, hats, decorative figurines, and folk remedies. Skins are used in dog chew toys and shoe leather.

The slaughter of these animals is violent and pitiless. Cats are strangled inside their cages as other cats look on. Dogs are noosed about the neck by metal wires, and then slashed across the groin. The wire noose cuts into their throats as they struggle in pain before finally losing consciousness. In Harbin China, HSUS investigators documented a German shepherd still blinking and conscious as he was being skinned. At a dog farm several hours north of Harbin, investigators documented dead dogs hanging from hooks as others, still alive, awaited their fate outside the same cold, dismal room.

An investigator from Swiss Animals Protection/East International said: 'Conditions on Chinese fur farms make a mockery of the most elementary animal welfare standards... In their lives and their unspeakable deaths, these animals have been denied even the simplest acts of kindness.'

A LIFE OF MISERY BEFORE THEIR BRUTAL DEATH:

Fur-bearing animals are killed by gassing, neck breaking, and electrocution, clubbing, trapping, and injection with poisons so as not to damage their pelts. These animals live horrendous existences when they are 'ranch-raised' on a 'fur farm,' or are brutally killed in the hands of trappers. On ranches, they spend their entire lives in tiny, filthy cages and suffer tremendously; many become deranged until they meet with brutal deaths. The U.S. produces about 10 percent of the cage-raised fur in the world; 60 to 75 percent of the fur in coats sold in the U.S. comes from cage-raised animals, and 90 percent of cage-raised foxes are used in fur trim. (HSUS 2004).

– AntiFurSociety.org

"It's baffling how any clothier with a conscience could ignore the fact that this year alone, more than 2 million animals – including cats and dogs exactly like those we share our homes with – will be shoved into wire cages so tightly that they can't move and be trucked across China to be slaughtered. Some of them will be dead by the time they arrive. They are the lucky ones.

Those who survive will feel their bones break when workers throw the crates around like rag dolls. They may be beaten and stomped on. Or they may have the skin ripped from their bodies while they scream and thrash in pain."

– People for the Ethical Treatment of Animals, PETA.org

"Considering what animals endure there is nothing fashionable about fur. Please shun it.

– Stella McCartney, fashion designer

"Although it was a fabulous hit with the fashion world at the time, I realized later, with sorrow, that a quarter-million leopards had been killed in order to enable this fashion trend.

Animals continue to be needlessly slaughtered to satisfy the demands of thoughtless people who themselves remain entrapped in unnecessary fashion."

– Oleg Cassini, designer who dressed Jackie Kennedy in a leopard-skin coat in the 1950s. *New York Post,* May 13, 1999

"Animal rights provokes hostility from the arrogant people who enjoy power over animals, from the insecure who boost themselves by demeaning and exploiting animals, and from the guilty who do not want to confront their ignorance and implication in violence against animals."

– Dr. Steve Best

"It's a matter of taking the side of the weak against the strong. Something the best people have always done."

– Harriet Beecher Stowe

"I know of no sight more sorrowful than that of these unoffending animals as they are seen in the torture grip of these traps. They sit drawn up into a little heap, as if collecting all their force of endurance to support agony; some sit in a half-torpid state induced by intense suffering."

– Charles Darwin

"Killing an animal to make a coat is a sin. It wasn't meant to be and we have no right to do it. A woman gains status when she refuses to see anything killed to be put on her back. Then she's truly beautiful."

– Doris Day

Anti-fur Society, AntiFurSociety.org
Coalition to Abolish the Fur Trade, CAFT.org.UK
International Anti-Fur Coalition, Anti-FurCoalition.org
People for the Ethical Treatment of Animals, PETA.org

WATERLIFE: THE COLLAPSE OF THE SEAS

> "All of life is interrelated. We are all caught in an inescapable
> network of mutuality, tied to a single garment of destiny. Whatever
> affects one directly affects all indirectly."
> – Dr. Martin Luther King, Jr.

EVERY sea mammal and every type of fish, crustacean, and mollusk
is on the critical list. So are the seabirds and the bears that depend
on fish for their survival. The microscopic animals of the seas are also in
trouble. This is because air and industrial pollution is changing the
acidity level of the oceans and poisoning sea life; because synthetic
farming chemicals and waste from farmed animals are causing massive
algae blooms that block light and choke off waterlife; because of fishing,
recreational, cruise line, industrial, and military watercraft; and because
plastic trash is both killing marine life and gathering in and leaching
chemicals into the rivers, lakes, and oceans. To put it mildly, what is
going on in the oceans threatens every form of sea life, every form of
life dependent on ocean life, and every human on every area of the
planet.

Since the middle of the 1800s, the amount of carbon dioxide (CO_2)
in the atmosphere has increased in relation to the use of fossil fuels
(coal, petroleum, and natural gas). The burning of fossil fuels releases
carbon dioxide into the atmosphere. Plants naturally absorb carbon
dioxide. But the amount of carbon dioxide being produced by humans is
far beyond the amount that could be absorbed by the plants on Earth.
The oceans, lakes, and rivers also absorb carbon dioxide. But the world's
bodies of water are absorbing far more carbon dioxide than they would
in a balanced atmosphere.

The industrial pollution and carbon dioxide from the use of fossil
fuels have greatly increased the acidity of the oceans. The oceans of the
world are experiencing the worst acid trips ever. Because pollution can
hang in the atmosphere for decades, the oceans keep absorbing more of
it, and humans keep creating more of it, there are no signs that the acid
trip of the seas is going to come down soon.

The increasingly acidic situation of the oceans doesn't damage the
marine life only at the surface, but impacts marine life miles below
water. Every part of the ocean, from the surface that is increasingly

polluted with floating bits of plastic and oil slicks, to the water that is increasing in acidity and in toxic chemicals, to the bottoms of the oceans, which are becoming coated with sediment pollution and pools of chemicals, and to every living thing in and around the oceans, from the coral reefs to fish and sea mammals and sea birds, and also the land animals reliant on the ocean life, is being impacted by how people live, the products they use, and what they do with water, soil, and garbage.

Consider that you play a role in the health of the oceans. Even if you live more than a thousand miles from an ocean, what you do impacts the water that flows into rivers and lakes, and eventually into oceans. The electricity you use may originate from coal-burning electricity generating plants, which spew pollution into the air. That pollution contains mercury, which ends up in the oceans, poisoning fish and sea mammals, and the birds and animals that feed off that sea life. Because of mercury pollution, every large fish and every mammal that eats the fish contains mercury – which is highly toxic and leads to birth deformities, miscarriages, cancers, learning disorders, and a variety of health problems in humans.

> "History will not only judge us by our mistakes, but by what we do to fix them."
> – Jacques Yves Cousteau

The oceans start where you live. It doesn't matter if you live on top of a mountain, or in the meadowlands in the center of a continent. What you do impacts the distant oceans.

The way you live, including the foods you choose to eat, the variety of cleansers you use, the types of medications you take, the type of transportation you use, and the sources of energy you use, impacts the aquifers, rivers, lakes, and oceans around the planet.

Whenever you eat, consider what types of labor, energy, chemicals, packaging, and other resources and products were used to grow and bring that food to your plate.

When you use electricity, consider what types of resources are being used to create the energy.

When you use cleaning products, consider what sorts of chemicals they contain.

When you breathe, consider that the oxygen you depend on is being produced by trees and plants in forests and meadows, and by sea and water plants, thousands of miles away.

When you see water, realize that you and all life on the planet consist mainly of water. If the water bodies of Earth are not healthy, neither is humanity. If life in and around the water bodies of Earth dies, so will humanity.

Books:
Extinction: The Death of Waterlife on Planet Earth, by John McCabe
The Great Lakes Water Wars, by Peter Annin
Sea of Slaughter, by Farley Mowat
When the Rivers Run Dry: Water – The Defining Crisis of the Twenty-first Century, by Fred Pearce

Documentaries:
The Big Fix, TheBigFixMovie.com
Flow, FlowTheFilm.com
Tapped, TappedTheMovie.com

Please watch this free 22-minute documentary produced by the Natural Resources Defense Council: Acid Test: The Global Challenge of Ocean Acidification;
nrdc.org/oceans/acidification/aboutthefilm.asp

The documentary is about the rising acidity of the oceans. Everyone should understand the dire consequences of this problem. If you don't understand what burning fossil fuels is doing to the oceans and all life in and around the oceans, this documentary will explain some of it to you. In 2009, scientists estimated that 22 million tons of carbon dioxide is being absorbed into the oceans every day. In the ocean, carbon dioxide turns into acid, and this interfered with all forms of life in and around the oceans. Because of rising acidity, tiny sea creatures are dying, including those that make up coral reefs. One in every four sea creatures lives in, on, or around coral reefs. When the small life-forms in the seas die, it impacts food sources of all fish, sea mammals, sea birds, bears, eagles, and other wildlife. If the microscopic sea life dies, we all die. The microscopic sea life is dying. Currently, only 25 percent of the sea coral in the oceans is left. The rest has died off in the past 100 years. The smallest forms of sea life, including pteropods and krill, are not as abundant as they were just a few decades ago, and many of them show forms of damage from acidic water that is the result of pollution. These small forms of sea life are food for larger forms of sea life, including whales.

Scientists from many institutions from throughout the world have estimated that the current loss in sea life will lead to a collapse of ocean life before the year 2050.

Other documentaries about sea life:
The End of the Line, EndOfTheLine.com/Film
Pirate of the Sea, PirateForTheSea.com
The Cove, TheCoveMovie.com

To protect the rivers, lakes, and oceans, and all life that depend on them:

1) Drastically reduce your use of fossil fuels, including petroleum, coal, and natural gas.

2) Choose to eat organically grown foods. Work to distance yourself from depending on foods that have been grown using synthetic chemical fertilizers, pesticides, herbicides, insecticides, miticides, and fungicides. Support local organic farmers. Grow some of your own food using organic gardening methods.

3) Eat low on the food chain: Don't eat fish, birds, mammals, amphibians, reptiles, eggs, or dairy. Follow a plant-based diet that is largely raw, organic, and local.

4) Compost your kitchen scraps. Don't send them to landfills, trash dumps, or incinerators. Get local restaurants, cafes, and food production facilities to do the same.

5) Use household products, including cleaning products that are plant-based and biodegradable. Don't use chlorine bleach, or cleaning products containing petroleum or coal extracts.

6) Reduce your use of plastic. Look for truly biodegradable plastics that consist of 100 percent plant substances, such as corn, sugar cane, and soy.

7) When you shop: Use a nonsynthetic cloth bag, not paper or plastic. Make and/or purchase nonsynthetic cloth bags and give them out to your friends, family, neighbors, fellow students, co-workers, and others.

8) Get your local stores and businesses to reduce and eliminate their use of plastics that end up as trash.

9) Plant and protect trees, restore and protect forests, and protect coastal wildlife habitat. Support organizations that do the same.

10) Legalize industrial hemp farming. Hemp and bamboo can provide the materials we commonly depend on trees to provide, including paper and lumber. Unlike trees, hemp and bamboo can also be made into fabric, food, and engine fuel. An acre of either hemp or bamboo absorbs more air pollution than trees, which helps to reverse global warming. Unlike cotton, which is the most fertilized and water-hungry crop, hemp and bamboo grow easily without fertilizer while providing material that creates fabric that is stronger, softer, and lasts longer than cotton. Visit: VoteHemp.com.

11) Reduce pollution. Reduce your use of products that pollute. Recycle.

12) Pedal instead of driving. Support and promote bike culture.

13) Shop less. Stop trying to replicate corporate imagery in your life. Avoid mimicking commercialized celebrity culture.

These organizations work to protect marine and forest life:

Algalita, Algalita.org
Ancient Trees, AncientTrees.org
Blue Voice, BlueVoice.org
Common Vision, CommonVision.org
EarthEcho.org
Earth First, EarthFirst.org
Earth Island, EarthIsland.org
Earth Garden Magazine, POB 2, Trentham, VIC 3458, Australia;
  earthgarden.com.au. Magazine for sustainable living
Environmental Justice Coalition for Water, EJCW.org
Fishing Hurts, FishingHurts.com
Forest Advocates, ForestAdvocate.org
Forest Council, ForestCouncil.org
Forest Ethics, ForestEthics.org
Forests Forever, ForestsForever.org
Forest Protection Portal, Forests.org
Global Water Policy Project, GlobalWaterPolicy.org
Great Lakes Water Wars, GreatLakesWaterWars.com
GreenPeace, GreenPeace.org
The Greywater Guerillas, SFUAS.org
Harp Seals, HarpSeals.org
International Rivers, InternationalRivers.org
Leatherback Trust, LeatherBack.org
Native Forest, NativeForest.or
Natural Resources Defense Council, NRDC.org
Ocean Alliance, OceanAlliance.org
The Ocean Project, TheOceanProject.org
Oceanic Preservation Society, OPSociety.org
Ocean Protection Coalition, oceanprotection.org
Oil Sands Truth, OilSandsTruth.org
Protect Our Woodland, ProtectOurWoodland.co.uk
Rainforest Action Network, RAN.org
Rainforest Web, RainForestWeb.org
Rainwater Harvesting, RainWaterHarvesting.org
Rainforest Action Network, RAN.org
Reef Resilience, ReefResilience.org
Rising Tide Australia, RisingTide.org.au
Rising Tide North America, RisingTideNorthAmerica.org
Rising Tide UK, RisingTide.org.uk
Sanctuary Forest, SanctuaryForest.org
Save Japan Dolphins, SaveJapanDolphins.org
Save Oaks, SaveOaks.com

Save the Manatee, SaveTheManatee.org
Save the Redwoods League, SaveTheRedwoods.org
Sea Otters, SeaOtters.org
Sea Turtle, SeaTurtle.org
Sea Shepherd, SeaShepherd.org
Sequoia Forest Keeper, SequoiaForestKeeper.org
Shark Savers, SharkSavers.org
Surfers for Cetaceans, S4CGlobal.org
Tas Forests, TasForests.green.net.au
Tree Musketeers, TreeMusketeers.org
Tree People, TreePeople.org
Trees for Life, TreesForLife.org
Trees for the Future, TreesFTF.org
Trees Foundation, TreesFoundation.org
Water Keeper Alliance, WaterKeeper.org
We Save Trees, WeSaveTrees.org
The Wilderness Society, Wilderness.org
Wildlands CPR, WildlandsCPR.org
World Watch, WorldWatch.org
World Water Council, WorldWaterCouncil.org

"Water is the driving force of all nature."
– Leonardo da Vinci

"It is imperative to maintain portions of the wilderness untouched so that a tree will rot where it falls, a waterfall will pour its curve without generating electricity, a trumpeter swan may float on uncontaminated water – and moderns may at least see what their ancestors knew in their nerves and blood."
– Bernand De Voto, *Fortune*, June 1947

HONEY AND BEES

Because the wild bee population has been on a dramatic decrease, farmers are depending more on beekeepers to pollinate their plants. Formerly, beekeepers would pay farmers for placing their hives in their fields, but now farmers are paying the beekeepers.

The bees kept by the beekeepers are not enough to make up for the loss in the native bee populations. In the 1940s there were an estimated five million bee colonies being kept by American beekeepers. By 2004, that figure had decreased by half.

Honeybees aren't the only type of bee needed. Some native bees harvest from plants that honeybees do not. Because of the reduction in wild bee populations, farmers increasingly rely on bees brought in from other parts of the world. This bee importing increases the risk of transferring infectious diseases among bee populations. At least one Native American bee species, *Bombus occidentalis*, has been devastated by an infectious disease brought to North American soil by bees imported from Belgium.

In an attempt to bring back and preserve native bee populations, some farmers plant parts of their fields with native flowering plants.

Because bees are so sensitive to pesticides, nobody knows how long some of the fields sprayed with pesticides will be poisonous to bees. Increased urban and government sprawl will continue to reduce bee habitat.

Some live foodists use raw honey as a sweetener, and others avoid it. If honey is to be used, raw honey is a better choice than processed sugars and heated honey. However, some people are not comfortable with using honey and other bee products, including bee pollen, propolis, and royal jelly, because these people feel they are robbing the bees of foods the bees are gathering for their own communities (true).

People who consider themselves vegan based on the concept that their diet is free from the use of bees to gather their food may want to consider the fact that a large amount of food they eat originates from farms using managed hives to pollinate the crops. Some people will say that all of the food we eat is the result of bees pollinating plants, and that is not true. Nor is it true that bee pollination results in 80 percent of the foods we eat, which is another frequent claim. It is much lower than that, but bees are certainly used on farms to help pollinate crops, and the amount of bee influence varies depending on the crop.

People may avoid bee products because they feel the actions involved in collecting honey and other products are dangerous for the bees – such as bees being killed during harvest. Also, some beekeepers kill wildlife to protect their hives, but others do not engage in that practice. If you choose to consume bee products, please seek out the products from beekeepers that don't kill other wildlife.

A spoonful of honey or an equal amount of grains of bee pollen requires a lot of work done by the bees to gather food for their communities. A teaspoon of either is the result of hundreds of foraging trips. A jar filled with honey requires tens of thousands of foraging trips.

Humans have been keeping honeybees for thousands of years. Images of beekeeping have been found drawn on cave walls, illustrated on ancient pottery, and on architectural ruins. Ancient texts often mention bees, sweet honey, and bee pollen. Mud structures in Africa have been found with areas built into their walls for beehives. Apiaries were built into walls surrounding castles. Houses built in Europe in the last few hundred years feature coves on exterior walls for beehives to be kept. Bees provided honey for food and wax for candles. What we know today as cookies were originally sweet breads made of grain and honey, which were a part of ancient ceremonies and celebrations.

Bees that produce enough honey to make it worthwhile to keep apiaries comprise a small percentage of the types of bees that exist. Bees native to the North American continent didn't make enough honey for the settlements of Europeans who moved here. "Domesticated" European honeybees were brought to America by the seventeenth-century Spanish missionaries and by the colonists of Jamestown and Williamsburg. Within a hundred years after their introduction to the American continent, honeybees had established colonies throughout much of North America. Bees brought to the U.S. from Italy in the 1800s quickly became the most common type of honeybee to keep because they tend to gather more honey than other types of bees.

I use the term "domesticated honeybees" because that is the term most often used to describe the bees kept by beekeepers. But bees aren't trainable, and can't be changed from their natural behavior and social structures. What can be done is to provide bees with places to build their hives, and these hives can be kept by the beekeepers.

Both wild and "domesticated" bees are only one form of wildlife that pollinates plants resulting in the crops that humans and animals eat and flowers that they enjoy. Other pollinators include butterflies, flies, moths, wasps, snails, snakes, worms, lizards, frogs, bats, and hummingbirds and other types of birds, as well as some animals that inadvertently spread pollen as they move from place to place. The wind and rain also spread certain types of pollen. Tragically, because the populations of so many types of wildlife have been damaged by human activity, there has been a worldwide decline of all types of "wild pollinators."

Bees typically gather nectar and pollen from an area within four miles of the hive. Their eyes can decipher movement about six times faster than humans can, which means it is harder for them to recognize slow movement. They also see ultraviolet colors. Both of these help bees to determine whether or not to stop at a flower to gather nectar, pollen, and even water.

Inside the nest different types of dances performed by the bees communicate what needs to be done, including sending out an announcement for others to gather. When a bee finds a good source of nectar, she returns to the nest and performs a dance to announce to the others that she has found a source, where the source is according to the angle of Sun, and the type of nectar it holds.

The foraging bees gather the nectar or water in their honey-stomach. They store pollen in little holding bags naturally formed on their hind legs. These harvested goods can be over twice the weight of the bee.

When bees fly, their bodies build static electricity. When they land on a flower, the bee's vibrating body shakes pollen from the flower. The pollen showers and clings onto the bee because of the static. The bee uses her numerous comb-like legs to gather the pollen from her body and put it into the collection pouches on her hind legs.

On a single foraging trip bees typically stick to one type of flower. As bees move from plant to plant, they inadvertently spread the pollen from the male to the female structures of the plants, which results in some of the food in the form of produce that humans eat. On their return to the nest the foraging bees regurgitate the nectar or water, and unload the pollen.

The nectar is taken by the middle-aged bees that either distribute it as food, or process it into honey by regurgitating it and dehydrating it by fanning it with their wings. They then store it in the nest cells for food. One bee colony may process two pounds of honey per day.

The nurse bees use the water to dilute honey to feed the others, or use it to cool the hive by spreading water on the comb and allowing it to evaporate.

While nectar, after it is turned into honey, is the colony's source for carbohydrates, the pollen provides nutrients such as amino acids, fats, and vitamins. Some of the pollen is consumed by the bees as it is first gathered. The rest is stored in special pollen cells, which the nurse bees access to feed the larvae. During the winter the worker bees may eat over two pounds of honey per week.

Bees are especially sensitive to chemical poisons that are used on farms, around homes, on golf courses, and on the property of campuses and other public and private land. Pesticides are chemicals designed to poison living things. When pesticides are spread across farm fields, bees are particularly susceptible to poisoning because bees harvest from the flowers at the tops of plants, where the pesticides settle. When the bees unknowingly carry the poisons back to the hives, more bees, and their larvae, are poisoned, and many die.

When you support organic agriculture, and nongenetically engineered agriculture, you are protecting the bee populations of the world.

Nonstop urban sprawl and industrial agriculture has also damaged bee terrain. Huge amounts of land have been covered by buildings, homes, sidewalks, roads, freeways, and parking lots. This construction along with agriculture has wiped out many of the flowering plants the bees depend on. The situation now exists where over 4,000 different species of bees (not honeybees) in America are in danger. Similar situations exist for the worldwide bee species that are estimated to be over 30,000. It is important to have a diverse population of bees because some bees will only pollinate certain plants – which then support other wildlife, help to clean the air, clean the water, and produce oxygen.

You can help the bee populations in your region by planting native flowering plants and trees, by protecting fields of native weeds, by stopping urban sprawl, and by never using pesticides.

Some honey processors heat their honey to break down the sugar crystals. If you purchase honey, make sure it says "raw" or "unheated" on the label. Otherwise you will likely be purchasing honey that has been heated, which damages the enzymes.

In addition to enzymes, raw honey contains vitamins (especially pantothenic acid, riboflavin, thiamin, and vitamin B6), minerals (calcium, copper, iron, magnesium, manganese, phosphorus, potassium, sodium, and zinc), amino acids (the building blocks of protein), antioxidants (especially pinocembrin), and other trace nutrients.

Honey is an inverted sugar, doesn't ferment in the digestive tract, and doesn't encourage bacterial growth. Raw honey contains an antibacterial substance called inhibine, as well as anti-inflammatory, antifungal, and antiallergy properties.

With all of that said, practices of beekeepers may also turn you off of honey products. Some beekeepers clip the wings of the queen bee to prevent her from leaving, some kill the queen every year, many rely on getting queens from companies that use the sperm of male bees that had been killed to obtain the sperm.

For more on whether or not you will feel right about consuming bee products, do research that will help you make a choice with which you feel most comfortable. You may wish to read this article: Why Honey is Not Vegan: http://www.vegetus.org/honey/honey.htm.

Plenty of books have been written about bees and honey. Some of the first books published after the invention of the printing press were on the topic of bees and honey.

Backyard Hive, BackyardHive.com
Bee Culture magazine, BeeCulture.com
Bees Wax Co, BeesWaxco.com/HowBeesMakeHoney.htm
Phillip Chandler, biobees.com. He is the author of *Barefoot Beekeeper.*
Scientific Bee Keeping, ScientificBeeKeeping.com
Vanishing Bees, VanishingBees.com
Wild Flowers, Wild-Flowers.com

RESONATION OF INSTINCT

"'It's just the way things are.' Take a moment to consider this statement. Really think about it. We send one species to the butcher and give our love and kindness to another apparently for no reason other than because it's the way things are. When our attitudes and behaviors towards animals are so inconsistent, and this inconsistency is so unexamined, we can safely say we have been fed absurdities."
– Dr. Melanie Joy

"How can you eat anything with eyes?"
– William Kellogg

When I was ten, walking alone on my way home from school one early spring day, I stepped on the last bits of ice that were undermined by water running in the street gutter. As I stepped on these little shelves of ice they collapsed into the thin stream of water. Those that wouldn't easily break got stomped on. As they collapsed, they splashed water onto me – which was part of the fun of it.

"Look deep into the eyes of any animal, and then for a moment, trade places, their life becomes as precious as yours and you become as vulnerable as them. Now smile if you believe all animals deserve our respect and our protection, for in a way, they are us, and we are them."
– Philip Ochoa

As I walked along I noticed that the water was turning pink. Looking ahead I saw a thin stream of red that had slowed alongside the street gutter. I wondered why someone had spilled a bunch of red paint. With my eyes I followed the streak of red and saw that it was running in a very thin line down the middle of a driveway of a neighbor's house. Walking up to the driveway, I stopped. My breath left me.

The only time I had seen large animals was at the zoo and on my relatives' dairy farm. But I had never seen a deer up close.

That day I did.

My absent neighbors had returned from a hunting trip. Maybe they were inside taking showers.

I stood alone trying to understand what my eyes were seeing.

Hanging by its hind legs from the backyard tree next to the driveway was a large deer. Its limp body had given up the ghost. Someone had slit through its neck so deeply that its head looked to be hanging from a bit of flesh. Its face on the nearly decapitated head looked to be painted red. Its snout dripped with blood into a puddle of gore on the lawn.

With my eyes, I followed the blood from the puddle, down the driveway, past my feet, and into the street gutter, where it turned the water from the melting ice a bloody pink.

I walked away with a memory I knew I would never forget.

"I am the voice of the voiceless. Through me the dumb shall speak. Till the deaf world's ear be made to hear. The cry of the wordless weak."
– Ella Wheeler Wilcox

"As long as humans continue to be the ruthless destroyer of other beings, we will never know health or peace. For as long as people massacre animals, they will kill each other. Indeed, those who sow the seed of murder and pain will never reap joy or love."
– Pythagoras of Samos

"Each and every animal on Earth has as much right to be here as you and me."
– Anthony Douglas Williams

Where I grew up there were wild berry bushes and cherry and other fruit trees. I often saw birds eating the berries and cherries, and they seemed to do so with great pleasure. When you see animals enjoying themselves by doing such things as feasting on wild berries, or playing with their young, you realize that they are beings that feel pleasure, establish relationships, and care for each other. Observing these social behaviors displayed in wild animals has helped to make me want to protect them from harm.

"When animals are in pain, do they not cry out? When animals are cut, do they not bleed their precious life out? When animals see their children taken from them, do they not follow after and anxiously want their children back? When animals are mortally wounded, do they not die? Just like humans, they suffer, they bleed, they love, they die. We are all connected."
– Marla Stormwolf-Patty

"In ways that matter, we are all the same. I have yet to find an emotion that is normally attributed to humans that is not displayed by animals. Just because they don't speak our words doesn't mean

284

they are not communicating. They are constantly communicating. Once you click in, you can see it. If we let go of the unconscious limits we normally impose on animals and simply look at them, listen to them, and pay attention, they have a whole lot to say, and they say it clearly."
   – Kathy Stevens, founder of Catskill Animal Sanctuary

"The more we come in contact with animals and observe their behavior, the more we love them, for we see how great is their care of the young."
   – Immanuel Kant

"All animals are made of flesh, blood and bone – including us, the human animal. All animals have the same five senses, value their families, form friendships, have individual personalities and don't want to die. Other animals are more like humans than they are unlike humans."
   – Benjamin Zephaniah

"I believe animals should be respected as citizens of this earth. They should have the right to their own freedom, their own families, and their own life."
   – John Feldmann

"Mankind's real moral test, a test so radical and so deep that it escapes our gaze, is probably the one of its relations with those that are the most at its mercy: the animals."
   – Milan Kundera

Animals are not simple stimulus response mechanisms. It has been proved that the brains of animals release hormones in relation to the thoughts they are displaying; this is similar to how human brains function.

"The very fact that an animal is going to be eaten seems to remove it from the category of intelligent beings, and causes it to be regarded as mere animated 'meat.'"
   – Henry S. Salt

"To my mind, the life of a lamb is no less precious than that of a human being. The more helpless the creature, the more that it is entitled to protection by man from the cruelty of man."
   – Mahatma Gandhi

Ethologists are scientists who study animal behavior. Throughout the years those working in this field have conducted numerous studies concluding that animals have memories, show affection, romance their lovers, establish community standards, and role play among themselves; are aware of their behavior as compared to others; experience moods and express emotions of eagerness, jealousy, excitement, compassion, distress, guilt, sadness, depression, and joy; mourn for their dead; have preferences; understand reasoning; are able to remember where they buried things; can experience post-traumatic stress; show favoritism, socialize, teach their young, form intention, practice intimidation tactics, anticipate needs, are cautious, display an understanding of cause and effect, gather observations and make conclusions from them, are able to do simple math; cooperate with the agreements of others; communicate desires; plan strategies, and sometimes hide things from others. They not only form friendships, but their health deteriorates if they do not experience physical and mental stimulation. From ants that cultivate fungus farms, to animals that protect and care for the young of other species, and to dolphin that guard humans from sharks, to New Caledonian crows that fashion hooks to forage for bugs, to bee birds in Africa that know how to lead badgers and humans to beehives, wildlife is made up of active thinkers who display individual personalities and various levels of understanding, and clearly show that they each have a consciousness.

Koko, a gorilla living at the Gorilla Foundation in Northern California, has learned sign language to the point of recognizing over 1,000 signs, as well as thousands of English words. She displays an IQ that may be higher than some people.

Animals deserve to live freely on this planet we share. Free from animal farming, free from being experimented on in laboratories, and free from environmental disasters caused by petroleum spills, fracking chemicals, mountaintop removal, rainforest destruction, genetic engineering, toxic farming chemicals, nuclear waste, war, and ocean acidification. Their habitat needs to be protected, and large parts of it need to be restored so they can survive and prosper.

> "The sun, the moon, and the stars would have disappeared long ago – had they happened to be within the reach of predatory human hands."
> – Havelock Ellis, *The Dance of Life*

Witnessing the damage humans have done to wildlife sickens me. Vast areas of Earth and wildlife have been violated by humans in the pursuit of making money, conducting warfare, and simply selfishly disrespecting the treasures of Earth and nature. All throughout the world humans have violated the animal kingdom. Within human society many more billions of animals are violated by the mass breeding, incarceration, and slaughter that is the animal farming and meat industry; by the fishing industry; by rodeos; by the fur industry; by the exotic animal trade; by zoos and circuses; and by use in scientific experimentation. All of these activities create bad energy and damage all forms of life on Earth.

"The art of angling: the cruelest, the coldest, and the stupidest of pretended sports."
– Lord George Byron

"Suffering is suffering, whether experienced by animals or humans. The physiological process is identical."
– Professor Mirko Bagaric, Head of Deakin Law School

The way factory farm animals are treated, how they are mechanically raped to breed them, the drugs they are given, the unnatural foods they are fed, the toxic chemicals they are treated with, and the crowded and caged conditions they live in make them stressed, depressed, confused, angry, frightened, and diseased. It is no wonder why the rates of degenerative and chronic diseases are so high in countries where the most factory-farmed meat, dairy, and eggs are consumed. People who are eating factory farmed meat, dairy, and eggs are eating the toxins from the chemically grown food fed to the animals and traces of the mass quantities of chemical drugs and sprays the animals are treated with. People who are eating meat are eating the hormones that had rushed through the tissues of the animals as they were slaughtered. They are also eating the molecules of emotion associated with stress, confinement, depression, frustration, confusion, repression, sorrow, anger, fright, poison, and disease.

"Eating meat is a learned behavior and habit. Do not confuse that with nature. It is not natural to keep animals in cages, breed them and mutilate their bodies, and drug them up so much that they are fully grown when they are still babies. It is not natural to drink the breast milk of another species, in adulthood. It is not natural to use animals as machines and void them of any resemblance of life."
– Kady Singer

By consuming a diet that consists of plants in the form of a vegan diet, a human can release the energies and illness they have absorbed into their system through their previous consumption of meat, eggs, and dairy products. The longer people consume a diet that is free of meat, eggs, and dairy, but that consists of a variety of fresh fruits, vegetables, and raw nuts and seeds, the more they will improve not only their own life, but also those of the people and animals around them. As their body absorbs a higher quality of nutrients it spins a new fabric of molecules and they resonate with a new level of energy that is attuned to and that will attract vibrant health.

287

The book *Old MacDonald's Factory Farm*, by C. David Coats, contains a preface about the absurdity of man. It tells of how it is an odd world where humans inflict so much pain on animals, then kill and eat the animals, which makes humans ill, then, in an attempt to "cure" themselves of the diseases created by eating the animals, they turn to toxic chemical drugs produced by the pharmaceutical industry, which spends hundreds of millions of dollars developing the drugs and testing them on tortured animals in outrageous and horrible laboratory experiments. Many of the drugs people take also contain ingredients that are derived from farmed animals killed in slaughterhouses. (Read: *Naked Empress*, by Hans Ruesch. Access: PETA.Org. Read the books *Mad Cowboy* and *No More Bull*, by Howard Lyman. Access: MadCowboy.Com.)

> "Going vegan is a double-edged sword: it has shown me the true beauty in animals – and the true ugliness in humans."
> – Tracey Anderson

Not only does following a completely or almost totally raw vegan diet protect animals from exploitation, it also protects wildlife, wildlands, the oceans, lakes, marshes, and rivers, and Earth. This is because a raw vegan diet has a much lower impact on Earth than that of the standard American diet consisting of meat, dairy, eggs, and highly polluting junk food. It starts with the fact that most food grown on the planet is being fed to billions of mass-bred farmed animals, including billions of farmed fish. This may come as a surprise to those who thought that there is a food shortage on the planet. Humans could not possibly consume all of the food that is growing on Earth. There is more than enough food to feed every human on the planet. The largest part of the problem is that most food grown on the planet is used to feed billions of farmed animals so that the rich countries can have their meat, dairy, and eggs.

> "Credit crunch? The real crisis is global hunger. And if you care, eat less meat: A food recession is under way. Biofuels are a crime against humanity, but – take it from a flesh eater – flesh eating is worse… While 100m tonnes of food will be diverted this year to feed cars, 760m tonnes will be snatched from the mouths of humans to feed animals – which could cover the global food deficit 14 times. If you care about hunger, eat less meat."
> – Journalist George Monbiot, London's *Guardian*, April 15, 2008

> "Industrial agriculture has told the world a big lie, which means the corporations that run it have told the people a big lie, including the governments who have supported them. The lie is that industrial agriculture feeds people. Industrial agriculture feeds profits. People are going hungry. A billion people are hungry today because

chemical farming does not let them eat the food they grow; instead they have to pay back the debt."
– Vandana Shiva, author of *Soil Not Oil* and *Earth Democracy*

Not only is most of the food grown on the planet fed to farmed animals, an increasing amount of seafood is also turned into feed for farm animals. The animal farming industry has turned into one of the chief problems relating to overfishing and the collapse of ocean life. Also, because it causes so much land pollution, which ends up in the rivers, lakes, and oceans, the animal farming industry is damaging water-life in a variety of ways.

As I mention earlier, the human dietary need for animal protein is absolutely zero. The human body flourishes in vibrant health on a vegan diet consisting largely of raw fruits and raw vegetables combined with adequate exercise and regular sleep.

"Plant protein can meet requirements when a variety of plant foods is consumed and energy needs are met. Research indicates that an assortment of plant foods eaten over the course of a day can provide all essential amino acids and ensure adequate nitrogen retention and use in healthy adults, thus complementary proteins do not need to be consumed at the same meal."
– American Dietetic Association, 2009

When we refuse to eat animals, dairy products, and eggs, and instead subsist on a plant-based diet rich in raw fruits and vegetables, we are agreeing to live more in tune with Nature. We are not participating in the terrible resource-heavy and pollution-rich animal-killing industries of factory farms, farmed fish, fishing trawlers, and slaughterhouses. We are not part of the tremendously fossil fuel-dependent monocropped GMO grain farming industry using mass quantities of toxic farming chemicals to grow more than 75 percent of its products to feed unnatural diets to billions of incarcerated and drugged animals on meat farms. We are not a part of the fishing industry that kills billions of fish and millions of sea mammals and birds every year. We are not supporting fish farms that are decimating coastal areas, killing wildlife, and using a variety of drugs and toxic chemicals to grow billions of catfish, tilapia, salmon, carp, and other harmless creatures in crammed pens. We are not supporting the rape of the oceans to provide unnaturally high-protein feed for farmed animals that are naturally vegan and that would never eat ocean creatures. We are not part of the egg industry, which kills billions of male chicks soon after birth simply because they can't produce eggs. We are not part of the dairy industry, which kills millions of baby bulls every year so that the mothers' milk can be taken and sold as human food. We

289

are not part of the ranching industry that collectively kills millions of wolves, bears, lions, foxes, groundhogs, raccoons, predator birds, and other wild animals every year. We are not part of an industry that is cutting down the rainforests, sending species into extinction, and ruining the lives of poor people to provide land for cattle-grazing and growing more grain to feed to farmed animals to support the global fast food industry that greatly contributes to human disease and various forms of pollution – including medical pollution. We are not supporting the killing of billions of animals every year. We are cutting down on our use of fossil fuels, water, and land. We are less dependent on corporations and their supermarketing. We are more likely to be of a healthy weight, and to experience fewer of the common chronic and degenerative diseases – which means, not depending on toxic synthetic chemical drugs that end up in the environment, poisoning wildlife, and us. When we follow a diet that does not contain anything that was born or hatched, and especially if we grow some of our food and we compost our kitchen scraps into soil, we are helping to protect wildlife, wildlands, forests, the oceans, lakes, marshes, streams and rivers, and Earth.

"Honestly, I would eat cardboard rather than go back to eating animals."
– Ellen Degeneres

Nature and animals can teach us things simply by being part of our existence.

"There are some barbarians who will take this dog, that so greatly excels man in capacity for friendship, who will nail him to a table, and dissect him alive. And what you discover in him are the same organs of sensation you have in yourself."
– Voltaire, *Philosophical Dictionary*

Centuries of writing from all areas of the planet, among the people who didn't know that others existed, and who had no way of communicating with people on other continents, have recorded events where humans have communicated with animals. Native people from various continents even include their communicative thoughts with animals and nature as part of their spiritual practices. An example is that of the Native Americans who include in their prayers an acknowledgment of a spiritual connection to animals such as deer, bears, wolves, wildcats, serpents, fish, and birds. Writers of novels and songs often include references of communicating with animals and nature in their works.

Animals and insects are tuned in to an energy that humans ignore, don't seem to consider, think of as impossible, or don't believe they can tune into.

Where hope falters, possibilities fail.

Migratory birds often fly thousands of miles at the same time of year, returning to the same spots year after year. Fish, such as salmon, also migrate hundreds and even thousands of miles, only to return to where they were born. Whales, sea turtles, tuna, and even butterflies do the same. Animals seem to know where they are and where they are going. Dogs and cats removed from their owners often find their owners, even when the owners move to new homes miles away. Farm animals have escaped from their confinement only to be found later at distant farms where they had never been, but to where their babies had been sold off.

A magnetic field that wraps the Earth, the alignment of the stars, the angle of sun and the moon, the smells of different regions of Earth, polarized ultraviolet light patterns, and other factors may play a part in migration. But there are also factors that guide living things that seem to be tuned into a resonance or energy – an invisible power.

Is this energy field, or a connection to instinct and nature, something humans are missing out on by eating such unhealthful foods and living in a way that is disconnected from nature? I believe so.

"Would Nature have placed our very means of survival – food – in mobile animals, another mammal's skin, and under a hen, or in 260,000 varieties of plants spread over Earth?"
– Rex Bowlby, author of *Plant Roots: 101 reasons why the human diet is rooted exclusively in plants*

"If you don't want to be beaten, imprisoned, mutilated, killed or tortured then you shouldn't condone such behavior towards anyone, be they human or not."
– Moby

"My refusal to eat meat has occasioned inconvenience, and I have been frequently chided for my singularity. But my light repast allows for greater progress, greater clearness of head, and quicker comprehension."
– Benjamin Franklin

"Besides agreeing with the aims of vegetarianism for aesthetic and moral reasons, it is my view that a vegetarian manner of living, by its purely physical effect on the human temperament, would most beneficially influence the lot of mankind."
– Albert Einstein

Plant-Based Foods and Health: Nature Provides Our Food

INADEQUATE nutrition and the consumption of junk food contribute to everything from skin problems to heart disease, and from depression to birth defects. Eating whole foods, such as unprocessed fruits and vegetables and whole grains, provides the body with important nutrients such as vitamins, minerals, fiber, amino acids, essential fatty acids, and enzymes; and phytochemicals, including isoflavonoids and lignans.

Tremendous health benefits can be gained by consuming a diet rich in substances originating in raw, edible plants – and especially so if the diet is free of the health-damaging substances contained in meat, milk, and eggs. These beneficial plant substances are natural chemicals called antioxidants. These chemicals only exist in animals in trace amounts, and only because the animal ate plants containing the antioxidants. It is antioxidants that shield us from free radicals that naturally occur in our bodies, and also that are introduced to our systems through low-quality foods, including meat, dairy, and eggs, and also by way of substance abuse, such as by smoking and drinking alcohol. Free radicals damage body tissues, including the muscles, cardiovascular system, skin, and the mechanisms within the eyes. This is one reason why antioxidants called carotenoids, which are found in carrots and other vegetables and fruits, are said to help the eyes. Free radicals also play a role in cancer. Antioxidants are so centric to good nutrition that they are a basic key to maintaining vibrant health and a strong immune system. Without a diet rich in raw plant matter, you are lacking in the spectrum of beneficial antioxidants that can only be obtained through the consumption of plants.

Someone may say that there are some antioxidants in meat. They are not incorrect in saying this. But it is like comparing a raindrop to a lake, with a piece of meat being the raindrop, and an apple or other raw fruit or vegetable being a lake of beneficial nutrients. Any antioxidants in the meat got there only by way of the animal eating plants. Animals, including humans, do not conduct photosynthesis, which is the process that takes place in plant cells when they absorb sun energy and store it, forming the colors in the plants. Therefore, antioxidants, which are in the natural colors of plants, are vastly more available in edible, raw plant substances, and much less present in meat, dairy, and eggs. Consuming animal protein to try to access antioxidants is less effective than licking the juice from a knife that just cut through a piece of fruit, instead of simply eating the fruit itself.

By consuming animal protein, you are also consuming free radicals, which exist and form in meat, milk, and eggs. So, even if you are consuming some trace amounts of certain antioxidants in the animal protein, you are countering it by also consuming the damaging free radicals in that animal flesh, dairy, or eggs. This scenario does not equal good nutrition – especially considering that meat, dairy, and eggs also contain saturated fat, cholesterol, and a variety of other substances that work against health.

Studies are constantly revealing how certain fruits and vegetables (broccoli, peppers, onions, garlic, carrots, cranberries, apples, pomegranates, cucumbers, tomatoes, beets, squash, ginger, beans, broccoli, sprouts, spinach, collards, cauliflower, chard, kale, dandelion, cilantro, berries, etc.) not only provide needed nutrients that are beneficial to health, but also that they contain and provide properties that prevent certain serious ailments, such as diabetes, cancer, Alzheimer's, MS, and heart disease; limit intestinal exposure to carcinogens; and help the body to contain, transport, and eliminate toxins.

Eat a vegetarian diet and you will be doing what many world-class athletes are doing. For instance, Dave Scott, who has won the Hawaiian Ironman contest six times and is considered to be among the best athletes who ever lived, is a complete vegetarian.

In July 2011, Michael Arnstein, a low-fat raw vegan who has the site TheFruitarian.com, won the Vermont 100 Ultra Marathon. For the past two years, he and his wife, Victoria, have thrown the Woodstock Fruit Festival, which is a week of seminars, sports, and good times in upstate New York. In 2012, Michael and Victoria both ran the Vermont 100, days after Michael ran the Badwater race in California.

Ultramarathon champion Scott Jurek won the Western States race seven straight times. In 2005 Jurek also won the grueling 135-mile Badwater race, which begins at the lowest elevation in the Western Hemisphere, in Death Valley, California, and ends 8,300 feet up a mountain, and he did it faster than anyone in the history of the race. Then he won it again in 2006. He did this all while following a vegan diet.

On October 16, 2011, Fauja Singh finished the Toronto Waterfront Marathon in about eight hours. You may think that eight hours is a slow time for completing a marathon. Well, consider that at the time of the race, he was 100 years old! He credited a vegetarian diet as being key to his longevity, stamina, and ability.

Vegan athletes include Australian Division One biker and marathon runner, Harley "Durianrider" Johnstone of 30BananasADay.com; Can-

293

adian triathlete Brendan Brazier of MyVega.com; Ironwoman Ruth Heidrich; tennis pro Martina Navratilova; heavyweight boxing champion Peter Hussig; karate champion Ridgely Abele; Heisman trophy winner Desmond Howard; the exceptional running back, Montell Owens; Olympic wrestler Chris Campbell; Mr. Universe Bill Pearl; gymnast Dan Millman; bodybuilders Evan Connelly Novacek and Kristopher Flannery; marathon champion Jane Wetzel; Olympic skater Surya Bonaly; boxer Keith Holmes; world mixed martial arts champ Mac Danzig; and many more. In 2011, boxer Mike Tyson said he had been following a vegan diet for a couple of years, and that it has helped him to heal on many levels. In 2012, Lance Armstrong spoke of the benefits of increased energy experienced by switching to a lower-fat, organic, mostly vegan diet – a better choice than performance drugs. Armstrong had been training with Rip Esselstyn, an athlete and the author of *The Engine 2 Diet*, which advocates a 100 percent vegan, low-fat diet.

"Even when you're training really hard, it's normal that you would have certain things for lunch or certain things for breakfast, and then have this dip, or almost like a food coma. I don't experience that anymore. My energy level has never been this consistent, and not just consistent, but high. I'm a big napper – I couldn't even take a nap these days if I wanted to.

The other thing – I expected to get rid of that dip, but I didn't expect the mental side of it, and the sharpness and the focus that I've noticed. And I was the biggest nonbeliever, I was like 'whatever, man,' and I'm in. I'm not doing dinners yet, but breakfast and lunch, I'm in."
    – Lance Armstrong, speaking of following a largely low-fat vegan diet while training for a marathon, March 2012

"I have been a vegan for almost two years now and the benefits have been tremendous. I have more stamina and it helps keep me in a positive state of mind. I didn't realize how weighed down I was when I ate meat. I never really felt 100 percent until I freed it from my diet. Now, I can't imagine going back to meat. I feel incredible."
    – Mike Tyson, World heavyweight boxing champion; quotation 2011

"Today you have processed meats and a lot of animals suffering unnecessarily for it. Now, some people just blow that off and don't have a conscience about it, or they just don't care. They wouldn't eat their dog, but they feel that way about other animals. But for me, I decided to stop eating meat. I didn't want to contribute to all of that. I'm not trying to change the world, or wear that on my sleeve, or make a political statement, because that just turns people away. I

only have control over one person, and that's myself. And I feel good about it."
– Mac Danzig, vegan mixed martial arts champ

"I've found that a person does not need protein from meat to be a successful athlete. In fact, my best year of track competition was the first year I ate a vegan diet."
– Carl Lewis, nine-time Olympic gold medal winner

Although it is reasonable to assume that there have always been people who have followed a diet consisting of only plant substances, the modern vegan diet is often attributed to the teachings of Donald Watson, who died at age 95 in Cumbria on November 16, 2005. He became a vegetarian after seeing his Uncle George involved in the slaughter of a pig. Hearing the pig's screams haunted him. "I decided that farms – and uncles – had to be reassessed: The idyllic scene was nothing more than death row, where every creature's days were numbered."

"Animals and humans suffer and die alike. Violence causes the same pain, the same spilling of blood, the same stench of death, the same arrogant, cruel, and brutal taking of life. We don't have to be a part of it."
– Dick Gregory

Eventually, Watson eliminated dairy from his diet. When his elder brother and a sister also became vegetarians, his mother, who was not a vegetarian, made the comment that she felt like a hen who had hatched a clutch of duck eggs.

"We may be sure that should anything so much as a pimple ever appear to mar the beauty of our physical form, it will be entirely due in the eyes of the world to our own silly fault for not eating 'proper food.' Against such a pimple the great plagues of diseases now ravaging nearly all members of civilized society (who eat 'proper food') will pass unnoticed."
– Donald Watson, founder of "veganism," acknowledging the critical microscope vegans were put under by those who consume the so-called "proper foods" of milk, eggs, and meat

As an adult, Watson became a woodworking instructor. In 1939 he registered as a conscientious objector and refused to go to war. At the end of the war he formed a group of "nondairy vegetarians." The group advocated the health benefits of such a diet, and taught that animal agriculture was likely to spread diseases, such as the tuberculosis that was identified in Britain's dairy cows. He concocted the term "vegan" by taking the beginning and end of the word "vegetarian." Terms that he and his group considered included "beaumangeur," "benevor," "dairyban," "sanivore," and "vitan." The first edition of The Vegan Society's *Vegan News* was published in 1944 and consisted of 12 typed pages.

When you consume a diet that consists of what nature provides, and the closer it is to its natural state, the nearer your body will be to its natural state.

> "My doctor told me to stop having intimate dinners for four. Unless there are three other people present."
> – Orson Welles

The natural state of the body is to be healthy and free from toxins and disease. The keys to health are healthful thought pattern, exercise regimen, diet, relationships, and atmosphere. You can't follow a more healthful diet than one consisting purely of a variety of quality organically grown vegetables, fruits, herbs, nuts, seeds, and water vegetables – especially if some are homegrown.

To experience the abundance that nature can provide for you, abundantly take advantage of what nature provides. What nature provides is a pathway to pristine health paved with nutritious foods consisting of plant substances. These are the substances that our bodies are genetically designed to eat. Anything else, such as processed foods, and those that contain artificial coloring, flavoring, textures, scents, preservatives, and so forth are not natural and should not be put into the body.

Don't try to get too complicated in regard to your food choices. Refuse to buy into the false information about various food companies trying to sell products that are filled with chemicals and chemically grown foods. Simply choose what is presented to us in nature. Fruits, vegetables, nuts, and seeds are in tune with nature, and this is especially true if they are organically grown, and not genetically altered.

Eating what is in tune with nature tunes us into nature and our natural state of being. That is the truth about food.

> "When I buy cookies I eat just four and throw the rest away. But first I spray them with Raid so I won't dig them out of the garbage later. Be careful, though, because Raid really doesn't taste that bad."
> – Janette Barber, writer and stand-up comic

It is simple. If you eat a healthful diet, you will experience better health than if you eat a diet of junk. This concept isn't part of the pop commercial diets promoted in books and through fad diet plans, which are based on ignorance, laziness, and greed. That is because people can't make money by simply telling you to eat organic fruits and vegetables – other than organic produce farmers, who deserve to be paid for their work. The most expensive diet plans out there consist of manufactured foods that have been deadened through cooking and processing. They lead to diseases of affluence, such as obesity, heart disease, Type-2 diabetes, Alzheimer's, Crohn's, MS., osteoporosis, and various cancers.

Many diet book authors are selling manufactured and processed food products and supplements that go with their "diet plan." But this book is not selling you any food products, pills, potions, or supplements. I am simply telling you to eat organically grown plant substances. I'm also suggesting that you grow as much of your own food as reasonable, and use organic growing methods to do so. It is best not to be completely reliant on stores and restaurants for your most basic needs, such as food. (Access: KitchenGardeners.org, UrbanHomestead.org, FoodNotLawns.com, VegetableGardener.com, and Yards to Gardens: Y2G.org. See the book: *The Edible Front Yard: The Mow-Less, Grow-More Plan for a Beautiful, Bountiful Garden,* by Ivette Soler.)

While acknowledging that people may not care to limit themselves to just a few types of fruits for their nourishment, it is still interesting to consider that just a few healthy fruit trees can supply a person with a lot more food than he or she could possibly eat in a lifetime. I have friends whose homes are surrounded by fruit trees producing so much fruit that they can't give away the fruit fast enough. They get as much as they need and abundantly more. And they aren't considered farmers.

If you want to have a lively, vibrant body, then you should be eating living, vibrant foods. The liveliest foods you can give to your body are those found in nature: vibrantly alive plant substances that have not been degraded by high temperatures, chemicals, or genetic engineering.

If you are confused by all the diet and health information you have heard and read about in pop culture, there is a reason you are confused, because nature is not confusing. Only the information put out by man is confusing. Forget about what advertising and fad diet plans have told you about nutrition. When choosing food, simply stick to nature. What nature provides for you will not do you wrong.

Learn to eat naturally, and rely on foods that are as close to their natural state as possible. When you do so, your body will begin to conform to its natural state.

Stop allowing yourself to be caught up in all of the complex diets promoted by the various pop culture diet gurus and multinational food companies that want you to buy and eat their products so that they can make more money. Ignore food advertising. Skip over all of the processed foods you face at the supermarket. Go straight to the produce section. Request that your local market sell more organic produce. Shop at farmers' markets. Join or start a CSA, or an organic food co-op. (Consider the Rawfully Organic Food Co-op in Houston that was started by Kristina Carillo-Bucaram. Access: RawFullyOrganic.com.)

Teach children how to grow food gardens, to forage wild edibles, and to prepare foods from scratch in alignment with a plant-based diet.

"When I was old enough to realize that all meat was killed, I saw it as an irrational power, to take a weaker thing and mutilate it. It was like bullies would take control of younger kids in the school yard."
– River Phoenix

"Chickens, pigs, and other animals are interesting individuals with personalities and intelligence. What people need to understand is that if they're eating animals, they are promoting cruelty to animals."
– Pamela Anderson

"I think something is odd about eating another living anything."
– Shania Twain

"I feel there is no need to cause another living thing pain or harm. There are so many other things we can eat. I have never eaten meat in my life and I'm five feet ten inches – and not exactly wasting away. A wise man once said 'animals are my friends, and I'm not in the habit of eating my friends.' That is exactly how I feel."
– Joss Stone

"I am a very strict vegetarian. I just really, really love animals, and I act on my values."
– Natalie Portman

"I stopped eating beef at 13, and stopped eating all meat a few years ago. I would feel guilty knowing that what was on my plate was walking around yesterday. Either I could live with that, or stop eating meat. I chose the latter, and I'm happier for it."
– Carrie Underwood

"A man can live and be healthy without killing animals for food; therefore, if he eats meat, he participates in taking animal life for the sake of his appetite. And to act so is immoral."
– Leo Tolstoy

"The real struggle in being vegan doesn't involve food. The hardest part about being vegan is coming face-to-face with the darker side of humanity and trying to remain hopeful. It's trying to understand why otherwise good and caring people continue to participate in the needless violence against animals just for the sake of their own pleasure or convenience."
– Joe Tyler

PLANT-BASED DIET IS THE WAY TO HEALTH

"I regard animals as persons of another species. And I don't eat their flesh for the same reasons that I don't eat the flesh of people. I know that nonhuman animals value their lives and their freedom and their families. And I know that life is as much an adventure and a joy for them as it can be for us. I wish to honor their interests as well as my own and help create a more peaceful place where we can all live."
– Don Robertson

"It is the hidden horror that the egg industry does not want you to see. In egg production male chicks are surplus to requirements, which means that they are sorted from the females in vast warehouses and then killed by the thousand at just a day or two old. Identical to the chicks you see on Easter greeting cards, these uncomprehending young birds are either sent on a conveyor belt to be gassed or thrown alive into electric mincers. The same system is used to sort those which move to barn, free range, or even most organic egg farms. It is an unimaginable waste of life – and all just to bring an egg to your morning table."
– Justin Kerswell

"It seems rather bizarre to me, and somewhat Jekyll and Hyde, to be sitting at your table devouring a creature while at the same time lovingly stroking another as your pet. But then again, when one's raised that way, I guess the irony (some would say hypocrisy) isn't so easily seen."
– Lance Landall

"When a vegan is talking to a meat-eater about these issues, he or she is not 'preaching,' 'trying to convert,' or any such thing. We're not telling you what to eat. We're telling you what you're eating. Since animals can't speak a language humans can understand (though I think the screams and terrified moans that fill slaughterhouses should be pretty much universal – all living beings want to live), it's up to us to tell their stories and inform people of the suffering that goes on conveniently out of the public eye. If as a

299

meat eater, being exposed to this reality bothers you, it is not the fault of the vegan."
    – Ari Solomon

Putting meat, dairy, and eggs out of your life clears your spirit and detoxifies your body from the heinously bad energy associated with the entrapment, confinement, suffering, and killing of farm animals; from the horrors of the slaughterhouse; and from the sickly energy of the caged farm animals that are fed lousy, unnatural diets, are treated with drugs, and are sprayed with chemicals. A plant-based diet releases you from the bad energy of misusing Earth's resources in the way it is done by the mass breeding and killing of animals. And it releases you from the support and/or involvement of the packaging, marketing, cooking, and consumption of meat from billions of farmed animals (mammals, birds, and farmed fish).

"Once we recognize how poor the reasons are for killing 'food animals,' we glimpse the deeper explanation of why so few people actually visit slaughterhouses – and why so many want to remain blissfully ignorant of what transpires there. Every thoughtful person understands the truth of Emerson's observations: 'You have just dined, and however scrupulously the slaughterhouse is concealed in the graceful distance of miles, there is complicity.' That sense of our own complicity is what, deep down, we hope to shield from ourselves by refusing to look the death of animals in the eye. Before any rational reflection begins we understand that, if we looked, we would see the animals' blood on our hands. We would be aghast at ourselves for what we have done. And for what we are doing. So we look, not inside but aside, in search of every excuse not to face our involvement in the needless massacre (for that is what it is) of millions upon millions of animals, day in and day out. Opaque walls make good neighbors."
    – Tom Regan

When you work your life in tune with the energy of nature and follow a plant-based, natural diet, you are tuned into your natural instinct. Your body and brain will function better. You will be able to think more clearly. You will be healthier and have more energy. You will experience a synchronicity with your thoughts, actions, feelings, goals, and talents. A healthier you will manifest from inside as you shed the physical and spiritual residues you carried from living and eating unhealthfully.

When you follow a diet consisting of only or mostly raw plant substances, you are eating what is grown in nature and what will be synchronized with the patterns of the microscopic structures of your body tissues. As you sustain a diet consisting of totally or almost completely raw plants you will be infusing your system with the wavelengths of light and life that infuse all life forms.

The longer you maintain a diet of healthful foods rich in raw fruits and vegetables, the sooner you will be able to detect the changes in your body when you don't eat the best quality of foods. When you are eating a healthful, plant-based diet rich in raw fruits and vegetables, your body can better communicate what is good and healthful and what is not. As you become attuned to how your body feels after you consume certain foods, you will naturally want to stick with the foods that make you feel good. Your body will acclimate to eating and desiring that which is healthy.

Following a sunfood diet increases your vibrancy. By eliminating the deadness of cooked food from your diet, you will be subsisting on the unadulterated nutrients of plant matter radiant with the vibrational patterns of Sun and Nature. You will experience a new health destination and your life will align in accordance with it.

On a vegan diet rich in raw fruits and raw vegetables your life becomes alive.

Once you get a taste of how good your life can become, you will instinctively want to increase the good. Your perceptions of what you are capable of accomplishing and your abilities to do so awaken and become clear to you.

By working with the natural resources within you that give you the desire to succeed and experience happiness, and guiding yourself with those desires through goal setting and intentional daily actions, your life can improve in ways you previously may have thought were not possible.

Realize that life is full of possibilities for those who believe in their divinity, and who seek and believe and work toward making things happen through intentional actions using intellect, goal setting, talents, skill, and craft.

Be daring, brave, and wise. Bring yourself out of the box you have kept yourself in. Break down the walls of dullness. Decide now to enliven your energy. Stop eating dead foods. Allow yourself to experience the benefits of the sunfood diet rich in raw fruits and vegetables that infuse health. It will ignite your life and propel you into experiencing amazing things.

For more about radically transforming your life, read my book *Igniting Your Life: Pathways to the Zenith of Health and Success.*

"The planet does not need more 'successful' people. But it does desperately need more peacemakers, healers, restorers, storytellers, and lovers of every shape and form. It needs people who live well in their places. It needs people of moral courage willing to join the fight to make the world habitable and humane. And these needs have little to do with success as our culture has defined it."
– David Orr

"Animals are not humans with reduced capacities. They have their own capacities, their own spectrum of aptitudes and behaviors."
– Jean Kazaz

"I try to remember how I thought before I was vegan.
I thought of animals as a big group rather than a big group of individual beings. I was disconnected from the fact that animals are individual beings.
Now I know every nonvegan choice has an individual being on the other end of that choice. And the individual being typically suffers pain, both physical and emotional, beyond our worst nightmare.
So please think of the individual beings, and change your nonvegan choices into vegan choices. And the next thing you know, you are vegan, you are connected, you are at peace."
– Sarah Woodcock

"One day the absurdity of the almost universal human belief in the slavery of other animals will be palpable. We shall then have discovered our souls and become worthier of sharing this planet with them."
– Martin Luther King, Jr.

"I enjoy the health benefits of a vegan life and the knowledge that I am drastically lowering my carbon footprint, of course, it's the ethical principle of not subsidizing cruelty to animals that means the most to me."
– Dan Piraro

"When animals express their feelings they pour out like water from a spout. Animals' emotions are raw, unfiltered, and uncontrolled. Their joy is the purest and most contagious of joys and their grief the deepest and most devastating. Their passions bring us to our knees in delight and sorrow."
– Mark Bekoff

COLORS IN PLANTS: SPECTRAL NUTRITION

"Beauty and vitality are gifts from nature, for those who live by her laws."
– Leonardo da Vinci

I like to visit and support animal sanctuaries where animals that were once sickly from being caged or mistreated are able to live in natural surroundings and reclaim their health by eating a natural diet. Many of the animals that I have visited on these sanctuaries were once on the brink of death and have truly been transformed into healthy beings with a zest for life.

Just as the animals that have been rescued from the horrible living and diet conditions of factory farms can become healthier through improved nutrition and more healthful surroundings, the human body that has been mistreated and/or neglected can also regain much of its luster and vigor. This is obvious in those who have gone from obesity to a healthy weight simply by changing their food choices, increasing their physical activity, improving their atmosphere, and restructuring their thought processes to become more positive and successful.

"That which we persist in doing becomes easier for us to do; not that the nature of the thing itself is changed, but that our power to do is increased."
– Ralph Waldo Emerson

The body works to generate health. The microscopic activities deep in the cells work toward health in the best way possible using whatever nutrients are provided.

"Food is that material which can be incorporated into and become a part of the cells and fluids of the body. Nonuseful materials, such as chemical additives and drugs, are all poisons. To be a true food, the substance must not contain useless or harmful ingredients."
– Dr. Herbert Shelton, author of *Food Combining Made Easy*

Health comes from within. To assist this activity, it is wise to supply the body with the best form of nutrients available. Doing less than that is limiting the ability of the body to produce vibrant health.

"Bring the power of plants into your body. There's nothing like freshly made juices to nurture your 100 trillion cells."
– Jay Kordich, the juiceman

According to the U.S. Centers for Disease Control, in 2009 only 26.3 percent of Americans were eating vegetables three or more times per day, and only 32.5 percent were eating fruit two or more times per day. Through its Healthy People 2010 program, the CDC set a goal of getting 50 percent of people aged two and older to consume three or more servings of vegetables per day, and 75 percent of people aged two and over to consume two or more servings of fruit per day. While increasing the consumption of fruits and vegetables is a good thing, for the best of health, the goals set by the CDC didn't go far enough.

"A diet high in fruits and vegetables can reduce the risk for many leading causes of death."
– U.S. Centers for Disease Control and Prevention, 2010

Raw fruits and vegetables are what the body needs, and especially for those wanting to experience the best health.

Consider the colors of fruits and vegetables that capture our attention when selecting them. Would you consider the unadulterated, vibrant botanical colors to be nutrients? There is more than meets the eyes to the colors among the plants that we eat.

The spectrum of botanical pigments existing inside plant cells contain molecules that absorb specific wavelengths of sunlight energy. In turn, the cells of the plant store and carry different levels of vibrational energy fields, including tiny specks of light called biophotons. These frequencies contained in the unheated substances of plants have a function when consumed. There are photoreceptor proteins in the brain that are similar to those in the eyes, and they also exist throughout the body. The biophotons that exist within all living cells are part of the cellular communication system. Some people refer to biophotons as our *life force energy*. As you may expect, those following a diet largely consisting of a variety of raw plant matter have been found to contain richer banks of biophotons in their tissues than those following a diet that is cooked and otherwise highly processed.

"Nothing will benefit human health or increase the chances for survival of life on earth as the evolution to a vegetarian diet."
– Albert Einstein

A diet rich in raw plant matter is also rich in antioxidants.

Your body wants and desires to be around certain colors of nature. You automatically are attracted to the piece of fruit that has reached its peak level of ripeness, be it the radiant peach, the passionately red strawberry, the gleaming plumpness of melon, the practically glowing colors of fresh bananas, tomatoes, cherries, grapes, persimmons, citrus, and apples, or the richness of green vegetables. Once fruits and vegetables have passed their prime and their colors have begun to fade, they don't elicit the same response from us.

The pigments synthesized within plants often work as defense mechanisms for the plants much in the same way the immune system of the human body works to protect health. The plant chemicals have been described as "plant antibiotics." They work to protect plants from the elements, such as fungi, bacteria, tissue damage, extreme temperatures, and ultraviolet light. It is understood that there is some interaction between the plant and a pathogen that will trigger the manufacture of certain chemicals within the plant to defend it against the pathogen. Plants will also manufacture certain chemicals when the plant is exposed to certain stresses, such as wind, temperatures, moisture, and dryness.

Plants that are not provided with sufficient nutrients and conditions through soil, light, water, and temperature become weak and do not produce the chemicals they need to protect themselves from pathogens and environmental stresses.

Amazingly, when humans consume plants, the very same natural chemicals that protect the plants have been found to protect human health. They lower cholesterol, prevent heart disease, regulate blood sugar, and function as antioxidants. A diet rich in raw plant matter is also rich in antioxidants.

Similar to plants, a human body that is not provided with the right combination of nutrients and atmosphere will also fail to defend itself from pathogens and stresses.

There are hundreds of thousands of plant chemicals that benefit human health. Probably the most commonly known beneficial plant color is the beta-carotene that is found in apricots, cantaloupe, carrots, peaches, pumpkin, and spinach. There is also alpha-carotene that is found in carrots, red and yellow peppers, and in pumpkins. Lutein, a carotenoid that is found in avocado, corn, kale, and spinach, has been found to prevent cataracts. Zeaxanthin is a carotenoid that helps give color to corn and saffron, and has been found to protect vision. Then there is lycopene in pink grapefruit, guava, tomatoes, and watermelon, and many other plant colors. These are only a few of over 600 identified plant chemicals that give plants their colors. Many more are being identified and studied. Because there are at least thousands in each plant, the identifying and study process can go on for many, many years. With each new discovery comes research that looks into the health benefits of the phytochemical, how the chemical works with others, and how the enzymatic systems of the human organs metabolize them.

By the process of photosynthesis, antioxidants form in plants, not in animals. To experience the best of health, we need to consume a diet rich in antioxidants, and there are more of them in raw plant matter than in heated plant matter. As mentioned in the previous chapter, there are only slight amounts of antioxidants in meat, milk, and eggs, and they are only there because the animal consumed plants. What meat, milk, and eggs do contain much more abundantly are free radicals, and you don't want to be putting foods rich in free radicals into your body, especially when they are accompanied by the saturated fat and cholesterol and other health-depleting substances contained in meat, milk, and eggs.

While all areas of the body are reliant on antioxidants, one area that relies on antioxidants in a very specific way is the macula of the eyes. The continual chemical changes in and around the macula are what brings us sight. It is in the macula that light waves are turned into energy recognized by our nerves. The light waves also continually react with the fatty acids of the macula, which is a process that creates low levels of free radicals. To counteract this free radical activity, we need antioxidants, which we obtain from eating fresh plant matter. Raw fruits and vegetables like mangoes, apricots, melon, citrus fruits, berries, red and yellow peppers, carrots, broccoli, broccoli leaves, squash, spinach, and collard greens contain the carotenoids that are particularly beneficial to eye function. Green leafy vegetables contain an antioxidant called lutein, which is specifically beneficial to the lenses of the eyes. As mentioned earlier, lutein helps to prevent cataracts – another condition associated with long-term diets lacking in antioxidants. Raw edible plant matter also happens to contain the essential fatty acids we need to obtain from food, and some of these fatty acids are utilized by the macula and the nerves servicing the eyes. These are more reasons why it is good to consume raw fruits and raw vegetables, sprouts and germinates, and raw seaweeds, as they all contain essential fatty acids. Those who consume a diet rich in raw fruits and vegetables have been found to experience better vision later in life.

Animal protein, including eggs, dairy, and meat of all varieties, contain free radicals, saturated fats, and foreign cholesterol, all of which are not good for the eyes. Meat, dairy, and eggs also lack antioxidants, making them a quadruple threat to long-term eye health. The condition labeled "age-related blindness" is largely the degeneration of the macula, the leading cause of blindness, and you do not need to experience it. Eliminate meat, dairy, and eggs, and foods that contain them, from your diet, follow a diet rich in raw fruits, vegetables, sprouts, and germinates, and you are more likely to avoid macular degeneration and cataracts.

While some people believe they are protecting their vision by taking vitamins specifically identified as being beneficial to sight, such as vitamins C and E, they would be much better off consuming raw fruits and vegetables that naturally contain the vitamins, essential fatty acids, amino acids, antioxidants, and likely an unknown number of substances beneficial to eye health, brain health, heart health, muscle and bone health, skin health, and whole body health. Pills containing one vitamin and not the whole host of substances contained in edible plant matter may not provide the benefits the marketing material may claim. In other words, for true nutrition, eat raw fruits and vegetables.

One plant chemical that has received a lot of attention as an antioxidant is one given the tongue-twisting name pterostilbene (pronounced tero-still-bean). This chemical is present in colorful fruits like blueberries. It is sensitive to light and air, which means it is present in fruits that have not been processed or heated.

Another plant chemical that is rightly touted as a health-enhancer is resveratrol. This chemical is present in the skin of grapes, cranberries, and in some berries. It has been shown to improve liver and neuron tissue health, and may contribute to a longer life among those who consume an abundance of plants containing it.

Resveratrol survives the winemaking process, and is present in red wine, which is a raw food. (If you purchase wine, make sure it is organic and that the company does not use any animal by-products in their processing. Some wines will indicate on the label that they are "vegan." Please stay away from alcohol if you have any problems with it.)

Each edible plant consists of a different variety of healthful, natural chemicals that work as nutrients when consumed by humans. To gain the benefits of these chemicals, eat a variety of unheated, raw, organically grown vegetables, fruits, nuts, seeds, sea vegetables, and edible flowers. Allow your diet to consist of a kaleidoscope of colors. The biological functions the colors play within the plants will also play a part in maintaining your health.

Many nutrients are transported into the system by way of dietary fats. Carotenoids are fat-soluble. With a belief that including oil in the diet helps to assimilate nutrients, many raw foodists add olive oil, hemp oil, grapeseed oil, flax oil, or coconut oil to their foods. However, oil is present in all plant substances because each cell naturally contains some oil. You may notice that when you squeeze lemon into water, there will be natural oil from the lemon floating on top of the water. It is true that the oils in olives, avocado, nuts, and all plant substances work to help the body absorb the nutrients of the foods accompanying those plant substances. But there is no need to be concerned with getting enough oil, because all of the raw plant substances you eat naturally contain some oil. Even lettuce contains oils within its cells. Raw seeds, such as hemp, flax, and sesame are oil-rich and can be ground first in a coffee grinder to increase the availability of the nutrients.

We know that humans respond both emotionally and physically to colors. Being around certain colors can trigger emotional responses, such as alarm or calm, which elicit changes among the molecules within body tissues. The molecules within living plants carry specific color ratios and these are resonations of energy. There is an interaction going on between the frequencies of the molecules within the plants and the molecules within your body.

The energy frequency of the foods you eat is reflected in your body tissues, from your skin to your bones. It becomes obvious who is eating a deadening diet consisting of highly cooked matter and heated oils and meats and little to no fresh plant matter as much as it is obvious who is eating an abundantly nutritious diet that is rich in fresh, raw, edible plant matter.

When you cook plants, the colors throughout the plant tissues change, the order of the molecules changes, and the energy fields fade. When you are putting deadened plants inside a body that relies on living plants to bring in nutrients, you are not getting the full benefit of the plants.

In other words, plants collect substances from the soil, air, atmosphere, and light and turn these into their structures, which nourish us when we eat them – especially if we eat them when they are unheated and fresh. The raw plant matter carries a resonating energy that is in tune with the quality of nourishment they received as they grew.

"The answer to the American health crisis is the food that each of us chooses to put in our mouths each day. It's as simple as that."
– T. Colin Campbell, Ph.D., Cornell Univeristy, author of *The China Study* and *Whole;* TColinCampbell.org

To experience vibrant health, partake of foods containing their full spectrum of colors and living frequencies of energy. Eat vibrant, radiant, raw, living, edible plant matter that has been organically grown in healthy soil.

"There is more to us than we know. If we can be made to see it, perhaps for the rest of our lives we will be unwilling to settle for less."
– Kurt Hahn

To make this process of consuming fresh fruits and vegetables more easily available to you, get involved in growing food, and in composting your food scraps to make rich soil for growing your garden. By doing so, you will be participating in one of the most basic human experiences, and that is: growing and harvesting your own food.

"For many years, researchers have been studying how foods affect arthritis. Some of the early studies were not of the best quality, but by 1991, the issue was settled beyond any reasonable doubt. In *The Lancet*, a prominent British medical journal, researchers reported that a specially designed vegetarian diet can greatly reduce the signs and symptoms of arthritis. In the study, researchers found that a vegetarian diet lessened joint stiffness, swelling, and tenderness, and improved grip strength. The benefits lasted long after the study was over.

Here is why it works: Certain foods act as an arthritis trigger, stimulating the inflammatory process that attacks the tender synovial lining that is inside joints. The most common trigger foods are dairy products. Because it appears that a dairy protein is the culprit, even fat-free versions can trigger the inflammation that causes pain. A switch to soy milk or rice milk can help. Eggs and meat can contribute to joint pain for some people, which is why researchers are especially fond of vegan diets."

– Dr. Neal Barnard, author of *Foods That Fight Pain;* NealBarnard.org

ESSENTIAL FATTY ACIDS

"On average, we consume 35-40 percent of our total calories as fat. We have been consuming high-fat diets like this since the late nineteenth century, at the onset of our industrial revolution. Because we had more money, we began consuming more meat and diary, which are relatively high in fat. We were demonstrating our affluence by consuming such foods."
– T. Colin Campbell, Ph.D., Cornell University; author of *The China Study* and *Whole: Rethinking the Science of Nutrition*; TColinCampbell.org

If we are to experience vibrant health, we need essential fatty acids. Unfortunately, the fats that most people are consuming through industrial processed foods are of low-quality, negate health, and are damaging – especially fats that have been fried, sautéed, microwaved, or otherwise heated to high temperatures. We are also consuming too many fats. While a healthful level of fat intake would be about 10 percent of total calories, many Americans are consuming two or three times that much fat, with 30 percent or more of their calories from fatty snack foods, like chips, French fries, and cookies, donuts, scones, and rolls.

We sometimes are drawn to fatty foods, and especially at times of emotional upset. When our nerves are feeling frazzled, we often turn to fatty foods. Those who are in abusive relationships, neglectful relationships, or unsatisfying relationships, or who are not dealing well with life issues, often binge on fatty foods. This is interesting, especially because nerve health is highly reliant on quality dietary fats. Even the brain largely consists of fat.

A diet rich in oil slows the metabolic process. One reason is because it alters cell membrane function, slowing the ability of insulin to transfer nutrients into the cells. That is not good for people with diabetic conditions. A fatty diet also slows the ability of cells to excrete waste products, and leads to the accumulation of toxins that gather in the fat cells, including environmental toxins, such as heavy metals and synthetic chemicals. Regularly eating fatty foods leads to weight gain, slothfulness, a slower metabolism, and alters the ability of the body to absorb nutrients. However, those aren't the only adverse effects of consuming a high-fat diet.

Within minutes after being consumed, signs of a high-fat meal show up in the bloodstream. There, the oil slows the function of the endothelial cells, which line the walls of all of the veins, arteries, capillaries, and heart. The endothelial cells produce nitric oxide, which keeps the arteries open and the blood flowing smoothly. The longer a person consumes a fatty diet, the more clogged the blood system can become, and that can lead to the accumulation of plaque in the walls of the veins and arteries, which is what leads to adverse health events like heart attacks and strokes. Research shows that high-fat diets raise bad cholesterol, and increase the incidence of cancer, diabetes, and in men, erectile dysfunction.

Within days, omitting fatty foods and added oils from the diet increases the metabolism, improves the flow of the blood system, lowers cholesterol, brings blood sugar levels into better balance, and improves the function of the pancreas. How do we accomplish this? Don't eat fried foods, or foods sautéed in oil. Don't add bottled oils, including olive oil, to any foods. Avoid or greatly restrict the consumption of coconut, avocadoes, and nuts. Eliminate meat from the diet, including fish and fowl. Don't consume milk, or anything made from dairy, including cheese, creamer, ice cream, butter, yogurt, kefir, whey, and casein. Don't eat eggs, or anything containing eggs.

Relying on the trace but adequate amounts of oils that are naturally present in all raw fruits, vegetables, nuts, seeds, and seaweeds provides the body with the essential fatty acids it needs to function at a high level.

When switching from an unhealthful diet to one that is rich in raw fruits and vegetables, the body will release old, low-quality and sticky cooked oils, and will utilize the quality raw oils in the raw plant matter. The body will begin to function in a way it was meant to, with food being fuel, structural, and operational materials, rather than clogging and toxic residues and plaque.

Eliminating unhealthful fatty foods, such as meat, milk, eggs, fried foods, and highly heated oils, improves health in more ways than one. It helps the body get to an ideal weight, removes the physio-emotional shield a person may have been brandishing to avoid facing troubles or issues in life, allows people to focus more clearly on those things in their life that need their attention, and provides the oils that benefit the nerves: raw plant oils consisting of the essential fatty acids.

"In those parts of the world where coronary artery disease is rare, diets are low in fat and serum cholesterol levels are consistently below 150 mg/dL. In the United States, where vascular disease is the leading killer, the average citizen eats sixty-five pounds of fat per year – consuming two tons of suet by the age of sixty – and average cholesterol levels hover around 200 mg/dL."

– Dr. Caldwell B. Esselstyn, author of *Prevent and Reverse Heart Disease*; HeartAttackProof.com

Food choices can be a powerful tool in preventing and reversing common diseases, like cardiovascular disease, kidney disorders, osteoporosis, and diabetes. As research has revealed how this works, and also how disease processes take place and progress, dietary approaches to adjusting health have changed.

"The traditional approach to diabetes focuses on limiting refined sugars and foods that release sugars during digestion – starches, breads, fruits, pasta, etc. With carbohydrates reduced, the diet may contain an unhealthful amount of fat and protein. So diabetes experts have taken care to limit fats – especially saturated fats that can raise cholesterol levels – and to limit protein for people with impaired kidney function.

The new approach focuses more attention on fat. Fat is a problem for people with diabetes. The more fat there is in the diet, the harder time insulin has in getting glucose into the cells. Conversely, minimizing fat intake and reducing body fat help insulin do its job much better. Newer treatment programs drastically reduce meats, high-fat dairy products, and oils. At the same time, they increase grains, legumes, fruits, and vegetables. One study found that 21 of 23 patients on oral medications and 13 of 17 patients on insulin were able to get off of their medications after 26 days on a near-vegetarian diet and exercise program. During two- and three-year follow-ups, most people with diabetes treated with this regimen have retained their gains. The dietary changes are simple, but profound, and they work. Low-fat, vegetarian diets are ideal for people with diabetes."

– Dr. Neal Barnard, author of, *Dr. Neal Barnard's Program for Reversing Diabetes: The Scientifically Proven System for Reversing Diabetes without Drugs*; PCRM.org

While some may tell you that you can get quality fats by eating salmon, or from cod, or fish liver oil, what they may be overlooking is that you also get a whole slew of other substances when you rely on fish as a source of quality oils. Fish are constantly taking in water, just as we take in air. Fish work as filters of all sorts of toxins from whatever water they are in. Unfortunately, even the distant seas are polluted with substances like mercury, farming chemicals, military and cruise ship pollution, industrial and city runoff, and toxins absorbed into the oceans from airplanes and from air pollution drifting from distant cities and from coal-powered electricity generating plants and cement kilns. Pollutants tend to accumulate in fat.

If you choose to eat salmon or cod liver oil, or other fatty fish, or any sea creature, what you are getting is a collection of toxins found in the water where that creature lived. Since many of the sea creatures that humans tend to eat are also creatures that eat smaller creatures, the larger fish are consuming the toxins that exist in the smaller fish, and onward up the food chain, one concentrating the toxins of the other. The toxins accumulate in the fat of the fish – and especially in the liver.

Cod liver oil is also not good to consume. While all cells of the body engage in detox processes, the liver is the body detoxification center. All toxins in the fish pass through the liver. If you choose to consume cod liver oil you are getting the most concentrated amount of toxins, such as heavy metals and chemical pollution that exist within that fish. Unfortunately, even people living on islands and who rely on fish for food are being exposed to pollution spreading throughout the oceans. As I write this, tuna off the California coast are testing positive for radiation from Japan's ongoing Fukushima nuclear disaster. People living in areas where food can be grown would benefit by avoiding eating fish.

Besides the toxins in their fats, fish may also be harboring parasites that make people sick and/or rob them of nutrients. Fish also contain cholesterol and saturated fat, which are not good for the cardiovascular system, and increase the incidence of various chronic and degenerative diseases, including cancer. Fish do not contain fiber, carbohydrates, vitamin C, reliable stores of antioxidant, or many nutrients the human body needs for vibrant health.

You can exist on fish for years at a time. But your bones will suffer. A high-protein diet increases the likelihood of osteoporosis (weak bones from bone tissue loss).

At this stage in the industrialization of the world, when you eat fish you may be poisoning yourself with pollutants that can cause neurological disorders, birth defects, miscarriages, hormonal imbalances, and cancers. If you are a pregnant or nursing mother, your child can be harmed if you are consuming fish containing heavy metals and industrial pollutants – which, unfortunately, most fish do contain.

For those who advocate taking fish oil for heart health, I strongly advise that you avoid taking fish oil, because:

1) The fish and sea life populations have suffered greatly because of industrial fishing, loss of habitat, and from pollution. Sea life around the planet has been decimated and is at a fraction of what it was just a few decades ago. Many types of sea life are regionally extinct, or are on the edge of complete extinction.

We also don't need to be harvesting krill from the seas and killing it for its body oil. Krill is a shrimp-like crustacean and is the food for sea life, such as baleen whales, mantas, and whale sharks, which are suffering from what humans have done to the seas.

2) Ingesting fish and extracts of sea creatures increases your exposure to mercury, PCBs, and other environmental toxins from industrial pollution the creatures are exposed to in the increasingly polluted streams, lakes, rivers, marshes, and oceans. Consuming these contaminates leads to an accumulation of them in your cells, which then increases your risk of cancer and other health disorders.

Some people may say that the fish oil products they purchase are from uncontaminated waters free of industrial pollution. Keep dreaming. Unfortunately, there is no longer such a thing. Industrial pollution flows into lakes and rivers and into the oceans, and it also ends up in the air, which is then absorbed into the rivers, lakes, marshes, and oceans around the world. Mercury from coal-fired electric generating plants and cement kilns travels in the atmosphere, and is absorbed into the oceans thousands of miles from where it was released into the air. The main reason polar bears are now so contaminated with industrial pollution, such as fire retardants and heavy metals, is that they are getting these toxins by eating fish containing residue of industrial pollution. These toxins are impacting polar bears to such an extent that the toxins are damaging their bones, their nerves, and their ability to reproduce.

3) The benefit of taking fish oil is to obtain the omega-3 essential fatty acids. Instead of taking fish oil to get omega-3s, you can take algae supplements (which is where the fish get the omega-3s), and/or also include things like hemp seed powder, germinated chia, germinated buckwheat, soaked flax seeds, and other plant sources rich in essential fatty acids in your diet, including raw fruits and vegetables, and especially leafy green vegetables, including the common weed, purslane, which is rich in a variety of nutrients, including omega-3s and antioxidants.

The chicken eggs that are advertised as being rich in omega-3s are simply from chickens that have been fed raw flax seeds and/or meal containing fish oil or fish meal from fish that are being so overfished that many forms of life, including humans, are endangered.

Skip the eggs. Skip the fish oil and the fishmeal. Instead, eat the raw, freshly ground flax – and other plant sources of omega-3s.

The beef that is marketed as rich in omega-3s is from cattle that have grazed in meadows, eating raw greens. Skip eating the cow, simply eat fresh green salad. Raw greens are rich in omega-3s.

Quality fat sources: All must be eaten raw to get the best quality fats undamaged by heat.

As is mentioned elsewhere, it may be beneficial to your health to avoid adding oil to you foods. (See Dr. Esselstyn's book _Prevent and Reverse Heart Disease;_ HeartAttackProof.com.)

Raw seeds can be ground in a coffee grinder and used in dressings, smoothies, dips, hummus, pâtés, and other foods. They can also be germinated or sprouted and used in salads or as garnishes.

- **Buckwheat:** Germinated for one to two days.
- **Chia seeds:** Germinated for 20 minutes to 24 hours.
- **Coconut:** Fresh coconut meat, or fresh coconut water.
- **Fruit:** All raw fruit contains some trace, but adequate amounts, of quality fats. (Avoid cooked fruit: pies, jams, jellies, and pasteurized fruit juice.) Eat raw fruit.
- **Grapes:** Get seeded grapes and eat the crunchy seeds.
- **Green-leafed vegetables:** All raw vegetables contain some trace amounts of essential fatty acids.
- **Flax seeds:** Freshly ground raw seeds.
- **Hemp seeds:** Buy raw hemp seeds. Use a food processor to fracture them, or a coffee grinder to turn them into powder. There are also raw hemp seed powders and fractured hemp seeds sold in natural foods stores. Keep them refrigerated.
- **Olives:** Find raw olives.
- **Pumpkin seeds:** Or raw pumpkin seed butter.
- **Purslane:** Also known as pigweed, it is rich in omega-3 fatty acids, including eicosapentaenoic acid (EPA). Grow it.
- **Quinoa:** Germinate for several hours, or up to 24 hours to increase the essential fatty acids and other nutrients.
- **Sesame seeds:** Raw whole seeds or ground seeds, such as truly raw tahini.
- **Soy beans:** Raw, uncooked, organic, fresh. Eat sparingly.
- **Sunflower seeds:** Sprouts, soaked, or germinated.
- **Vegetables:** All raw vegetables contain trace, but adequate amounts of quality fats.
- **Walnuts:** Raw walnuts. If you eat nuts, eat few of them, and avoid those that have been heated, such as roasted, toasted, fried, kiln-dried, etc. While not always convenient, it is better to soak the raw nuts in water for an hour or so before eating.

The way food is prepared affects the quality of the fat. Heating fat degrades it, and turns it into something that can be damaging to health.

Fats are important in the digestion of sugars because fats slow down their absorption into the digestive tract. This allows for a more even flow of energy obtained by the sugars. Dietary fats also are important because they lubricate the tissues; insulate nerve tissues; transport nutrients to the tissues; and feed the fat cells that pad and support the organs.

The cells of all fruits and all vegetables contain some oil. As mentioned earlier, consuming a diet rich in raw fruits and vegetables provides adequate amounts of quality oils that help to reverse cell damage caused by the consumption of cooked oils. Cooked oils play a role in obesity, organ diseases, and cardiovascular disorders. The lipase enzyme that is present in raw plant oils helps to metabolize the cooked oils that clog the blood and lymph systems, and that interfere with the function of cell membranes. Within the membrane of cells, the quality raw oils replace the transfatty acids that hinder cell respiration.

The fats in raw fruits and vegetables stabilize and ground the system and provide structural material, nutrient transport, and fuel. In comparison, cooked and low-quality fats destabilize the system, collect and prevent the release of toxins, interfere with cell respiration, clog and slow body systems, slow the function of the endothelial cells, weaken the immune system, and pave the way for slothfulness and illness to set in.

The source of the fat is one factor that determines its quality. Because toxins collect in fats; foods that are grown with the use of toxic farming chemicals may contain traces of the chemicals in the plant oils. We know that these farming chemicals alter our hormonal balances, can play a role in nerve and other systemic disorders, and can trigger skin disorders, learning and behavioral problems, tumor growth, and birth defects. Therefore, organically grown fruits, nuts, seeds, and vegetables are better sources for dietary fats.

Fat is made up of glycerin and fatty acids. The type and number of fatty acids that are attached to the glycerin molecule are what determine the type of fat.

Because the body cannot manufacture certain types of fats called linoleic and linolenic, these fats are called "essential fatty acids." These fats, grouped into omega-3 and omega-6 fatty acids, exist in all raw fruits, vegetables, nuts, seeds, sprouts, germinates, and seaweeds, including the algaes spirulina and chlorella. Raw hemp seeds and flax seeds are often given as examples of foods containing omega-3s, with hemp seeds being the better choice over flax. It is omega-3s that are seriously lacking in the modern diet, and that is because people have become reliant on processed and manufactured foods for their calories, which are foods deficient in omega-3s. Raw walnuts are often mentioned as an excellent source, as are germinated chia and buckwheat. Leafy green vegetables and fresh sprouts are excellent sources of omega-3s.

More specifically, there is alpha-linolenic acid (ALA), which is an omega-3 good fat, when it is raw. It is polyunsaturated and, because it is beneficial in nerve function and blood pressure, is called "heart and brain healthy." It also is involved with nutrient transport and delivery.

There is also docosahexaenoic acid, or DHA, which is also an omega-3 fat or oil. It can be obtained from fish.

And, there is eicosapentaenoic acid, or EPA, which also can be obtained from fish, and fish obtain it from algae.

EPA is also found in what many people consider a common garden or invasive weed called purslane, or pigweed. The excellent nutrient profile contained in purlsane is the reason why you may hear people speak of adding purslane to their salads, smoothies, and other foods.

You may hear people say that you need to eat fish so that you get DHA. However, the human body can convert ALA into EPA. EPA is a precursor to DHA, and the body makes the DHA that it needs.

Because it takes less work to get EPA and DHA by eating fish, the body simply will obtain them from the diet when a person eats fish, rather than converting ALA into EPA and DHA. Something to consider is: Does less metabolic activity make the system lazy? Could this little bit of effort by the metabolic process taking place in the vegans burn the calories so that it helps vegans to end up being a more healthful weight?

It is said that older people may have a decreased ability to convert ALA into EPA and DHA. But when making blanket statements like this, one may consider that the animal studies used to come to this conclusion may not apply to humans. And human studies with the same conclusion may not apply to vegans or raw vegans with a history of following low-fat diets rich in raw fruits and raw vegetables containing unheated oils and not containing synthetic chemicals.

The ability of the metabolism to utilize and/or metabolize any nutrient can be impaired by unhealthful living, such as substance abuse, smoking, lack of exercise, bad sleeping patterns, stress, consumption of low-quality foods, synthetic food additives, and a diet rich in animal protein. Understanding that, it can be clear that a study using only humans that have a lifetime of eating animal protein and ingesting other health-damaging substances and/or leading unhealthful lives may not be the most reliant study to apply to those humans who have followed a vegan diet rich in raw fruits and vegetables.

Certainly, there are a variety of people who have been vegan for decades, and many more children are now being raised on vegan diets. This pretty much kicks out the concept that we need to eat fish, or take fish-oil supplements to get DHA. Our bodies make the DHA that we need, and they do it by utilizing the ALA in the raw fruits, vegetables, sprouts, and other plant matter that we consume.

"I recommend adding flaxseed to your diet regularly. Flaxseeds have a tough outer coating and should be freshly ground in order to receive the most nutritional benefit. You can grind whole seeds with a coffee grinder or in a VitaMix blender dry container. I recommend adding one or two tablespoons of ground flax meal to your salads, soups, or smoothies. Flaxseed is also a good source of omega-3 fatty acids, and it is by far nature's richest source of plant lignin, an important anticancer phytonutrient."
– Victoria Boutenko in her book *Green for Life*; RawFamily.Com

Fats from animals, including meat, milk, and eggs, are saturated, are nutritionally lower quality, are damaging to cell walls, trigger the production of cholesterol, alter cell membrane function, are rich in free radicals that damage tissues, have been connected to a variety of chronic and degenerative diseases, including diabetes, cardiovascular disease, Alzheimer's, MS, macular degeneration, cancers, and other ailments, and should be avoided.

Fats from animals contain residues of the toxic chemicals the animal was exposed to (including from the chemically grown and GMO foods the animals ate), as well as the hormonal chemistry of the animal.

"When the levels of fats in the bloodstream become elevated, everything begins to change. Gradually, the endothelium (lining of the blood and lymph vessels and heart), the white blood cells, and the platelets, the blood cells that cause clotting, all become sticky. Eventually, a white blood cell adheres to and eventually penetrates the endothelium, where it attempts to ingest the rising numbers of LDL cholesterol molecules that are being oxidized from the fatty diet. That white blood cell sends out a call for help to other white blood cells. More and more of them converge on the site, becoming engorged with bad cholesterol and eventually forming a bubble of fatty pus – an atheroma, or 'plaque,' the chief characteristic of atherosclerosis."
– Dr. Caldwell B. Esselstyn, author of *Prevent and Reverse Heart Disease*; HeartAttackProof.com

One environmental toxin that accumulates in animal fat is dioxin. This is a long-lasting, hormonal-disrupting compound that has been linked to cancers, birth defects, and developmental problems. Dioxin is commonly found in all animal products that are sold as food, including meat of all varieties (including seafood and birds), eggs, and dairy. Foods likely to contain dioxin residues should especially be avoided by women planning on becoming pregnant, by expectant mothers, and by nursing mothers.

Animal fats are less likely to be eaten raw because milk products are usually heated (pasteurized), and meat and eggs are usually cooked in some manner. The heating of the animal fat destroys most of what could be considered to be the beneficial dietary qualities of the fat, and turns it into a substance that is harsh on the human system.

It should be very clear that I don't advocate eating meat, milk, or eggs in any form, raw or cooked. They all contain the fat and cholesterol that increase blood lipids, leading to plaque in the cardiovascular system, and raising risk of heart attacks and strokes. They also all raise blood cholesterol levels, and increase the risk of diabetes, arthritis, macular degeneration, cataracts, atherosclerosis, Alzheimer's, Parkinson's, Crohn's, multiple sclerosis, osteoporosis, obesity, kidney disease, liver cancer, colon cancer, rectal cancer, breast cancer, brain cancer, lymph cancer, lung cancer, blood cancer, eczema, varicose veins, and, in women, uterine cancer and ovarian cancer, and, in men, prostate cancer and erectile dysfunction.

If you do choose to consume milk, it is much better to get it raw, unheated, and from an organic dairy where the cows graze in open fields, and to consume that milk raw, and not pasteurized or heated. Milk from cows that graze in open fields, and that are not treated with common drugs, contains higher levels of beneficial essential fatty acids, including omega-3 and the omega-6 conjugated linoleic acid. However, we do not need milk from another animal in our diet. The milk we need is what we get as a baby, from our mothers. After the toddler stage in life, we no longer need milk. Children who consume dairy are more likely to experience diabetes.

"Cow's milk is adapted for the rapid growth of a calf into a large herbivorous animal, and is not suited for the slower growth of a smaller human being. The gain in weight must therefore be at the expense of vitality."
– Dugald Semple, in his 1956 book *The Sunfood Way to Health*

The process of getting milk from cows involves taking the baby cow or bull from its mother soon after birth (often within a day), and then taking the mother's milk to sell for human consumption, including as milk, butter, ice cream, creamer, cheese, yogurt, kefir, whey, and casein. The female calves are kept for future milk production. Very few, if any, of the male calves are kept for stud service. More than likely the baby bull is sold and soon killed for its tender meat, which is marketed as veal = meat of slaughtered baby calves (Access: NoVeal.org), or the male calf is raised for slaughter to sell its meat. This is one of the dark secrets of the dairy industry. As the female cows age and lose their ability to produce enough milk to pay for their keep and to make a profit by

319

selling their milk, they are also sold off to slaughter. Their bodies are cut up and the meat is made into such things as hamburgers, processed meats, and canned chili and stew meat. Those meats contain all the residues of the toxic farming chemicals the cow was exposed to and consumed through a diet of grains grown using massive amounts of farming chemicals – which then end up in the human system, triggering nerve disorders, immune system disorders, hormonal imbalances, and cancer growth. Raising all of the many millions of mass-bred farmed cows uses a tremendous amount of resources, including fuel, steel, concrete, land, and water to grow food to feed the millions of cattle.

"Cows are amongst the gentlest of breathing creatures; none show more passionate tenderness to their young when deprived of them; and, in short, I am not ashamed to profess a deep love for these quiet creatures."
– Thomas de Quincey

A main problem with fats from animal flesh is that it is saturated and contains cholesterol. The consumption of saturated fat in the human body triggers the production of cholesterol. This overload of cholesterol leads to the scenario of cardiovascular disease, strokes, gallstones, and many chronic and degenerative conditions, including vision problems.

Plant oils do not contain cholesterol. Although cholesterol is needed in the human body, it does not need to be obtained from food. The only cholesterol the body needs is naturally made by the liver. Beyond that, ingesting extra cholesterol leads to the health problems that keep hospitals busy, and drug companies making billions. Foreign cholesterol introduced into the body through the consumption of meat, dairy, and eggs is not needed, and is problematic for the body to eliminate.

The only people who need cholesterol in their diets are infants and babies, who need it for proper brain formation. Ideally they get their cholesterol from their mother's milk. They also produce cholesterol in their liver.

Those who are experiencing heart disease, who have had a stroke or a heart attack, have been told their arteries are clogged, or have been told they are at a risk of heart attack or stroke, would be very wise to remove all animal products from their diet, as well as heated oils, all oil extracts (including olive, flax, corn, canola, sunflower, soy, palm, safflower, and other bottled oils), all fried foods, all foods sautéed in oil, and all foods containing processed salt, processed sweeteners (such as white or brown sugar, corn syrup, and agave), and all synthetic dyes, flavors, scents, and preservatives, and MSG. They will benefit by transitioning to an all or nearly all raw vegan diet consisting of organically grown foods. Then the body can go about the process of removing the accumulation of cholesterol in the system. (See books about reversing heart disease written by Dr. Dean Ornish, Dr. John McDougall, Dr. Neal Barnard, and Dr. Caldwell Esselstyn. Please, watch the documentaries *Forks over Knives* and *Fat, Sick, and Nearly Dead*. Don't eat animals.)

Although the process of ridding the body of cholesterol plaque from the tissues can take years, benefits can be experienced within days of eliminating from the diet all meat, dairy, and eggs, and foods that contain them. Especially if all fried and sautéed food, all foods containing processed salts, all processed sugars, all bleached and gluten grains, and all bottled oils are also eliminated while increasing the consumption of raw fruits and vegetables.

As mentioned earlier, fats that are naturally present in all raw fruits and vegetables play a role in the distribution of nutrients throughout the body, including minerals, vitamins, and antioxidants to the bones and tissues. Raw plant fats also effectively increase the electric tension on cell membranes, making the cells more permeable to oxygen and nutrients. Unhealthful fats damage the cell walls, interfere with nutrient absorption, allow toxins to enter and collect, and limit the cells' ability to rid waste products and to maintain health.

Eating foods containing cooked fat, especially foods that have been cooked at high temperatures, is damaging to the body. These fats are the undesirable transfatty acids. They clog the system; slow the blood and lymph systems; irritate the alimentary tract; and interfere with the function of the power generators of every cell within the body.

Those power-generating structures within the cells are called the mitochondria. They become less effective in the cells of a person eating a junk diet, and especially of a diet containing cooked or fried fat, animal fat, and processed sugars, salts, and synthetic chemicals.

All fats that have been heated to high temperatures, hydrogenated, pasteurized, or oxidized should be avoided. They are damaging to health, and cause the body to accumulate toxins. They lead to obesity, low energy, and degenerative diseases.

Oils naturally present in raw plants are much less likely to lead to the accumulation of toxins in the system. This is because the cells accommodate, work with, and need the essential fatty acids of raw plants. Unlike cooked fats, which are sticky, raw plant oils are fluid. Anyone who has scrubbed sticky cooked fat from kitchen pots and pans knows how stubborn cooked oil can be to wash away. Compare that to washing away raw nut, seed, and avocado oils from a salad bowl, and you get the idea of how much easier the body cells have it when they are dealing with raw plant oil as compared to sticky, cooked oils.

Eliminating all cooked fats and animal fats from the diet and allowing in only raw fruits and vegetables leads to weight loss when a person is overweight. This is because the toxic fats will begin to be eliminated, and the cells will release the toxins that were contained in those unhealthful fats. Then the cells can begin to work more efficiently as their respiration improves and the cell walls and mitochondria function healthfully.

Raw plant fats contain lipase enzymes, which play a part in the "burning" of fats for body fuel. This fat-splitting enzyme is typically lacking in the bodies of overweight people, and in the bodies of those consuming unhealthful foods. The enzymes help the body metabolize collections of cooked fat residue in the bodies of cooked-food eaters.

As people transition into a raw vegan diet from that of a cooked diet – and especially from a diet that contained meat, dairy, and eggs – they may mistake the empty feeling they have for a lack of protein. Some may try to fill this feeling with cooked vegetables, or cooked starches. Eating a good variety of raw fruits and vegetables will provide an abundance of the amino acids the body needs to form protein. All fruits and vegetables contain the amino acids the human body uses to form protein.

Nuts are a fatty food more than they are a protein food. They (almonds, cashews, hazelnuts, macadamias, pecans, Brazil nuts, pine nuts, walnuts, etc.) should be eaten raw, and never heated, roasted, baked, sautéed, toasted, fried, or microwaved.

Eating too many nuts can be a bit harsh on the digestive tract; they carry a lot of calories; are acid-forming in large quantities; and, because they are acidic, eating too many can trigger mucus formation as the body works to be alkaline. To keep the calories from fat low, avoid consuming a lot of nuts.

The consumption of nuts is best balanced with raw greens and fruits. Raw walnuts go well in green and fruit salads.

The consumption of greens with nuts counteracts the acid of the nuts, and prevents a mucus-forming reaction. Greens are alkaline.

Soaking raw nuts for two to ten hours in water can reduce the enzyme inhibitors that exist in them and that work to prevent their growth into a plant. People who follow a living foods diet typically soak raw nuts in water for a matter of hours before using them.

It is good to use little or no oil in recipes. When using oil, add very little raw hemp seed oil or raw tahini. Or, try raw coconut oil. I figure that I get enough essential fatty acids from the raw fruits, vegetables, sprouts, seeds, germinates, and few seaweeds that I consume. Eating at raw restaurants or the food of private chefs catering an event can be a different experience, as they tend to make foods that contain more oils and nuts than I'm used to eating at home.

Many seeds contain more fat than protein, and are considered to be fat-dominant. Raw seeds that are fat-dominant and have high-quality oils are the previously mentioned flax, hemp, chia, pumpkin, grapeseed, and sesame. Coconuts are fat-dominant seeds containing high-quality oils. (Those who consume coconut should be sure that it is raw, not heated, roasted, toasted, baked, fried, or microwaved.)

There are three types of dietary fats: saturated, monounsaturated, and polyunsaturated. Fats, when obtained from raw plants, are beneficial to health. Only when plant fats are heated, or eaten in abundance, are they damaging. Otherwise, raw plant fats are good for the body – but best from whole fruits, vegetables, sprouts, germinates, and seaweeds.

Coconuts contain a form of saturated fat that is of medium-chain triglycerides that can trigger the liver to metabolize ketones, which have been found to feed brain nerve cells. Raw coconut oil has been found to raise good cholesterol and to improve brain function in people suffering from Alzheimer's disease (see the book _Alzheimer's Disease: What if there was a cure?_ by Mary T. Newport). If you use coconut oil, please don't heat it. Use it raw, and purchase the organic coconut oil. Or, instead of using the coconut oil, simply get coconuts, drink the water, and scrape out the meat.

Avocados, raw olives, olive oil, and nuts contain monounsaturated fat. Polyunsaturated fat is found in walnuts, and in sunflower, flax, hemp, sesame, and other seeds.

Raw plant fats contain antioxidants and help to prevent free radicals from damaging the tissues. Meat, eggs, and dairy are rich in free radicals. Free radicals are electron-deficient molecules that are produced by oxygen and cooked fats in the body. Free radicals damage amino acids, enzymes, and other substances of the cells by taking electrons. Raw plant fats have long-chain fatty acids and carry an abundance of electrons, and this allows for free radicals to obtain the electrons from the fat without robbing the cell.

Fats that have been cooked, and meat, dairy, and eggs allow for, and cause free radical damage. But raw plant fats, especially those that are in the polyunsaturated fat class, prevent free radical damage. This is because raw plant fats contain nutrients, such as vitamins C and E, as well as carotene and selenium. In addition, various other raw foods contain antioxidants, such as bioflavonoids in citrus and beta-carotene in certain vegetables – especially green leafy vegetables. So the abundance of electrons provided by the raw plant fats saturates the body with spare electrons, and this essentially deactivates free radicals, allowing the cells of the body to remain healthier, and preventing aging and degeneration of the eyes, brain, skin, and other organs and tissues.

Some people think that they are eating healthfully if they are staying away from cooked foods containing animal fats, and instead, eating cooked foods that contain plant fats, such as olive, sunflower, canola, palm, soy, corn, or safflower oils. While eating plant fats is better than eating fats from animals, cooking any kind of fat damages nutrients and changes the chemistry of the fat, making it into something that is not good for the body.

As mentioned earlier, fats from animals carry environmental and farm toxins the animals were exposed to; are saturated and trigger the production of cholesterol in the body; contain cholesterol from the animals that overloads the human system, causing plaque to form within the blood passageways; interfere with the endothelial cell production of nitric oxide that keeps the veins and arteries open; contain free radicals that damage cell tissues; contain the hormonal chemistry of the animals; and carry energy and emotion chemicals that are not good for human health. Animal fats are toxic to the human system, lead to fat buildup, contain toxic residues, build the terrain for degenerative and chronic diseases, and otherwise result in compromised health.

Again, I clearly do not advise anyone to consume milk, other than human milk for human babies. Those who consume cow milk are exposing themselves to the toxins, cholesterol, and unhealthful body chemistry of the animal – especially if that animal was raised in a factory farm. The conditions, food, sounds, atmosphere, and drugs and chemicals used on factory farms are horrible for animals, and create a body chemistry of fright, stress, anger, and illness. People who drink milk are also consuming the Neu5Gc molecule (N-glycolyeneuraminic acid) in the milk, which is also in meat, is produced by nonhuman mammals, can't be synthesized by humans, causes inflammation, is found in human cancers, and can make cancer more aggressive (anyone with cancer should absolutely eliminate all meat, milk, and eggs from their diet).

While milk fat is a healthier animal fat than the fat from meat, it does not carry the health benefits many people believe it has. Raw milk fat is also better than cooked milk fat. Milk from animals that are raised eating organic foods where they graze in open fields, and raised in a way that does not expose them to toxic farming chemicals and drugs, is healthier than milk from factory farms, where the animals are fed unnatural diets; exposed to unhealthful conditions that cause stress and disease; treated with growth hormones and other drugs; and exposed to various chemicals. (Access: MilkIsCruel.com)

Goat milk and goat cheese are also consumed by some people. I don't advocate drinking goat milk, or anything made or derived from it, as it is best for baby goats. But if goat milk is consumed, it should be from an organic farm source where animals graze in open fields, and should be raw, not pasteurized. As with cow milk, the way goat milk is produced for human consumption involves getting the goat pregnant, killing the baby male goats, then taking the mother's milk that would have fed the baby male goat. The females are raised for milk production. Some of the flesh from the baby goats is sold as meat, but most of them are simply disposed of. In other words, the lives of the baby male goats are of no monetary value, so they are killed.

It may surprise those who have lived in a milk-consuming society that people in many parts of the world frown on drinking milk and on eating cheese, and consider consuming animal milk as disgusting.

The main reason people drink milk is for the calcium. At least, that is what they have been brainwashed into believing by the dairy industry. A vastly better choice for getting minerals in the diet is raw green vegetables, which is what the cows eat. There is no reason to eat the cow to get the minerals that the cow gets from eating greens. Simply eat a salad consisting largely of green leafy vegetables.

Kale is especially rich in the minerals your body uses to build strong bones. Kale is also a better source of protein than beef. If you want even more minerals, add some seaweed flakes to that salad. Seaweeds, such as kelp and dulse, are rich in a variety of minerals. Unlike milk, which contains saturated fat, cholesterol, and free radicals, in addition to minerals, greens are rich in antioxidants, fiber, and a variety of nutrients that are lacking in milk. Again, skip the cow, eat a salad.

Pasteurization of milk is a heating process, which damages the fats and creates a product that leads to degenerative conditions in the human body, such as heart disease and arthritis. Milk is already damaging enough, because it contains casein. As T. Colin Campbell explains, as far as food substances, "casein is the most relevant cancer promoter ever discovered." The lactose in milk also causes problems, as humans have no need for milk after the toddler stage, when they are naturally weaned from their mother's milk. And the cholesterol in milk is not needed for human health, but contributes to cardiovascular disease.

Men who eat more dairy and/or eggs have higher rates of prostate cancer than men who eat little or no dairy and/or eggs.

Some people that have found out about the problems with a fat-rich diet, and how it can increase the incidence of cancers and cardiovascular disease, have switched to nonfat and low-fat milk. However, nonfat and low-fat milk have also been linked to prostate cancer. People consuming nonfat and low-fat milk are still getting the animal protein, which has been proven to be a cancer trigger. And, they are getting the N-glycolylneuraminic acid, the problematic sugar molecule that is found in dairy and in nonhuman mammal meat, and that is found on human cancer cells. And they are increasing their risk of osteoporosis, diabetes, arthritis, and other health problems linked to diets rich in dairy products, which are rich in tissue-damaging free radicals.

Researchers at the University of Hawaii analyzed data from the Multiethnic Cohort Study that was conducted between 1993 and 2002 and identified low-fat and nonfat dairy products as problematic in that they increase the risk of localized and nonaggressive tumors. In addition to this, the December 1, 2008, issue of the *American Journal of Epidemiology* reported that researchers at the National Cancer Institute at the National Institutes of Health found that the consumption of skim milk was linked to advanced prostate cancer. They also found that calcium from plant foods was linked to a reduced risk of nonadvanced prostate cancer.

"In 1997, the World Cancer Research Fund and the American Institute for Cancer Research concluded that dairy products should be considered a possible contributor to prostate cancer. And yet another research study came out in April 2000 pointing to a link between dairy and prostate cancer: Harvard's Physicians' Health Study followed 20,885 men for 11 years, finding that having two and one-half dairy servings each day boosted prostate cancer risk by 34 percent, compared to having less than one-half serving daily.

Researchers are looking not only at whether milk increases cancer risk, but how. The answer, apparently, is in the way milk affects a man's hormones. Dairy products boost the amount of insulin-like growth factor (IGF-I) in the blood. In turn, IGF-I promotes cancer cell growth. A small amount is normally in the bloodstream, but several recent studies have linked increased IGF-I levels to prostate cancer and possibly to breast cancer as well.

Milk does other mischief. Its load of calcium depletes the body's vitamin D, which, in turn, may add to cancer risk. Most dairy products are also high in fat, which affects the activity of sex hormones that play a major role in cancer.

And it would come as no surprise that milk might affect the growth of cancer cells. After all, its biological purpose is to support rapid growth in all parts of a calf's body. After the age of weaning, calves (like all mammals) have no need for milk at all, and there is never a need to drink the milk of another species."

– *Milk and Prostate Cancer: The Evidence Mounts*, by Neal D. Barnard, M.D., Physicians Committee for Responsible Medicine, PCRM.org

The casein protein in milk can also cause mood swings, depression, and anxiety. Those who experience depression and/or anxiety would be wise to avoid milk, processed sugar (including agave, corn syrup, and white and brown sugar), salt, fried foods, sautéed foods, and gluten

grains (including all types of wheat, barley, and rye), and increase the
ratio of raw green vegetables and raw fruit in their diet.

Raw dairy may provide some substances beneficial to establishing a
base of healthy intestinal flora. But if dairy is consumed, it should be
minimally. Ideally, a person would obtain minerals and flora from raw
plant sources and not depend on dairy, which is mucus forming, acidifying, can leach minerals from the system, and carries a negative energy
into the system. (For more information about the negative impact dairy
products have on human health and the health of the environment, read
The Food Revolution, by John Robbins. Also, access: NotMilk.com.)

"Cows' milk is a high-fat food exquisitely designed for turning a
65-pound calf into a 400-pound cow in a year. That is what cows'
milk is for."
– Dr. Michael Klaper, author of *Vegan Nutrition*

For more on essential fatty acids, read *Becoming Raw: The Essential
Guide to Raw Vegan Diets*, by Davis, Melina, and Berry; Dr. Caldwell
Esselstyn's *Prevent and Reverse Heart Disease*; and *Whole*, by T. Colin
Campbell. Another book containing helpful information about raw fats
is Victoria Boutenko's *Green for Life*.

"What is one of the most striking differences between a
hummingbird and a hibernating bear? Their metabolism. One
moves extremely fast and the other is extremely slow, largely due to
differences in the composition of fat in their bodies. According to
recent scientific research on factors affecting metabolism, 'the fats
of high-speed animals such as the hummingbird are loaded with the
omega-3 fatty acids.' Contrary to that, bears have to accumulate a lot
of omega-6 fatty acids in their fat before they can go into
hibernation. Omega-3s and omega-6s are seemingly alike substances
and are even united under one name: essential polyunsaturated fatty
acids. However, there are major differences between them.

The omega-3 molecule is unique in its ability to rapidly change
its shape. This exceptional flexibility of omega-3s is passed to organs
that absorb it. Omega-3s thin the blood of humans and animals as
well as the sap of plants. As a result of these qualities, omega-3s are
utilized by the fastest functioning organs in the body. For example,
omega-3s enable our hearts to beat properly, our blood to flow
freely, our eyes to see, and our brains to make decisions faster and
more clearly.

The omega-6 fatty acids, on the other hand, serve the opposite
function: they thicken the blood of humans and animals as well as
the juices of plants. Omega-6s solidify and cause inflammation of

327

the tissues. Some scientists link an excess of omega-6s in the human diet with such conditions as heart disease, stroke, arthritis, asthma, menstrual cramps, diabetes, headaches, and tumor metastases."
– Victoria Boutenko, author of *Green for Life*. RawFamily.com

Those new to raw veganism may notice that some raw foodists spell nondairy cream as *kreme*, and nondairy milk as *mylk*. The spelling is also something you may notice on the menus of vegan restaurants and cafes.

"The truth is I feel humbled being vegan rather than superior to those who aren't. I have no cause to be self-righteous. There was a time when I ate animals and made excuses, and I feel grateful to be armed with knowledge and awareness and to be able to act on my values of compassion and kindness. Rather than feel morally superior to people who eat animals, I feel great sorrow for animals who suffer and for the humans who inflict that suffering. If we keep this big picture in mind, we can create the compassionate world we all envision."
– Colleen Patrick-Goudreau

"Humans who enslave, castrate, experiment on, and filet other animals have had an understandable penchant for pretending animals do not feel pain. A sharp distinction between humans and 'animals' is essential if we are to bend them to our will, make them work for us, wear them, eat them without any disquieting tinges of guilt or regret. It is unseemly of us, who often behave so unfeeling toward other animals, to contend that only humans can suffer. The behavior of other animals renders such pretensions specious. They are just too much like us."
– Carl Sagan

"Many cultures view one of these animals as a friend, a companion, even part of the family to be doted upon, whilst the other is considered an unfeeling machine, a slave bred to generate meat or milk for our breakfast, lunch and dinner. Both of these beings can equally feel joy or pain and both can equally experience or express love. In a world where humans could easily survive without inflicting harm of any kind upon either, we begin by imposing the most rudimentary harm; which is to stamp the labels of 'pet' and 'livestock' upon them, respectively."
– Anthony Damiano

The best way to prevent disease is to avoid doing things that help create the terrain for diseases to take hold. Following a vibrant diet consisting largely of raw fruits and vegetables is one major key in maintaining vibrant health.

Foods that damage enzymatic activity within the body include meat, milk, eggs, and products made with them, which are all rich in free radicals. Enzyme-damaging foods also include fried and sautéed foods, and others containing highly heated oils, and foods containing MSG, gluten grains, bleached foods, and artificial sweeteners, dyes, and flavors, as well as other artificial ingredients. Eating these deadened foods clutters the system and puts the body out of tune with nature.

The good news is that a system that has been damaged by unhealthful eating can be made healthier by cutting out deadened foods, and by eating a healthful, vibrant diet rich in raw fruits and vegetables. Because the biological factory that exists within the body is designed to function in a certain way, it will always work better if it is given the proper fuel.

Your body cannot function at its highest level if you are not feeding it what it needs to function at that level. You can change that now, today, with your food choices. Make a conscious decision to select and eat food that is high-quality, and preferably consisting of raw, organically grown fruits, vegetables, sprouts, herbs, nuts, seeds, and water plants.

Make a list of organic farms in your region. Locate local organic fruit wholesalers. Find the closest organic food co-op, or start one. Grow a food garden. Plant native fruiting trees and bushes.

B-12 VITAMIN
(COBALAMIN, CYANOCOBALAMIN, METHYLCOBALAMIN)

B-12 comes from microorganisms and is present in meat, milk, and eggs.

While the claim is often made that vegans and vegetarians don't get enough B-12 in their diet, this depends on what type of veggie diet the vegan or vegetarian is following. While vegans and vegetarians often test lower for B-12 than do people who consume animal protein, many people who consume meat and dairy have been found with low levels of B-12.

The health of the stomach and intestinal tract play a major role in the presence of B-12 in the body. The quality of the food also is key to getting and maintaining sufficient amounts of B-12. Those who take diabetes medications, painkillers, and some other medications may experience low B-12 absorption.

It may be good to include several sources of B-12 in the diet so that there is no possibility of B-12 deficiency.

Cyanocobalamin is a cheap form of B-12, in which a cyanide molecule is used as a binding agent. Because cyanide isn't exactly something you want in your body, it is advisable to avoid cyanocobalamin. To remove the cyanide from your body through your liver, the body's natural resources of methyl group molecules are used, which can interfere with the system's ability to metabolize homocysteine. Too much homocysteine can play a role in heart disease.

A better choice for a B-12 supplement is to take methylcobalamin in sublingual form (a tablet placed under the tongue and dissolvee there). There are also methylcobalamin skin patch products that deliver B-12 through the skin, such as by placing the patch on the skin behind an ear. The skin patches also usually contain the B vitamin folic acid, which also plays a role in heart health. Methylcobalamine is a coenzyme form of B-12 that is more bioavailable than cyanocobalamin, and is more easily absorbed into the system.

B-12 plays a role in cell replication, in the construction of DNA, and in the formation of red blood cells in the bone marrow. It is the red blood cells that bring oxygen to the body tissues. B-12 is also needed to maintain healthy nerve fiber sheaths, and for converting carbohydrates, fat, and protein into sources of energy.

A diet lacking in B-12 could lead a person to experience hyperhomocystemia, which is a condition defined by an elevated level of homocystine in the blood. Homocystine is an amino acid that is produced normally in the process of breaking down methionine, an amino acid. Too much homocystine can damage the walls of the arteries, cause the accumulation of atherosclerotic plaque, and lead to cardiovascular disease and stroke, and damage the eyes, kidneys, and other organs.

Vitamin B-12 deficiency can also cause weakness, dizziness, fatigue, shortness of breath, depression, paranoia, delusions, intestinal upset, upper respiratory infection, nerve damage, macrocytic anemia, sore tongue, indigestion, diarrhea, slow reflexes, and numbness and tingling in the fingers and toes. A woman with low levels of B-12 is more likely to have a baby with birth defects. Women who are breastfeeding and who have low levels of B-12 may produce nutritionally weak breast milk, which can stunt brain and nerve cell growth.

Where do vegans get B-12?

- **Algae**: Spirulina, chlorella, wild blue green algae. Not the most reliable sources. Chlorella does contain cobalt, which is at the center of the B-12 molecule, and may be a source of B-12, but it should not be the only thing a person consumes to rely on obtaining adequate amounts of B-12. Wild blue green algae can also help to maintain B-12 levels. Seaweeds may also contain inactive B-12 analogs that can take up the same receptor sites as true B-12, and give a false positive on the serum B-12 test.
- **Fermented seed or nut cheeses**: When they contain Red Star Vegetarian Support Formula nutritional yeast, which is available in most natural foods stores.
- **Intestinal flora**: The good bacteria in your digestive tract, including the mouth. While the bacteria in the large intestine does manufacture B-12, that ends up leaving the body. The receptor sites are in the small intestine.

  You can increase the amount of intestinal flora in your system by taking a vegan probiotic supplement. They are sold in either capsule or powder form in the refrigerated section in the nutrition departments of natural foods stores.
- **Kimchi:** A fermented vegetable salad. Best if made using raw, unheated, organically grown ingredients. It is much more likely to contain B-12 if it is made in a wooden vat rather than a ceramic or

steel container, or if a reusable wooden compression weight is used within the nonwooden container. See Sauerkraut, below.

- **Mushrooms**: Specifically, cultivated white button and flush mushrooms. In 2009, the *Journal of Agricultural and Food Chemistry* published a study conducted at the Centre for Plant and Food Science, College of Health and Science, University of Western Sydney, concluding that B-12 was found on and in white button and flush mushrooms from a variety of farms. Because B-12 was found to be more present in the peel than other structures of the mushrooms, the study suggested that the B-12 is likely bacteria derived from bacteria originating in the soil.

- **Noma shoyu:** A raw, fermented, soy sauce-like product made with wheat, soybeans, salt, and a bacterial starter. Only purchase if it says it is raw, and has not been heated. Although the product is made using cooked wheat and soy, the sauce is the product of months of fermentation, which results in a vat of enzymes, amino acids, good bacteria, and other nutrients, usually including B-12. For a variety of reasons, including because of the salt content and the processing, many raw foodists do not consume Noma Shoyu. Those who are avoiding gluten-containing foods may also wish to avoid Noma Shoyu.

- **Nutritional yeast:** Grown on mineral-enriched molasses. Red Star Vegetarian Support Formula nutritional yeast is available in most natural foods stores, either in bulk form, or in a container. It is also rich in other B-complex vitamins as well as in amino acids. Nutritional yeast is NOT baker's yeast, which is different. It has been found to be beneficial in helping to reverse B-12 deficiency, but not as helpful as B-12 supplements. Regularly using nutritional yeast is one way of helping to maintain healthful B-12 levels. Nutritional yeast should be stored in a covered container kept in a cool, dry place (not frozen), and in a place where it isn't exposed to constant light. Cooking it will damage the nutrients. It can be added to salads, hummus, dips, dressings, spreads, and patés, and to nut and seed cheeses.

"A number of reliable vegan food sources for vitamin B-12 are known. One brand of nutritional yeast, Red Star T-6635+, has been tested and shown to contain active vitamin B-12. This brand of yeast is often labeled as Vegetarian Support Formula with or without T-6635+ in parentheses following this new name. It is a reliable source of vitamin B-12. Nutritional yeast, Saccharomyces cerevisiae, is a food yeast, grown on a molasses solution, which comes as yellow flakes or powder. It has a cheesy taste. Nutritional yeast is different from brewer's yeast or torula yeast. Those sensitive to other yeasts can often use it."

– Vitamin B-12 in the Vegan Diet, by Reed Mangels, Ph.D., R.D.; Vegetarian Resource Group

- **Rejuvelac:** While some bacteria in rejuvelac may produce B-12, it should not be considered a reliable source. If it is made using the water from soaking organically grown wheat berries or other seeds to the sprouting stage, rejuvelac may contain more B-12. Rejuvelac is often used in raw vegan cheese recipes, including those that also contain B-12-rich nutritional yeast and/or vegan probiotic powder.

- **Organically grown raw fruits and vegetables**: Soil organisms are on the leaves and skins of these. It can be reasoned that some B-12 is obtained from the bacteria. An organic garden using composted kitchen scraps from organic fruits and vegetables can contain more soil organisms that form B-12 than a garden grown using chemical fertilizers.

- **Probiotic powder**: Vegan probiotic powder is often used in raw foods, such as in cheeses, dressings, spreads, and sauces. It provides healthy doses of beneficial flora for the intestines, but it should not be considered a way of obtaining adequate amounts of B-12.

- **Recycled B-12:** The body does reclaim and reuse some B-12. The bile extracts B-12 that has been absorbed into the small intestines, and then reabsorbs the vitamin again in the small intestine. Some people's systems are more able to do this than others, but this should not be considered as a reliable source of adequate amounts of B-12. Those who consume a diet that is free of heated oils, including sautéed foods and fried foods, and those who stay away from gluten, dairy, eggs, meat, bleached grains, processed sugars, and synthetic food chemicals while consuming a diet rich in fresh fruits and vegetables are more likely to have a more healthful alimentary tract that is able to absorb nutrients, including B-12.

- **Sauerkraut:** A fermented cabbage salad that may also contain other vegetables. It should be made using raw, unheated, organically grown ingredients. Sauerkraut sold in your market is likely to have been pasteurized, which kills the enzymes and bacteria. Sauerkraut is relatively easy to make. Some natural foods stores and vegan restaurants now sell raw sauerkraut. It is more likely to contain B-12 if it is made in a wood container, rather than a ceramic, glass, or metal container. A reusable wooden compression weight used inside a nonwooden container can also increase the presence of B-12.

- **Sea vegetables:** The seaweeds dulse, nori, kelp, and wakame, may contain little or no B-12. The algaes chlorella and spirulina may be a more reliable source of B-12. While they may contain some B-12, they may also contain inactive B-12 analogs, which can use the same receptor sites as B-12, and may lead to a false positive on a B-12 blood test.
- **Sprouts:** Not a reliable source, but some beneficial organisms producing B-12 may be obtained from these, particularly sprouts grown in organic soil, such as sunflower seed sprouts used for salads and also sprouted grasses used for juicing.
- **Wheat, barley, and other grass juices** made from grass grown in organic soil.
- **Vegan B-12 supplements**: For those who have any concern at all that they are not getting enough B-12 through their food choices. Companies making vegan B-12 supplements include Freeda, Nature's Bounty, Solgar, and Veg Life. As mentioned above, if you purchase B-12 supplements, make sure they are methylcobalamin, and not cyanocobalamin. Get the sublingual methylcobalamin B-12 tablets or liquid. There are also injectable B-12 products, and, as mentioned above, the skin patch B-12 delivery products that work by placing the patch on the skin behind an ear.

While a vitamin B-12-rich diet isn't necessarily required every day, or even every week, and stores of B-12 can last months in the body, some people use their stores more quickly than others. While little of it is needed, B-12 is truly an essential nutrient, and people should be sure to get adequate amounts of it in their diet. Taking a quality B-12 supplement of at least 10 micrograms (10 mcg) is a reliable way to guarantee that your system receives adequate amounts of B-12. Many people advise taking a sublingual B-12 supplement, which is one that is held under the tongue until it is dissolved.

Expectant mothers, women who are breastfeeding, and women expecting to become pregnant should be sure to get sufficient amounts of vitamin B-12 (and a wide variety of other nutrients, especially those present in raw fruits and raw vegetables).

"Some people on raw diets include raw animal products in an effort to get vitamin B-12. With age, the body's ability to absorb the form of vitamin B-12 that is present in animal products diminishes. In animal products, vitamin B-12 is attached to a protein, and as people get older, production of the stomach acid that can split this complex of vitamin B-12 and protein diminishes. The recommendations for vitamin B-12 take into account that up to one in three of all individuals age fifty and older have low stomach-acid secretion. The form of vitamin B-12 that is present in fortified foods and supplements is not attached to protein; therefore, its absorption is not affected by a change in acid production. It is recommended that people over the age of fifty, regardless of their diet choice, rely either on foods fortified with vitamin B-12 or supplements to meet their recommended intakes."

> – *Becoming Raw: The Essential Guide to Raw Vegan Diets*, by Brenda Davis, Vesanto Melina, and Rynn Berry.

For more about B-12, read *Becoming Raw: The Essential Guide to Raw Vegan Diets*, by Brenda Davis, Vesanto Melina, and Rynn Berry.

FoodStudies.org
GoVeg.com
Dr. Michael Greger, DrGreger.Org and NutritionFacts.org
Dr. Michael Klaper, VegSource.Com/Klaper/
Vegan.com
VeganHealth.org
VeganHealthStudy.Com
Vegan.org
VeganOutreatch.org
VeganSociety.com
VeganSociety.Com/html/Food/Nutrition/B12/
Vegetarian Resource Group, VRG.org
VegInfo.org
VegSource.com

Earth, Air, Water, Bacteria, Fungi, Sun, and Vitamin D

All life on the planet relies on sun. Even the forms of life that are not directly exposed to sun are still dependent on sun. The plants that give us oxygen to breathe could not do so without sun. The photosynthesis that happens within the plants is powered by sun energy. That photosynthesis creates a variety of nutrients, including antioxidants, which we rely on for healthy tissues and to experience vibrant health.

It can be said that we are partially made up of sun. We are also made up of Earth, plants, water, air, fungi, and bacteria. If any one of these were missing, all life as we know it would die. We are truly all of these substances, and some others, transformed. Fungi and bacteria aid in the function of healthy soil and in transforming substances that can be absorbed into plants. Then, we eat the plants, infusing the nutrients into our bodies, and the nutrients become the fabric of our tissues. As plants are the transformed substances of fungi, bacteria, water, soil, sun, and air (which all consist of many substances), we and other animal life consist of these substances transformed into our structures.

Sun also triggers the formation of hormones in your brain and body tissues that lift the mood and spread throughout all of the tissues. Those who live in regions of the world where sunlight is limited often experience gloom, and all that goes along with that malady.

Exposure to sunlight and the consumption of raw fruits and vegetables go hand-in-hand. Beta-carotene and other carotenoids, which are substances in the fruits and vegetables we eat, protect us from damaging ultraviolet rays. They protect the cells of the plants, and within our bodies after we eat the plants, the carotenoids protect the cells of our tissues.

Just as sunlight helps to bring nutrients into the leaves of plants through evaporation of water from the leaves, which pulls more water with nutrients into the plant through the root and stem systems, sunlight creates nutrients in our bodies. Sunlight also triggers us to drink water, thus bringing that nutrient into our bodies. Sunlight also helps our body to metabolize sugar, which is interesting in that sweet fruits are more common in the sunny months when we also tend to get the most amount of sun exposure.

Sunlight also draws toxins out of the skin as the water evaporates from our skin during sun exposure. This is why you may feel like rinsing off after you sunbathe – your skin becomes coated with the toxins being brought to the surface. This is not to say that we should roast our bodies under sunlight to the point of damaging our skin.

Reasonable sun exposure can help to heal bruises, rashes, and other skin ailments and injuries. Sun exposure stimulates the flow of blood through the capillaries within the skin, and this works to eliminate discoloration within the skin caused by fungi, bruises, rashes, and other skin issues. Sunlight can also kill bacteria that exist in skin infections, such as ingrown nails, acne, and sties.

Those with candida benefit from reasonable amounts of sun exposure because it helps to both metabolize sugar and kill mold. Those with candida and/or yeast infections benefit from sunbathing while following a diet of a variety of raw fruits and vegetables.

If we don't get exposure to sun, our health suffers. Exposure to the ultraviolet rays of sun stimulates the creation of vitamin D 3 (cholecalciferols) in our skin, and vitamin D 2 (ergocalciferols) in plants. D vitamins are steroid compounds that absorb and transfer calcium, phosphorus, and magnesium through the intestines, and work to deposit these minerals in the bones. A lack of vitamin D results in rickets, a condition of undermineralized bones and teeth. Vitamin D also plays a part in maintaining healthy levels of calcium in the blood, and is vital for healthy kidney, parathyroid, and immune cell function, and also for a steady mood, and restful sleep.

Too much vitamin D can result in increased levels of calcium in the blood, which can result in kidney stones. It also can cause calcification (hardening) of the arteries, as well as general physical weakness, fatigue, bone pain, nausea, vomiting, and heart rhythm irregularities.

Through reasonable amounts of sun exposure, the body has an amazing ability to create and maintain healthy levels of vitamin D. It is when people take vitamin D supplements and eat lots of foods with added vitamin D that problems of an overdose may occur (rare).

> "Of 14 case studies that have been done on dairy and prostate cancer, 12 have shown a statistically significant relationship – and the other two just aren't strong enough to see anything – and they conclude that all of the predictors of prostate cancer, the consumption of dairy is the best predictor of prostate cancer."
> – T. Colin Campbell, Ph.D., Cornell University; author of *The China Study* and *Whole: Rethinking the Science of Nutrition*; TColinCampbell.org

People say, "Well, I drink milk, and there is my vitamin D source." Those countries where drinking lots of dairy products and eating foods containing added vitamin D, are also the countries with the highest levels of arteriosclerosis (thickening and hardening, and loss of elasticity, of the arteries). It is well established that the consumption of milk increases the incidence of prostate cancer. The cholesterol and saturated fat in milk also play a role in erectile dysfunction. Milk is clearly not something men should include in their diet. Nor should women be drinking milk (or eating cheese, ice cream, creamer, kefir, yogurt, butter, whey, casein, etc.), as dairy has also been linked to the development of breast cancer and cancers of the reproductive organs. Many studies have concluded that milk consumption plays a role in the development of diabetes.

"There is virtually no evidence that drinking two or three glasses of milk a day reduces the chances of breaking a bone."
– Walter C. Willet, MD, Chairman of the Department of Nutrition, Harvard School of Public Health

The sialic acid sugar protein molecule called Neu5Gc (N-glycolylneuraminic acid) is in nonhuman mammal milk. Neu5Gc is also in nonhuman mammal meat. It is produced by nonhuman mammals; can't be synthesized by humans – because they lack the enzymes to produce it; binds to cell surfaces; causes an immune response and inflammation; is often found in human cancers, such as of the breast, colon, and prostate; and can make cancer more aggressive. The only way Neu5Gc gets into the human system is by the consumption of mammal meat and nonhuman milk (including butter, cheese, whey, casein, yogurt, kefir, creamer, and ice cream). To avoid Neu5Gc, simply don't consume animal milk or mammal meat.

The only time you need milk is when you are a baby, and the best form is breast milk from your mother. There is no need to consume milk past the stage of infancy. Avoiding both meat and milk will also decrease your risk of experiencing heart attacks and strokes, and cardiovascular disease, diabetes, arthritis, kidney disease, Alzheimer's, Parkinson's, Crohn's, eczema, macular degeneration, osteoporosis, a variety of cancers, and other degenerative and chronic diseases.

The consumption of dairy creates an acidic condition in the blood, pulling calcium out of the bones, and causing a depletion of vitamin D, and acting hormonally to speed up growth of certain tissues, which can help trigger the growth of tumors. It is helpful to get your vitamin D in a natural manner, through sun exposure, and not to rely on food additives and vitamin D supplements. However, a quality, mushroom-based vitamin D supplement may be helpful to certain people.

Reasonable amounts of exposure to sunlight is important. As part of your health maintenance regime, be sure to get some exposure to sun.

Just remember, overexposure is not a good thing. Several minutes a day can be enough. Just as too much water and food, as well as too much sleep, or being awake too long, are not good for you, too much sun also works against you. Be reasonable about the amount of sun exposure you allow onto yourself. Even wild animals seek shade and are wise enough to limit their exposure to sunshine.

Eating citrus fruits, berries, vine fruits, fresh leafy greens, and other vitamin C-rich foods works in conjunction with sun exposure because vitamin C enhances vitamin D activity. It is a myth that citrus is the best source of vitamin C. As long as you are eating raw fruits, including berries, stone fruits, and vine fruits like tomatoes, and also vegetables, such as leafy greens, you are getting enough vitamin C.

In addition to getting vitamin D by direct sun exposure on the skin, vitamin D can also be had by eating edible mushrooms that have been exposed to sunlight, as it has been found that mushrooms also form vitamin D. Most mushrooms available in stores have been grown in the dark, and are not exposed to sun – and they lack vitamin D. There are some mushroom powder vitamin D products on the market. These are better than taking typical vitamin D supplements, which may have been derived from wool – meaning, the supplements aren't vegan. If you choose to take vitamin D supplements, use the mushroom supplements.

In the winter, a good source for vitamin C is rose hips. They can be gathered throughout the year from organically grown and wild rose bushes. It is important to avoid rose hips from bushes treated with chemical fertilizers, insecticides, fungicides, and/or herbicides.

One way to use rose hips is to split them open, put them into a bottle of water along with mint leaves and shavings of ginger root. Let the bottle remain in the sun for three or more hours when temperatures are above freezing, then drink this winter sun tea. (Be sure not to let the water freeze in the bottle as it can cause the glass to fracture.)

"You are not Atlas carrying the world on your shoulder. It is good to remember that the planet is carrying you."
– Vandana Shiva, VandanaShiva.org

WEIGHT MANAGEMENT

"The Oxford compoenent of the European Prospective Investigation into Cancer and Nutrition assessed changes in weight and BMI over a five-year period in meat eating, fish eating, vegetarian, and vegan men and women in the United Kingdom. During the five years of the study, mean annual weight gain was lowest among individuals who had changed to a diet containing fewer animal foods. The study also reported a significant difference in age-adjusted BMI, with the meat eaters having the highest BMI and vegans the lowest. Similar results were reported by the Adventist Health Study."
– Dr. Michael Greger, NutritionFacts.org

- Choose foods that are not concentrated. Concentrated foods include oils, clarified, sugars (including corn syrup and agave – which are best to avoid), nuts, bleached grains, baked products, and foods rich in fat and/or animal protein. Dried fruit is also a concentrated food. Cooking concentrates foods. Eat little to no cooked foods.
- If you choose cooked foods, choose steamed and boiled foods, such as steamed veggies (including spaghetti squash), no-oil vegan soups, or boiled wild rice, quinoa, lentils, millet, beans, or quinoa pasta.
- Don't eat foods that have been fried, sautéed, grilled, charred, char-broiled, roasted, barbecued, toasted, baked, or microwaved.
- Choose foods that are whole and provide bulk, such as raw greens, vegetables, vine fruits, tree fruits, berries, and sprouts.
- If you consume grains, choose unbleached, nongluten grains.
- Avoid synthetic chemical preservatives, dyes, flavors, scents, sweeteners, or substances that leach into foods, such as from can linings and plastic bottles.
- Include omega-3-rich foods: raw fruits, raw green vegetables, sprouts, raw hemp seeds, ground flax, and germinated chia and buckwheat.
- If you want something sweet, eat raw fruit. Consume no or very little cooked fruit. Eliminate jams and jellies, baked pies, and pasteurized, canned, bottled, or jarred fruit juices.
- Follow a regular sleep pattern.
- Exercise daily to break a sweat and keep the heartbeat up for a half hour or more. It is especially good to exercise in the morning.
- Drink water, not soda, colas, or "energy" or pasteurized drinks.

SEEDS: EMBRYONIC NUTRITION

Get them raw, unheated, unroasted, unblanched, organic, unsalted, uncoated. When you hear of "embryonic nutrition," people are speaking of eating raw germinated seeds. Nutrients contained in raw, unheated seeds include minerals, vitamins, amino acids, essential fatty acids, biophotons, and antioxidants. Seeds are also rich in fiber.

To get more nutrients out of whole, raw seeds, soak them for a few hours, or up to a day. This turns off the enzyme inhibitors, triggers enzyme production, and magnifies the number of nutrients.

Seeds contain properties that protect and nurture the cardiovascular and nerve systems. They also can aid in hormonal balance, reduce inflammation, and protect against cancer.

Raw seeds can be used freshly germinated, or you can spread about a half cup on a ceramic plate, or put in a screen straining bag, and leave to dry for later use.

Whole seeds can be scattered into salads, and used as ingredients in a variety of recipes, including raw pie crust and dehydrated vegetable pulp crackers.

Some seeds, such as flax, fenugreek, hemp, cilantro, pumpkin, and sesame can be ground and used as an ingredient in everything from smoothies to hummus and dressings. It is best to grind them right before using so that the nutrients, including the essential fatty acids, are fresh and don't degrade or, with oils, go rancid.

Flax seeds are particularly rich in lignans, and studies show that including a heaping spoonful of feshly ground flax seeds in your daily diet can improve blood pressure, reduce the incidence of diabetes, breast cancer, prostate cancer, and prostate gland enlargment. It is far better to eat feshly ground flax seeds than it is to eat flax oil.

Freshly ground seeds can also be used to make seed tea. Add a flavor, such as fresh lemon, mint, and/or freshly shaved ginger, and you have a nutrient-rich elixir tea.

Hemp seeds are rich in omega-3 fatty acids. They can be blended with dates, bananas, water, and cinnamon to make hemp milk.

• Apricot seeds
• Buckwheat seeds
• Chia seeds

- Cilantro seeds
- Cumin seeds
- Fenugreek seeds
- Flax seeds
- Grape seeds
- Hemp seeds
- Pomegranate seeds
- Poppy seeds
- Pumpkin seeds
- Quinoa
- Sesame seeds
- Sunflower seeds

GARDENING AND FARMING

"Let's not dissect the evils of corporate food – let's feed ourselves! The creation of a garden is as simple as you make it. Be it a barren patch of Earth newly liberated from the smothering embrace of concrete, a rooftop or a porch smattering of five-gallon buckets, it can take any form you desire. Be resourceful! Imagination can manifest square-foot primitive horticulture just about anywhere… Free yourself from wage slavery by eliminating the need to buy some or most of what you eat. Grow enough to feed the nomads among us. Ingesting fresh, native, seasonal plants gives us vibrant health. And how delicious it is to sink our fangs into a succulent squash that we first knew as a seed!"
– The Moment Is Ripe, aleksandra, *Earth First! Journal*, Dec.-Jan, 2002

IN addition to wild foods, the best way to get fresh food bursting with nutrients is to grow your own organic food garden.

Growing a food garden is good for the soul, for the mind, for the body, and for your life. Growing and harvesting your own food gives you exercise; connects you with nature; tunes you into the seasons; raises your frequency; bonds you with your environment; and provides you with the freshest food you can possibly have.

If you live in nearly any town or city you are living on land that was once farmland of some sort. Cities now cover most of the ancient farmland. This is because people originally settled on land that was good for growing food. As the settlements grew into towns and cities, houses, stores, schools, churches, jails, office buildings, streets, and parking lots covered the farmland. By planting food gardens in your area you are bringing back an ancient culture of growing and harvesting food.

"Today, 58 million Americans spend approximately $30 billion every year to maintain over 23 million acres of lawn. That's an average of over a third of an acre and $517 each. The same-size plot of land could still have a small lawn for recreation, plus produce all the vegetables needed to feed a family of six. The lawns in the United States consume around 270 billion gallons of water a week – enough to water 81 million acres of organic vegetables all summer long.

Lawns use ten times as many chemicals per acre as industrial farmland. These pesticides, fertilizers, and herbicides run off into our groundwater and evaporate into our air, causing widespread pollution and global warming, and greatly increasing our risk of cancer, heart disease, and birth defects. In addition, the pollution emitted from a power mower in just one hour is equal to the amount from a car being driven 350 miles. In fact, lawns use more equipment, labor, fuel, and agricultural toxins than industrial farming, making lawns the largest agricultural sector in the United States. But it's not just the residential lawns that are wasted on grass. There are around 700,000 athletic grounds and 14,500 golf courses in the United States, many of which used to be fertile, productive farmland that was lost to developers when the local markets bottomed out.

Turf is big business: $45 billion-a-year big. The University of Georgia has seven turf researchers studying genetics, soil science, plant pathology, nutrient uptake, and insect management. They issue undergraduate degrees in Turf. The turf industry is responsible for a large sector of the biotech (GMO) industry, and much of the genetic modification that is happening in laboratories across the nation is in the name of an eternally green, slow-growing, moss-free lawn."

– Heather Coburn, author of *Food Not Lawns: How to Turn Your Yard into a Garden and Your Neighborhood into a Community*; FoodNotLawns.org

By growing your food, you reduce pollution because you will be reducing the use of shipping, packaging, marketing, and all of the fuel, paper, plastics, and other resources and processes used to otherwise bring commercial food to your plate.

By maintaining your own organic food garden you can feel assured that there are no toxic farming chemicals on your food. Not only will you experience the benefit of getting food as fresh as possible, you will also benefit from food that is nutritionally and energetically stronger than food available at the store.

Chemically grown food is weaker in electrical frequency and has diminished nutritional properties. Studies have shown that organically grown food has a denser reserve of vitamins, minerals, and other nutrients than food that has been grown chemically. Perhaps this is because the organically grown plants have to fend for themselves, and don't rely on chemical fertilizers for nutrients, or depend on chemicals to protect them. Like people who become weak when they are pampered, plants also can become weak if they are grown in an atmosphere where too much is done for them.

In America today about 35 percent of all household water goes to tend lawns. Because there are so many lawns, including those on school campuses, golf courses, cemeteries, and around government buildings and office buildings, and even prisons, the number-one crop being produced in the U.S., and many other countries, is landscape clippings.

"When you use a manual push mower, you're cutting down on pollution and the only thing in danger of running out of gas is you!"
    – Grey Livingston

It is amazing how much time, energy, money, and water is spent in the U.S. and other wealthy countries to try to keep home lawns green. The people get nothing out of it but a green lawn. They don't have food gardens, even though they have the land to grow them, but instead buy all their food at grocery stores, snack shops, and restaurants. This scenario has helped create the situation that exists today where, on average, the typical meal in the U.S. has traveled 1,250 miles from farm to consumer. This is a terrific waste of resources and causes enormous amounts of pollution.

According to Ted Steinberg, author of *American Green: The Obsessive Quest for the Perfect Lawn*, there are 25 million acres of lawn in America, more land than what is used to grow cotton. To care for those lawns, there are more than 35 million gas-powered lawn mowers, over 25 million leaf blowers, and tons of lawn-treatment chemicals. And all this produces landscape clippings and polluted air, soil, and water. The leaf blowers alone produce more air pollution per engine cylinder than automobiles.

Think of how much better people would be if, instead of spending time, energy, water, and money, and using toxic fertilizers and weed killers to try to keep their lawns green and hedges perfectly trimmed, they would plant organic food gardens, including fruiting trees – and let the rest of the land grow wild and free. Not only would they not spend money and time on landscaping, they would save money on food as well. They would pollute less: A typical lawnmower can use enough gas in an hour to operate a small car for over 50 miles.

The products commonly used to keep a residential lawn green and weed-free contain many toxic chemicals. Glyphosate, a chemical in weed killer, which is poisonous to a variety of plants and wildlife, has been linked to non-Hodgkin's lymphoma, a cancer that is becoming more common. Other lawn chemicals are known to cause breast cancer, birth deformities, and learning disabilities. Lawn chemicals also cause health problems in pets and wildlife. Ironically, the companies that manufacture these toxic chemicals are often the same companies that manufacture cancer drugs.

345

When used as a well-organized food garden, a small plot of land the size of a common U.S. household lawn can produce more food in a season than a family of four can consume. The result would be that people would be sharing their food with neighbors, family, and friends. The people, their environment, and their community would be healthier.

Growing your own food may be a new concept for those who have lived their lives relying on commercial and restaurant food. It isn't new to a large percentage of the world's population that has always grown some or all their own food. Some countries that have relied on commercial food are now encouraging their citizens to grow more food gardens. Venezuela and Cuba are two countries that have been promoting self-sufficiency through home food gardens. The U.S. hasn't been involved in this type of program since the 1940s. At that time the government encouraged its citizens to grow "victory gardens." That was a revival of what went on during WWI when the U.S. encouraged people to grow "liberty gardens."

Even if you don't grow part, or all, of your own food, you can at least get involved with purchasing foods that have been organically grown locally. You can find these at your nearest farmers' markets.

You may also obtain locally grown food through "community supported agriculture" (CSA) co-ops that prepay local farmers for produce. This is an idea started in the 1970s, and has been growing in popularity in Europe, the U.S., and other regions.

Some people have the idea of moving the CSA and organic farming movement into the restaurant food sector. They want to gather people to gather the finances to open co-op vegetarian restaurants that use locally grown produce.

If you live in a city you may find that growing a garden in an abandoned lot to be a rewarding experience. Many people have done this throughout the years and it has spurred activism to create and maintain food gardens in the largest cities. The city or other government department may own the land, or it may be privately owned. Many communities have grown food on such land for many years without any problem from the landowner.

When New York's Mayor Giuliani announced that more than 100 city-owned lots where gardens had been planted were to be auctioned off to land developers in the spring of 1999, a citizen's campaign was organized to save the gardens. It was only a last-minute arrangement by entertainer Bette Midler and some others that the gardens were saved as they were purchased by the Trust for Public Land.

In Los Angeles, a plot of land that contained garden plots maintained by hundreds of families was bulldozed in 2006. The South Central Community Farm was planted with an enormous variety of food and medicinal plants and trees. It came into existence after the riots that took place after the 1992 Rodney King verdict. Originally purchased by the city through the eminent domain process, the city had planned to build trash incinerators on the site. The local community spoke out against this plan. The Concerned Citizens of South Central organized protests and the city eventually canceled its plan to build the incinerators. After the riots the city offered the land as space for community gardens. Many of the farmers were people who had moved to Los Angeles from Mexico and Central and South America. As the years went by, the farming gardens became a center of community with generations of families involved in planting and maintaining their gardens. Then, the person who originally owned the land wanted it back. In 2003 the land was transferred back to the original owner, who had plans to build warehouses on the property. As time passed, lawsuits were filed and the community organized protests. By the spring of 2006 the future of the farm was dismal. Community activists gathered to maintain a 24/7 presence. Julia Butterfly Hill, who once famously lived in a redwood tree for two years to save it from a lumber company, joined Darryl Hannah and other activists who camped on the farm. Finally, on a June morning hundreds of riot police were brought in to evict the protestors. Some, including Darryl Hannah, who were camping in a tree, were handcuffed and taken away. In the end the landowner won, bulldozing the gardens and placing people back in line at the supermarkets to purchase their food – forcing them deeper into poverty.

Wherever you are, get involved in growing some of your own food. If you don't have land, borrow some, or use pots, a roof, or window boxes. Be sure to plant some native flower species so that your garden attracts native bees and other helpful insects.

When you look for plants and seeds to plant in your garden, seek out those that have been organically grown, and that have not been genetically altered. You also may want to try "open pollinated" "heirloom" seeds, which have not been hybridized, and that can provide a better variety of food plants. Look into planting some food plants that you have never heard of.

There are many organizations involved in getting people to grow their own food. From the Slow Food movement that started in Italy to protest McDonald's opening at Rome's Spanish Steps in 1986, to city farming activists and organizations like Food Not Lawns, to EdibleSchoolyard.org, there is likely an organization that is near you and/or can help you get into growing food – and start your disconnect from total reliance on stores and restaurants.

Acres: The Voice for Eco-Agriculture, Austin, TX, 78709; 512-892-4400; AcresUSA.com. Sells books on organic gardening and farming.

Alternative Farming Systems Information Center, Community Supported Agriculture, NAL.USDA.gov/AFSIC/CSA

American Community Gardening Association, Council on the Environment, 51 Chambers St., Ste. 228; New York, NY 10007; CommunityGarden.org

American Farmland Trust, 1200 18th St., NW, Washington, DC 20036; Farmland.org

AppleLuscious Organic Orchards, AppleLuscious.com

Australian Community Gardens Network, communitygarden.org.au.

Avant Gardening, Avant-Gardening.com

Barefoot Farmer, BarefootFarmer.com

Big Barn, BigBarn.co.uk

Bio-Integral Resource Center, IGC.org

Black Farmers and Agriculturists Association, POB 61, Tillery, NC 27887; BFAA-US.org

Bountiful Gardens, 18001 Shafer Ranch Rd., Willits, CA 95490-9626; 707-459-6410; BountifulGardens.org

California Certified Organic Farmers, POB 8136, Santa Cruz, CA 95061; CCOF.org

California Rare Fruit Growers, CRFG.org

Canadian Organic Growers, COG.ca

Center for Food and Justice, 323-341-5099; Departments.Oxy.edu/UEPI/CFJ

Center for Informed Food Choices, InformedEating.org

Center for Rural Affairs, POB 136, Lyons, NE 68038-0136; CFRA.org

Center for Vegan Organic Education, POB 13217, Burton, WA 98013; 206-463-4520; VeganOrganicEd.org

City Farmer, Canada's Office of Urban Agriculture, Box 74561, Kitsilano RPO, Vancouver, BC V6K 4P4; Canada; CityFarmer.org

City Food Growers, Australia; cityfoodgrowers.com.au

City Repair Project, POB 42615, Portland, OR 97242; CityRepair.org

Coalition of Immokalee Workers, POB 603, Immokalee, FL 34143; CIW-Online.org

Common Ground Garden Program, CELosAngeles.UCDavis.edu/Garden

Community Farm Alliance, 614 Shelby St., Frankfort, KY 40601; CommunityFarmAlliance.org

Community Food Security Coalition, Venice, CA; FoodSecurity.org. Site contains listings of community gardening and urban farming resources.

The Cornucopia Institute, POB 126, Cornucopia, WI 54827; Cornucopia.org

CSA California, csacalifornia.org. Community Supported Agriculture is one way of supporting local farmers. Some may provide boxes or bags of locally grown produce that you pick up once a week at your farmers' market, at another location, or that gets delivered to you.

Desert Harvesters, DesertHarvesters.org

Dirty Girl Produce, Santa Cruz, CA; dirtygirlproduce.com. An organic produce farm.

Eat Grub, EatGrub.org

Earth Works Gardens, 1820 Mount Elliot, Detroit, MI 48207; Earth-Works.org

Eat the View, England, Countryside.gov.UK/LAR/Landscape/ETV/Index.asp

Ecological Farming Association, Watsonville, CA; Eco-Farm.org

Edible Estates Initiative, FritzHaeg.Com/Garden/Initiatives/EdibleEstates/Main.html

Edible Forest Gardens, EdibleForestGardens.com

Edible Schoolyard, EdibleSchoolyard.org

Environmental Working Group, 1436 U Street NW, Ste. 100, Washington DC 20009; EWG.org

Fair Trade Resource Network, POB 33772, Washington, DC 20033-3772; FairTradeResource.org

Family Farm Defenders, POB 1772, Madison, WI 53701; FamilyFarmDefenders.org

Farm Aid, 11 Ward St., Ste. 200, Somerville, MA 02143; FarmAid.org

Farmers' Legal Action Group, 360 N. Robert St., Ste. 500, St. Paul, MN 55101; FLAGInc.org

Farming Solutions, FarmingSolutions.org

Farm Labor Organizing Committee, 1221 Broadway St., Toledo, OH 43609; FLOC.com

Farm to Consumer Legal Defense Fund, FarmToConsumer.org

Farm Worker Justice Fund, 1010 Vermont Ave., NW, Ste. 915, Washington, DC 20005; FWJustice.org

FedCo Co-op Garden Supplies, POB 520, Waterville, ME 04903; 207-873-7333; fedcoseeds.com

Food First, Institute for Food and Development Policy, 398 60th St., Oakland, CA; FoodFirst.org

Food Not Bombs, POB 424, Arroyo Seco, NM 87514; 800-884-1136; FoodNotBombs.net

Food Not Lawns, POB 42174, Eugene, OR 97404; FoodNotLawns.com

The Food Project, POB 705, Lincoln, MA 01773; TheFoodProject.org

Free Wheelin Farm, Santa Cruz, CA; freewheelinfarm.com/home.html

The Future of Food, TheFutureOfFood.com

Garden Project, GardenProject.org

Garden Valley Seed Trust, GardenValleySeedTrust.org

Global Exchange, 2017 Mission St., 303, San Francisco, CA 94110; GlobalExchange.org

Going Organic, GoingOrganic.com

Goode Green, goodegreennyc.com. Green rooftop design and installation.

Green Earth Institute, Illinois; greenearthinstitute.org

Green Grid Roofs, greengridroofs.com

Green Guerillas, New York, NY; GreenGuerillas.org. Helping establish community gardens.

Green People, GreenPeople.org. Site contains a list of companies that sell organic seeds.

Green Roofs, greenroofs.org

Growing Gardens, 2003 NE 42nd Ave., #3, Portland, OR 97213; GrowingGardens.org

Growing Power, 5500 W. Silver Spring Rd., Milwaukee, WI 53218; GrowingPower.org

Guerrilla Gardening, GuerrillaGardening.org. A group of people in London who have late night planting parties to enliven previously neglected small plots of city land.

Heirloom Gardening Newsletter, 203-354-8756; HeirloomGardening.com

Home Orchard Society, HomeOrchardSociety.org

Institute for Community Economics, 57 School St., Springfield, MA 01105; ICECLT.org

International Confederation of Autonomous Chapters of the American Indian Movement, AmericanIndianMovement.org

International Culinary Tourism Association, 4110 SE Hawthorne Blvd., #440, Portland, OR 97214; CulinaryTourism.org

International Society for Ecology & Culture, ISEC.org.uk

Island Seed and Feed, Goleta, CA; IslandSeed.com

Kings Hill Farm, Wisconsin; kingshillfarm.com. An organic produce farm.

KitchenGardeners.org

The Land Institute, 2440 E. Water Well Rd., Salina, KS 67401; LandInstitute.org

Land Stewardship Project, 2200 4th St., White Bear Lake, MN 55110; LandStewardshipProject.org

Land Trust Alliance, 1331 H St., NW, Ste. 400, Washington, DC 20005; LTA.org

Leopold Center for Sustainable Agriculture, Iowa State University; Leopold.IAState.edu

Linking Environment and Farming, England; LeafMarque.com/LEAF

Local Harvest, LocalHarvest.org

Local Harvest, Santa Cruz, CA; LocalHarvest.org. Searchable database of farmers' markets, small farms, and related groups and businesses.

Lost Valley Educational Center, LostValley.org

Maine Organic Farmers and Gardeners Association, POB 170, Unity, ME 04988; MOFGA.org

Mindfully, Mindfully.org/Farm

Mindfully, Mindfully.org/Food

More Gardens Coalition, 376 E. 162nd St., #2, Bronx, NY 10451; MoreGardens.org

Mountain Gardens, MountainGardensHerbs.com. A botanical garden featuring the largest collection of native Appalachian and Chinese medicinal herbs in the eastern U.S.

Mycorrhizal Applications, Mycorrhizae.com. Information on beneficial fungi that improve soil health, plant health, and crop yields.

National Coalition for Pesticide-Free Lawns, BeyondPesticides.org/PesticideFreeLawns/DoorHanger/Index.htm. This organization offers door tags you can put on your neighborhood doors encouraging people to stop using pesticides on their lawns. The first 50 are free, and they ask only for a donation to handle the postage. You can also purchase more.

National Family Farm Coalition, 110 Maryland Ave., NE, Ste. 307; Washington, DC 20002; NFFC.net

National Farm to School Program, Center for Food and Justice, Occidental College, Los Angeles, CA; FarmToSchool.org

National Farm Transition Network, FarmTransition.org

National Immigrant Farming Initiative, 88 Atlantic Ave., #8, Brooklyn, NY 11201; ImmigrantFarming.org

Native Seeds, NativeSeeds.org

New England Small Farm Institute, 275 Jackson St., Belchertown, MA 01007; SmallFarm.org

New Farm, NewFarm.org. Sponsored by the Rodale Institute. Community Supported Agriculture information.

New World Publishing, Auburn, CA 95602; NWPub.net. Books on small-scale farming.

North American Fruit Explorers, NAFEX.org

North American Native Plant Society, NANPS.org

Northeast Organic Farming Association, Barre, MA; NOFA.org

Northern Nut Growers Association, ICSERV.com/NNGA/Index.html

Oakhill Organics, Dayton, OR; oakhillorganics.org. A 17-acre certified organic produce farm,

Organic Volunteers, OrganicVolunteers.org

Oregon Tilth, Tilth.org

Organic Gardening **magazine,** OrganicGardening.com

Osborn International Seed Co., osbornseed.com

Pennsylvania Association for Sustainable Agriculture, POB 419, Millheim, PA 16854; PASAFarming.org

Permaculture Institute, PortlandPermaculture.com

Pesticide Action Network, San Francisco, CA; PANNA.org

Planet Natural, 1612 Gold Ave., Bozeman, MT 59715; 800-289-6656; 406-587-5891; PlanetNatural.com

Plan Organic, PlanOrganic.com

Plants for a Future, 1 Lerryn View, Cornwall, United Kingdom; PFAF.org

Portland City Repair Project, CityRepair.org

Portland Permaculture Institute, PortlandPermaculture.com

Pro Active Ecology, ProActiveEcology.org

Real Goods RealGoods.com

Resource Centres on Urban Agriculture and Food Security, RUAF.org

Robin Van En Center for Community Supported Agriculture; Center for Sustainable Living, Wilson College, Chambersburg, PA; CSACenter.org

Roof Meadow, roofmeadow.com

Rooftop Farms, rooftopfarms.org

Sacred Earth Institute, SacredEarthInstitute.org

Safe Food and Fertilizer, SafeFoodAndFertilizer.org

Salt Springs Seeds, SaltSpringsSeeds.com

San Francisco League of Urban Gardeners (SLUG), Grass-Roots.org/USA/Slug.shtml

Seasonal Chef, SeasonalChef.com

Seattle Tilth Association, 4649 Sunnyside Ave. North, Rm. 120, Seattle, WA 98103; SeattleTilth.org

Seeds of Change, POB 15700, Santa Fe, NM 15700; 888-762-7333; SeedsOfChange.com

Seeds of Diversity, Seeds.ca/EN.php

Seedsaving and Seedsavers' Resources, Homepage.Eircom.net/%7Emerlyn/SeedSaving.html

Seed Savers Australia, seedsavers.net

Seed Savers Exchange, SeedSavers.org

Seed Savers Network, Australia; SeedSavers.net

Seeds Trust, Seedstrust.com

The School of Self-Reliance, Los Angeles, CA; Self-Reliance.net

Slow Food, SlowFood.com

Slow Food USA, SlowFoodUSA.org

Small Farm Association, England, Small-Farms-Association.co.uk

Snow Seed Organic, 831-758-9869; SnowSeedCo.com

Soil and Health Library, SoilAndHealth.org

Soil Food Web, Inc., SoildFoodWeb.com

South Central Farmers, SouthCentralFarmers.com

Sow Organic Seed, POB 527, Williams, OR 97544; 888-709-7333; OrganicSeed.com

Spiral Gardens Community Food Security Project, 2880 Sacramento, St., Berkeley, CA 94702; SpiralGardens.org

SunBowFarm, SunBowFarm.org

Sustainable Food, SustainableFood.com

Sustainable Table, New York, NY; SustainableTable.org

Sustain: The Alliance for Better Farming and Food, London, UK; SustainWeb.org

Tilth Producers, Washington; tilthproducers.org. Organic and sustainable farming association.

Toledo Garden, ToledoGarden.org

True Food Now Campaign, Greenpeace USA, TrueFoodNow.org

Trust for Public Land, 116 New Montgomery St., 4th Flr., San Francisco, CA 94105; TPL.org

United Plant Savers, UnitedPlantSavers.org

Via Campesina, ViaCampesina.org

Virginia Association for Biological Farming, Lexington, VA, VABF.org

Virginia Independent Consumers and Farmers Association, POB 915, Charlottesville, VA 22902; VICFA.net

Washington State University's Organic Agriculture Program, 888-468-6978; World-Class.WSU.edu/2006/Organic/Index.html. In 2006

Washington State University became the first university in the U.S. to offer a major in organic agriculture.

White Earth Land Recovery Project, 32033 E. Round Lake Rd., Ponsford, MN 54575; NativeHarvest.com

Wild Food Adventure, WildFoodAdventures.com

Willing Workers on Organic Farms, OrganicVolunteers.org

Women, Food, and Agriculture Network, 59624 Chicago Rd., Atlantic, IA 50022; WFAN.org

World Social Forum, Rua General Jardin, 660, 8th Flr., Sao Paulo, SP 01223-010; Brazil; WorldSocialForum.org

Worldwide Opportunities on Organic Farms, WWOOF.org

Worm Digest, POB 2654, Grants Pass, OR 97528; WormDigest.org

Yards to Gardens, y2g.org

Zenger Farm, ZengerFarm.org

"For too long we have occupied ourselves with responding to the consequences of cruelty and abuse and have neglected the important task of building up an ethical system in which justice for animals is regarded as the norm rather than the exception. Our only hope is to put our focus on educating the young."

– John Hoyt

THE PLIGHT OF THE FAMILY FARMERS

"Family farms are an important part of the American tradition of self-sufficiency, forming the bedrock for communities across the U.S.

Since 1935, the U.S. has lost 4.7 million farms. Fewer than one million Americans now claim farming as a primary occupation.

Farmers in 2002 earned their lowest real net cash income since 1940. Meanwhile, corporate agribusiness profits have nearly doubled (increased 98 percent) since 1990.

Large corporations increasingly dominate U.S. food production.

… Encourage your local grocery store and area restaurants to purchase more of their products from local farmers."

– FoodRoutes.Org, 2006

THERE was once a time when families ran the farms. They worked the land, grew a variety of crops, rotated the crops to manage a healthy soil, maintained seed supplies, and sold produce to the markets.

More recently, farms in the U.S. and an increasing number of farms in other countries, are being taken over by large multinational companies worth billions of dollars and that control many different levels of the food manufacturing and distribution processes. These monolithic companies buy up land and turn what were once many farms into one large complex involved in intensive monocropping (massive single-crop farms). They also contract with land-owning farmers and dictate what the farmers grow and how the farmers grow it. They use tons of chemical fertilizers, pesticides, fungicides, insecticides, and other toxic chemicals to grow, protect and process the grains, fruits, and vegetables.

"Monoculture is the original sin of agriculture."

– Michael Pollan

This has created a nightmare for family farmers, some of whom find themselves dealing with depression, life-threatening stress-related illnesses, and suicidal tendencies as they witness multigenerational farm life come to an abrupt halt. The family farm may have been all they and generations before them have ever known. The farmer can experience deep anguish when the farm is taken away instead of handed on to the next generation.

In the U.S., this change in the farm community has taken place because the government has been foreclosing on farmer loans and because corporations are taking over the farming industry. Several multinational corporations, such as Cargill, Continental Grain, and Archer Daniels Midland, control much of the U.S. food supply.

Mental depression related to economic stress among farmers is such a problem that one of the leading causes of death among farmers has been suicide. In 2003, the U.S. farmer suicide rate was five times the national average. Farmers sometimes make their deaths appear accidental so that their families can collect insurance to pay off family farming debts. Other countries have also been experiencing large numbers of farmer suicides. In India there have been thousands of suicides among farmers.

Kyung-Hae Lee, a farmer who was president of the Korean Advanced Farmers Federation, killed himself with a knife as a form of protest at the World Trade Organization's convention held in Cancun, Mexico, on September 10, 2003. He had written about the plight of the family farm and how "undesirable globalization" of multinational corporations is ruining the environment and killing farmers.

Farming in the U.S. changed rapidly starting in the Depression and Dustbowl periods. The government drew up a plan to help farmers by paying subsidies to those involved in growing corn, cotton, wheat, soybeans, and other crops under the farm subsidy program. Part of this involved paying farmers not to grow crops, or to destroy crops rather than to flood the market.

While the farm subsidy program may have been designed to keep family farmers in business, it quickly switched gears to benefit large industrialized agricultural businesses. These corporations began creating large, single-crop farms consisting of thousands of acres. This robbed the soil of nutrients, creating weaker plants susceptible to infestation. To improve crop harvests, farms began using tremendous amounts of synthetic pesticides, fertilizers, and other chemicals made of toxic substances developed during the World Wars. It is no coincidence that some of the farming chemicals can kill or explode, as that is why some of them were originally created – to be weapons of war.

The farm subsidy program turned into what is referred to as "corporate welfare" for the large agribusinesses. Today about 75 percent of the subsidies go to large corporate agribusinesses. These corporations rely on billions of dollars in U.S. government subsidies every year to support their damaging business practices. The huge amounts of food they produce flood the world market, putting the food on the market for less than it took to grow it, and less than what farmers in other countries can get for their own crops – ruining the livelihood of farmers globally.

The glut in American-produced grains and cottons has a negative impact on farmers and farm communities throughout the world that would be doing much better if this U.S. farm subsidy program were not so abused by corporate agriculture. Because of these subsidies, the corporations flourish, but the family farmers suffer, as does the environment from corporate farming practices relying on chemicals.

In another way, industrial agriculture subsidies also affect people of the inner cities of the U.S. When ways of cutting the budget of the U.S. Department of Agriculture are considered, often it isn't the farm subsidies that are the focus, but another part of the USDA, the school lunch programs, which largely serve unhealthful, chemically-saturated, corporate-farmed food.

Cities around the world are affected by the industrialization of agriculture. When farmers lose their farms, they often move to larger communities, such as cities. Often they travel to other countries to find a better way of life than they faced in their local towns, where many end up working in factories making products sold to wealthier countries. In the cities the immigrants become members of the working poor. In the country they often end up working as laborers for the industrial farms, for the factory animal farms, and for slaughterhouses. Some join the military to gain citizenship.

The corporate agribusinesses have a big influence on what the government does because these businesses often give donations to politicians and to political parties favoring the corporations. These corporations feed off and perpetuate the lie that writer George Pyle wrote of in his book, *Raising Less Corn, More Hell: The Case for the Independent Farm and Against Industrial Food*. It is the lie that the industrial agribusiness corporations are going to save the world from a food shortage. In truth, it is those corporations involved in industrial farming and the genetic engineering of food plants that are playing a major role in the world food problems, and especially in the problems being faced by family farmers and the environment surrounding them.

Rather than flooding the Third World countries with an overabundance of crops from American corporate farms, it would be better for the farmers to grow their own crops. If you give a person a piece of food, that person can eat for a day. If they are able to grow it, they can eat for a lifetime. The USDA doesn't seem to support this idea and keeps on promoting the idea that we need to bring more money into big business agriculture by exporting more and more crops.

On multiple levels the U.S. government has been no friend to family farmers – either domestically or internationally.

Historically, African-American farmers have had a rougher time of it than their lighter-skinned neighbors. The promise of land and a mule that was made when the slaves were freed never materialized. Throughout the years African-American farmers have been much less likely to benefit from government programs set up to help farmers. In 1999 a lawsuit was settled between the USDA and a group of African-American farmers in which a history of discrimination was acknowledged. But few have received any part of that settlement.

For many years, Japanese-Americans couldn't own farmland. If they wanted to farm they had to rent land. Compounding the deprivation, many of them had lost the rented farmland they were operating when they were forced into internment camps during World War II.

Not to be overlooked are the Native peoples, not only in what is now the U.S., but indigenous peoples on every continent, and on many islands. Indigenous peoples the world over have been forced from their lands, which was then given or sold to others, or kept by the new government. Some who have been allowed to keep their land have been taxed at stiff rates and/or subject to laws and regulations that create unreasonable hardship. Others who have had their prime farmland taken away have been moved to land difficult or impossible to farm.

More recently, many U.S. farmers went into debt to the federal government because the Farm Home Administration counseled farmers to take out loans in the 1970s when the value of the farms was inflating faster than the interest rates. Then the government raised interest rates on the farmers and foreclosed on family farms at record levels.

Under the massive takeover of farms by multinational corporations, family farmers are struggling to maintain and update equipment, pay for water, keep up with packing fees, pay for labor and transportation, and compete with pricing. This is a driving force in the formation of rural groups that have found good reason to mistrust the government.

In addition to losing their farms to the corporate farming industry takeover, farmers have been selling out to housing developers who offer more money for the farmland than the farm can make in several years of operating on a tight budget. So the housing tracts get built on the farmland and the streets are given pleasant country names like Wildflower Lane, Cherry Orchard Court, and Apple Blossom Road.

Some U.S. farmers have moved to other countries, including Brazil where they have started *fazendas* (Portuguese for farms). They arrive with the belief that the land there will be the next leader in world produce. What they are finding is land that costs a fraction of the farming land in the U.S. There, among the tens of millions of acres in Brazil's interior, with a long and favorable season, farmers can grow a wide assortment of crops, including bananas and tropical fruits as well as coffee and sugar. While corn is being used to make ethanol in the U.S., sugar cane in Brazil is a common crop used in producing the fuel. Brazil is the world's second-largest producer of soy beans, much of which goes to feed livestock in Brazil, and is exported to feed livestock in other countries.

357

Animal farming is huge business in Brazil, which has about 70 million cattle and an even larger population of chickens. The country exports about three billion dollars worth of beef per year to countries around the world, much of it raised on illegally cleared rainforest land. It is a country that has an enormous export industry supplying the world food market. Unfortunately, the farmers relocating from the U.S. also are finding the same multinational farming companies working their way into the Brazilian farming industry, promoting their toxic farming chemicals, and making big plans for expansion with mechanized mono-crop farming that employs very few people. Much of this farming is being done on land that was bulldozed, chainsawed, burned, or otherwise cleared of pristine rainforest – displacing indigenous peoples, fragmenting the land, drying out surrounding forests, inducing droughts, and decimating wildlife. Cultural and language differences can require some adjustment and learning for farmers moving to new lands. Other problems include people illegally harvesting crops; labor contracting problems; squatters; hired guns; illegal logging operations; an unreliable infrastructure; a different tax structure; dishonesty in suppliers, processors, and land sales and leasing; and government bureaucracy.

Those considering a move to distant lands to start a farm may want to stay put and move toward a different way of doing business.

Some U.S. farmers have found that cooperative selling and food processing organizations are a way to do business and increase income security. Under NGCs (New Generation Cooperatives), farmers join in and own food processing and marketing associations. Under CSA (Community-Supported Agriculture), member consumers, often from nearby towns and cities, buy into the upcoming season of vegetables and fruits grown on particular farms. It is "subscription farming," and it is helping small farmers, localizing what people eat, improving nutrition, reducing pollution, and creating sustainable agriculture. More and more farmers are finding the growing demand for organically grown produce as a way to create a brighter future for their small farms.

When you purchase organic foods, purchase non-GMO foods, purchase locally grown produce, and shop at farmers' markets, you are more likely to be supporting small farms, and less likely to be supporting the companies that have taken over family farms.

Becoming a member of a CSA is one way of supporting family farmers – as well as to get food that is locally and organically grown.

I once spoke with some residents of Eugene, Oregon, planning to organize an organic CSA by turning the yards of at least a dozen homes into gardens growing a variety of produce. They planned on selling their produce to local residents, to restaurants, and at farmers' markets.

"Government policies the world over tend to favor industrial-scale, chemical-dependent production of raw commodity crops at the expense of small-scale farmers and organic growers who produce real, nourishing food. The U.S. is no exception.

For too long, funding authorized under the U.S. Farm Bill has primarily benefited agribusiness and large, industrial-scale farm operations that aren't growing food people actually eat. Instead, they're growing genetically modified crops like corn, soybeans, and cotton that get turned into ingredients for animal feed, fuel, and highly processed food – at a high cost to Americans' health and the environment. Producers in developing countries often find it hard to compete against these heavily subsidized American [corporate] farmers.

Meanwhile, only meager public resources have been invested smartly in building dynamic, local food economies that help link small- and mid-sized family farms directly to local and regional markets. Rsearch done by the Environmental Working Group between 2008 and 2010 has found that the U.S. government, acting under the authority of the federal Farm Bill, spent $39.4 billion subsidizing a handful of grains and cotton, more than eight times what it paid out for programs to support research, promotion and purchasing of fruits, nuts, and vegetables.

The inequities were far greater when it came to supporting organic farming and small-scale farmers and helping expand local and regional markets. Over those same three years, the U.S. government spent just $159 million on organic agriculture and $300 million to build and strengthen local and regional food systems."

– Fairness for Small Farmers: A Missing Ingredient in the U.S. Farm Bill, by Kari Hamerschlag; Fair World Project magazine, Spring 2013; FairWorldProject.org

Community Alliance with Family Farmers, CAFF.org
Environmental Working Group, EWG.org
Fair World Project, FairWorldProject.org
Family Farm Defenders, FamilyFarmers.org
Farm Aid, FarmAid.org
Farm to Consumer Legal Defense Fund, FarmToConsumer.org
Food and Water Watch, FoodAndWaterWatch.org
Friends of Family Farmers, FriendsOfFamilyFarmers.org
Local Harvest, localharvest.org/store/local-csa.jsp
Organic Consumers Association, OrganicConsumers.org
Worldwide Opportunities on Organic Farms, WWOOF.org

ORGANIC FOODS

"We are witnessing a massive corporate genocide – the killing of people for super profits. To maintain these super profits, lies are told about how, without pesticides and genetically modified organisms (GMOs), there will be no food. In fact, the conclusions of International Assessment of Agricultural Science and Technology for Development, undertaken by the United Nations, shows that ecologically organic agriculture produces more food and better food at lower cost than either chemical agriculture or GMOs."
– Vandana Shiva, *The Killing Fields Of Multi-National Corporations*, *The Asian Age*, July 14, 2010. VandanaShiva.org

"Organic farming and ranching not only uses less fossil fuel and emits fewer climate-disrupting gases, but also can actually clean greenhouse gas pollution from the atmosphere, while at the same time feed the world, improve public health, and restore biodiversity. If we can move the world's 12 billion acres of farm and ranch lands into a transition to organic, and preserve and restore our 10 billion acres of forests, at least 50ppm of CO_2 can be drawn down from the atmosphere and stored naturally and safely in the soil. This is literally the difference between present and future climate stability or climate hell. Organic soil and land management can and must be scaled up now in order to buy us the time we need to make the long-term transition to radical energy efficiency and solar, wind, and geothermal power.

Obviously this Great Organic Transition is not going to be easy. Our energy-, chemical-, and GM-intensive food and farming system needs to shift from one where 125,000 megafarms produce 75 percent of the food, to a mass movement of millions of farmers, ranchers, and urban gardeners growing organic food for their local communities. Factory farms and feedlots belching methane and nitrous oxide must be phased out. Twenty-four billion pounds of synthetic nitrogen fertilizer needs to be replaced with organic compost and compost tea derived from food and yard waste.

This Great Transition will require a massive shift in public consciousness to wake up the majority of the population who are being force-fed a nutrition-poor diet of genetically engineered junk

food and animal products."
– Organic Consumers Association; OrganicConsumers.org

MANY studies have found that organically grown foods contain more nutrients than what is in the same foods that are grown using farming chemicals. A study by the University of California, Davis, found that organic tomatoes contain two times the amount of flavonoids. Organically grown fruits and vegetables also grow stronger, and are less likely to be susceptible to pest infestation. In other words, conventionally grown foods are weaker, less vibrant, and provide fewer nutrients.

Every minute enormous quantities of toxic pesticides, fertilizers, fungicides, insecticides, miticides, and other agricultural chemicals are being spread over farmland throughout the world. These chemicals are known to cause birth defects, hormonal imbalances, learning disabilities, cancers and other diseases in both humans and wildlife. Farming and industrial chemicals also accumulate in water, poisoning it, and resulting in large areas of the seas that are void of natural life. Inland, there are people who are told not to drink the tap water because it contains such high levels of chemical fertilizers that drinking the water can cause brain damage.

Low-paid farm laborers are exposed to toxic farming chemicals, and often get sick from them. Many farm workers have no idea what the dangers are of the chemicals they are being exposed to. For example, the fumigant chloropicrin that is used on farms contains the same active ingredient as tear gas. A chemical called Nemagon had been used for decades on sugar cane, pineapple, and banana farms. It caused cancers and a variety of terrible ailments among the farm workers. Women repeatedly exposed to it had miscarriages and stillbirths, and their babies that lived often were born with horrible deformities. Today there are similar chemicals being used that are poisoning workers on farms around the planet. When farm workers who are exposed to toxic chemicals do get sick they may not know what caused it. If they are able to visit a nurse or doctor they may be misdiagnosed, or their concerns are dismissed or become lost in translation. Long-term exposure can result in numerous health problems in the workers and in their children, and, as science has proved, in the third and later generations of the people poisoned by these chemicals.

Farming chemicals damage soil organisms, such as mycorrhizal soil fungi, which play a major role in soil health and help plant root systems obtain nutrients and water from the soil. There are many hundreds of trillions of natural chemical reactions taking place in a handful of soil as various forms of microorganisms live and interact through their life processes. If the genetically engineered plants and/or various toxic chemicals produced by industries begin to kill soil organisms or lead to a bacteria that largely damages or kills soil organisms, it could stop all plants from growing. If the obscene development of genetically engineered food plants isn't bad enough, there are companies that are developing genetically engineered bacteria. This should be stopped.

"Supporting local, ecologically sound agriculture is one step we can take toward achieving a more sustainable lifestyle. Buying locally grown food conserves fuel and reduces pollution by shortening shipping distances. Local food is also fresher, and therefore tastier and more nutritious. Choosing organically grown food provides for the conservation of our valuable agricultural soils. Supporting local farmers contributes toward preservation of the rural character of the New England landscape."
– FarmDirectCoOp.Org

"The amount of pesticides and nonorganic fertilizers used in farming today is shocking, and it is being ingested by us and Earth and damaging us both – for example, conventional strawberries use 300 pounds of synthetic pesticides, herbicides, fertilizer, and fungicides per acre."
– Terces Engelhart, co-author with Orchid of *I Am Grateful: Recipes & Lifestyle of Café Gratitude*; CafeGratitude.com

"Many new studies prove we can grow more food per acre on small organic farms than big chemically addicted agribusiness farms and that organic food is more nutrition than industrial food, so a lot of what we know instinctively is now backed by science. Which is great. What is good for our bodies and our communities is good for the planet."
– Deborah Koons Garcia, director of the documentaries *The Future of Food* and *In Good Heart: Soil and the Mystery of Fertility*

"GMOs (genetically modified organisms = genetically engineered foods) can't beat the capacity of organics for restoration, resilience, and abundance. Organic agriculture is the best way to remove billions of tons of greenhouse gases from the atmosphere and safely sequester them for centuries in the living soil of organic farms, pastures, and rangelands. If all the world's cropland were transitioned to organic, it would sequester 40 percent of current greenhouse gas emissions. Organic systems also produce higher yields than GMOs and are more resistant to droughts, floods, diseases and pests.

The organic solution to the climate crisis is threatened by contamination from GMOs. Organic agriculture relies on the diversity and resilience of the thousands of varieties of crops and food animals that humans have cultivated for every soil and climate on Earth. GMOs, also known as "recombinant DNA," are bizarre combinations of foreign genes forcefully inserted into "host organisms" from different species. Once you insert foreign genes into a food crop or animal, these mutant varieties breed and reproduce. These GE mutations are likely permanent, meaning that it is only a matter of time before natural and organic varieties are contaminated with GMO traits."

– The Organic Consumers Association, OrganicConsumers.org

Beyond Pesticides, BeyondPesticides.org
Bioneers, Bioneers.org
Co-op Directory, coopdorectory.org
Food Consumer, foodconsumer.org
Farm to Consumer Legal Defense Fund, FarmToConsumer.org
Gardenerd, gardenerd.com
Local Harvest, localharvest.org/store/local-csa.jsp
MolokaiMom.com
Monsanto Watch, MonsantoWatch.org
Non-GMO Shopping Guide, nongmoshoppingguide.com
Occupy Monsanto, OccupyMonsanto360.org
Organic Consumers Association, OrganicConsumers.org
Organic Foodee, OrganicFoodee.com
Organic Its Worth It, organicitsworthit.org
Organic Seed Alliance, SeedAlliance.org
Pesticide Action Network, PANNA.org
Real Food Challenge, RealFoodChallenge.org
Rodale Institute, RodaleInstitute.org
Say No to GMOs, SayNoToGMOs.org
The War on Bugs, TheWarOnBugsBook.com
Worldwide Opportunities on Organic Farms, WWOOF.org

GENETICALLY ENGINEERED FOODS

"Genetically modified foods are less nutritious, more likely to trigger an allergy, and contain higher levels of growth hormones and pesticides.

Common genetically modified food ingredients include corn syrup from GM corn, sugar from GM sugar beets, vegetable oils from GM soy, cotton and canola, and cheese, eggs, milk and meat from animals given GM feed or shot up with GM growth hormones and vaccines.

The same foods that are making people fat, sick, and undernourished are the ones that Monsanto has genetically engineered. High fructose corn syrup, transfats, fryer grease, chicken nuggets, and bacon cheeseburgers all contain GMOs.

The industrial-scale monocrop farms, factory farms and slaughterhouses that are abusing workers and animals, destroying the soil, poisoning the water, polluting the atmosphere with climate-destabilizing greenhouse gases, and creating a breeding ground for mad cow disease, E. coli, salmonella, and swine flu, are the best customers for Monsanto's RoundUp Ready and Bt-spliced crops. Agribusiness thrives off feeding taxpayer subsidized GMO crops, especially corn, soy and cotton seeds, to the chickens, pigs and cows they keep confined in cesspools of their own waste.

Companies like Monsanto and AquaBounty (the Frankenfish inventor) claim that GMOs are "sustainable" because they're going to feed the world as the global climate crisis accelerates. But genetic engineering companies' business model – mass-marketing techno-fixes for the industrialized food system – only perpetuates the waste and pollution that have already made agriculture the source of at least one-third of global greenhouse gas emissions.

GMO contamination could lead to the collapse of the industrialized food system. GMOs have the capacity to break the species barrier. Weeds that plague row crops have adopted the RoundUp Ready trait, creating super-weeds that are forcing farmers to turn to greater amounts of super-toxic herbicides and pesticides. The overuse of RoundUp, the most widely used pesticide in the history of agriculture, enhances the virulence of pathogens such as

Fusarium and may have dire consequences for agriculture, such as rendering soils infertile, crops nonproductive, and plants less nutritious."

    – The Organic Consumers Association; OrganicConsumers.org

PLEASE, read and learn about farmer Percy Schmeiser, who has been sued by Monsanto. Access his Website: PercySchmeiser.com.

"The companies that are genetically engineering and parenting seed are chemical companies. They have interest in selling more chemicals. They don't do genetic engineering to reduce chemical use; they do genetic engineering to increase chemical use."

    – Vandana Shiva, author of *Soil Not Oil*; VandanaShiva.org

"We are facing the ultimate takeover bully – genetic engineering on the cellular level and corporate control on the global scale – and, of course, there is a relationship. Corporate control of the genetic material of the planet by buying up the planet's seed supply and patenting everything they can patent has a major impact on the basic security of every person who eats. After all, having access to seeds and food is the foundation of security."

    – Deborah Koons Garcia, director of the documentaries *The Future of Food* and *In Good Heart: Soil and the Mystery of Fertility*

"In 1992, Monsanto successfully lobbied President George H.W. Bush's administration to deregulate its controversial and untested technology of genetic engineering or genetic modification. Vice President Dan Quayle made the announcement, saying, 'We will ensure that biotech products will receive the same oversight as other products, instead of being hampered by unnecessary regulation.'

The official policy is based on industry propaganda rather than peer-reviewed science; it claims that genetically engineered food, crops, and animals are "substantially equivalent" to conventional food and crops. No safety testing or labels are required.

The result is that GE foods are everywhere. People are unaware that they're eating them, and there isn't any scientific research that could tell us what effect this is having on human health. Study after study indicating serious damage to animals fed GMOs have been downplayed or ignored. Links to human hazards, such as the genetically engineered L-tryptophan disaster of 1989, which killed scores of Americans and permanently injured thousands more, or experiments in 1999 in the UK by renowned scientist Arpad Pusztai, have been literally suppressed."

    – Organic Consumers Association, July 2010; OrganicConsumers.org

"Four Simple Ways to Avoid GMOs

1. Buy organic – organic producers are not allowed to use GMOs

2. Look for "Non-GMO" labels

3. Avoid risky ingredients: corn, soy, vegetable oil (canola, cottonseed, and soy bean), sugarbeet sugar

4. Buy products listed in the Non-GMO Shopping Guide"
– Organic Consumers Association, OrganicConsumers.org

"I sat at meetings where (Monsanto) said, 'The reason we've got to do genetically modified organisms is because it's the only way we can claim a patent.' A patent is a claim to invention, a claim to creation. And it brings with it an exclusive right to exclude anyone else from using, having, distributing the patented product. They say the seed is no more a seed. It's an intellectual property. They make the society shift its thinking of what is at stake. Seed is the first link in the food chain. And therefore, when you control seed, you control food."
– Vandana Shiva; VandanaShiva.org

"Top 10 Reasons to Label Genetically Engineered Food

10. Almost all nonorganic processed food or animal products in the U.S. today contain ingredients that come from genetically engineered crops or from animals given genetically engineered feed, vaccines or growth hormones.

9. Genetically engineered foods have not been tested to determine whether they are safe for human consumption.

8. Genetically engineered foods ARE different from conventional and organic foods.

7. A single serving of genetically engineered soy can result in "horizontal gene transfer," where the bacteria in the human gut adopts the soy's DNA.

6. Animals fed genetically engineered feed ARE different from animals fed conventional and organic feed.

5. The third generation of hamsters fed genetically engineered soy suffered slower growth, a high mortality rate, and a bizarre birth defect: fur growing in their mouths. Many also lost the ability to produce pups.

4. The more genetically engineered corn fed to mice, the fewer babies they had and the smaller the babies were.

3. Biotech's scattershot technique of spraying plant cells with a buckshot of foreign genes that hit chromosomes in random spots would trigger the expression of new allergens and change the character of plant proteins.

2. Scientists reviewing data from Monsanto's own studies "have proven that genetically engineered foods are neither sufficiently healthy nor proper for commercialization."

1. The Convention on Biodiversity recognizes that genetic engineering is a threat to amount and variety of life on the planet."

– Organic Consumers Association, OrganicConsumers.org

Watch the documentary *The World According to Monsanto*, by accessing: FreeDocumentaries.org.

"Q. Hasn't research shown GM foods to be safe?

A. No. The only feeding study done with humans showed that GMOs survived inside the stomach of the people eating GMO food. No follow-up studies were done.

Various feeding studies in animals have resulted in potentially pre-cancerous cell growth, damaged immune systems, smaller brains, livers, and testicles, partial atrophy or increased density of the liver, odd-shaped cell nuclei and other unexplained anomalies, false pregnancies and higher death rates.

Q. But aren't the plants chemically the same, whether or not they are GM?

A. Most tests can't determine the differences at the level of the DNA. And, even if they appear to be the same, eyewitness reports from all over North America describe how several types of animals, including cows, pigs, geese, elk, deer, squirrels, and rats, when given a choice, avoid eating GM foods.

Q. Haven't people been eating GM foods without any ill effect?

A. The biotech industry says that millions have been eating GM foods without ill effect. This is misleading. No one monitors human health impacts of GM foods. If the foods were creating health problems in the U.S. population, it might take years or decades before we identify the cause.

Q. What indications are there that GM foods are causing problems?

A. Soon after GM soy was introduced to the UK, soy allergies skyrocketed by 50 percent.

In March 2001, the Centers for Disease Control reported that food is responsible for twice the number of illnesses in the U.S. compared to estimates just seven years earlier. This increase roughly corresponds to the period when Americans have been eating GM food.

Without follow-up tests, which neither the industry or government are doing, we can't be absolutely sure if genetic engineering was the cause.

Q. What about GM hormones in milk?

A. Milk from rbGH-treated cows contains an increased amount of the hormone IGF-1, which is one of the highest risk factors associated with breast and prostate cancer, but no one is tracking this in relation to cancer rates.

Q. Why do genetically engineered foods have antibiotic resistant genes in them?

A. The techniques used to transfer genes have a very low success rate, so the genetic engineers attach "marker genes" that are resistant to antibiotics to help them find out which cells have taken up the new DNA. That way scientists can then douse the experimental GMO in antibiotics and if it lives, they have successfully altered the genes. The marker genes are resistant to antibiotics that are commonly used in human and veterinary medicine. Some scientists believe that eating GE food containing these marker genes could encourage gut bacteria to develop antibiotic resistance."

– NonGMOShoppingGuide.com. From Jeffrey Smith's book *Genetic Roulette: The Documented Health Risks of Genetically Engineered Foods*

"Organic farming has been shown to provide major benefits for wildlife and the wider environment. The best that can be said about genetically engineered crops is that they will now be monitored to see how much damage they cause."

– Prince Charles

"Any politician or scientist who tells you these [GMO] products are safe is either very stupid or lying."

– David Suzuki, CC, OBC, PhD, UD, Geneticist

"Mexico is the center of origin for corn. Corn provides the primary source of calories for approximately 1.5 billion people in Latin America and Africa. In 2002 UC Berkeley environmental science professor Ignacio Chapela published in the journal *Science* that native varieties of corn had been contaminated by genetically modified corn."

– Trade Policy Special Report: Mexico by the Numbers: The Mexican Corn Issue Today, FairWorldProject.org

"82 percent of U.S. corn exports are controlled by three agribusiness firms: Cargill, Archer Daniels Midland (ADM), and Zen Noh. While family farmer incomes have plummeted during the first seven years of NAFTA, ADMs profits went from $110 million to $301 million, while ConAgra's grew from $143 million to $413 million."

– Global Exchange

Ban Terminator Seeds, BanTerminator.org
Bioneers, Bioneers.org
The Center for Food Safety, TrueFoodNow.org/Campaigns/Genetically-
Engineered-Foods/
The Corporation, TheCorporation.com
Earthlings, Earthlings.com
EarthSave, EarthSave.org
Farm to Consumer Legal Defense Fund, FarmToConsumer.org
Food Inc., FoodIncMovie.com. Please watch the documentary.
The Food Revolution, FoodRevolution.org
The Future of Food, TheFutureOfFood.com
GE Food Alert, GEFoodAlert.org
Genetically Engineered Food Dangers, HolisticMed.com/ge
Institute for Responsible Technology, ResponsibleTechnology.org
King Corn, KingCorn.net. Please watch the documentary, King Corn.
MolokaiMom.com
Monsanto Watch, MonsantoWatch.org
Mothers for Natural Law, Safe-Food.org
Non-GMO Shopping Guide, nongmoshoppingguide.com
Occupy Monsanto, OccupyMonsanto360.org
Organic Consumers Association, OrganicConsumers.org
Percy Schmeiser, PercySchmeiser.com
Rodale Institute, RodaleInstitute.org
Say No to GMOs, SayNoToGMOs.org
Seeds of Deception, SeedsOfDeception.com
Via Organica, Mexico, ViaOrganica.org

MAKE YOUR DIET SUSTAINABLE

"At a time when an estimated 20 million people die annually worldwide of hunger and its effects, 70 percent of the grain produced in the U.S. and over 40 percent of the grain produced worldwide is fed to animals destined for slaughter. Animal-based diets threaten to make global hunger worse in the future by contributing significantly to water shortages, global warming, and soil erosion. It takes up to 14 times as much water for an animal-based diet than for a plant-based diet. According to a 2006 UN FAO report, animal-based agriculture emits more greenhouse gases (in CO_2 equivalents) than all of the cars and other means of transportation worldwide combined (18 percent vs. 13.5 percent). Making matters worse, that same UN report projected a doubling of meat consumption in 50 years, worsening global warming and many other environmental problems. A major shift to plant-based diets is essential to move our imperiled planet to a sustainable path."
– Richard Schwartz; JewishVeg.com

"You, as a food buyer, have the distinct privilege of proactively participating in shaping the world your children will inherit."
– Joel Salatin

"It's phenomenal to me that groups come out with lists like '20 Things You Can Do to Change the Environment' and will list 'drive a fuel-efficient car' and 'change your light bulbs,' but won't say 'eat less meat.' They are omitting the single most powerful, most meaningful action you can take.
Let's say you take a shower every day and that these showers average seven minutes. That's 49 minutes of showering a week. Let's say that's 50 minutes a week, with flow rates of two gallons a minute (which is very strong). At that rate, you'd be using 100 gallons a week for showering. That's 5,200 gallons a year to shower. It takes 5,214 gallons of water to produce one pound of California beef (according to University of California Agricultural Extension). You'd save as much water by not eating one pound of beef as you would by not showering every day for one year."
– John Robbins, author of *The Food Revolution*; FoodRevolution.org

A diet consisting largely of fresh plant matter benefits the planet in many ways. Most significantly, it eliminates the dependence on the wasteful and environmentally damaging meat and dairy industries. And it greatly reduces reliance on processed and corporate foods.

"As human beings, our greatness lies not so much in being able to remake the world as in being able to remake ourselves."
– Mahatma Gandhi

Many people are consuming meat with no idea of the impact the meat industry has on the planet. The methane belched and otherwise emitted from a single cow amounts to about 145 pounds of methane annually. Methane is a greenhouse gas with 23 times the global warming capacity of carbon dioxide. Manure also emits methane.

Tremendous amounts of food are needed to feed the billions of farmed animals being raised throughout the world, including mammals, birds, and fish. More than 60 percent of the food grown on the planet is for feeding farmed animals. Additionally, an increasing amount of fish taken from the world's already depleted seas is going to feed farmed animals, including cows, pigs, lamb, birds, and fish, and for use as fertilizer to grow grains used to feed farmed animals.

Most commonly, the food grown for farmed animals is grown using nitrogen fertilizer, which is made from natural gas, a fossil fuel. The nitrogen fertilizer was developed using techniques used to develop nitrogen-based bombs during World War I. The fertilizers are manufactured in factories using large quantities of other fuels, including petroleum drilled from Earth and also electricity made by coal-burning generating plants – which use coal mined from Earth, which causes an extraordinary amount of environmental destruction, such as mountain-top removal and the obliteration of forests and river valleys. Nitrous oxide is a greenhouse gas with 296 times the global warming implications of carbon dioxide. It evaporates from fields where the nitrogen fertilizer is applied, and ends up contributing to lung-choking, high-particulate smog.

When most of the farmland on each continent is being used to grow food for farmed animals, which is the situation we have today, it means that most of the farm equipment is used to grow, harvest, store, and transport food for farmed animals. The equipment used on farms is largely powered by petroleum gasoline and diesel fuel, which emit massive amounts of carbon dioxide into the atmosphere.

Meat, dairy, egg, and seafood products need to be refrigerated, including in temperature controlled trucks, trains, and airplanes. The warehouses where they are stored use more fossil fuels to maintain the storage temperatures. Then the products are shipped inside refrigerated trucks, and taken to stores and restaurants where the products are stored in temperature-controlled rooms and/or put into temperature-controlled display cases. The purchaser must then store the products in a refrigerator or freezer. All of this refrigeration uses fossil fuels, contributing to global warming. More fossil fuels are used to cook the meat, seafood, and eggs, adding more to the global warming gasses.

Additionally, milk is most often pasteurized, which is a heating process involving the use of fossil fuels

"Our deeds determine us, as much as we determine our deeds."
– George Eliot

It is estimated that Americans throw away about 25 percent of the foods they purchase, either through leftovers or spoiled food. People who eat at home typically waste fewer food products, and people who eat out at restaurants waste more. Most of this wasted food ends up in landfills, where the throwaways are deprived of oxygen. This produces more greenhouse gasses in the form of carbon dioxide and methane. It is better to compost food in home gardens, which improves soil and reduces dependence on landfills.

An increasing amount of farmland around the planet is being used for raising farmed animals. This has been going on for many hundreds of years. This is happening not only on continents, but also on island countries.

As you can tell by my name, I am Scottish. My ancestors dealt with the Highland Clearances of 1800s Scotland. This was brought about by Britain's increased demand for meat. To provide land for cattle and sheep, many poor people were kicked off their land, their villages were demolished, and forests were cleared. This is just one small example of the impact cattle ranching has had on poorer people.

As I have traveled around North America, I never fail to be disappointed by the amount of land being used for livestock, and especially by the amount of land and resources used to grow food for farmed animals.

What happened in Scotland years ago has been happening for the past several decades in North, South, and Central America. An increasing amount of land is being cleared to grow food for cattle, and to provide grazing land for cattle. Many thousands of poor people are being forced from their land so that the land can be cleared for the world meat industry. Just as poor people in Scotland were kicked off the land so that the Brits could have more meat, in Central and South America poor people are being forced from the land to provide space to grow food for farmed animals and land for grazing farmed animals so that meat can be provided for the wealthier people of the planet. All over North America there have been smaller farms taken over by larger, corporate farms, and much of this has been to expand the amount of land being used to grow food for farmed animals.

"According to the United Nations Food and Agriculture Organization, 756 million tons of grain plus most of the world's soy bean crop are fed to animals and that amount has increased sharply in recent years as Asian nations have become more prosperous and their populations have started eating more meat."
– Peter Singer

A few years back NASA conducted a study concluding that the most fertile soil in the U.S. is now covered by cities. Although cities only take up a little over 3 percent of the continental land area, that land can produce as much food as the 29 percent used for agriculture. The study concluded that the land being used for agriculture is less fertile and this increases the use of fertilizers and other farming chemicals.

"If it came from a plant, eat it; if it was made in a plant, don't."
– Michael Pollan

The fresh food diet is not something that comes in a can, bottle, or plastic bag. It is a diet that consists of edible plant substances that can be grown in your yard, harvested in the wilds, and/or purchased from local organic farmers. The fresh food diet requires more fruiting trees and bushes and other culinary plants to be grown. More plants clean the air, provide oxygen, filter water, create homes for wildlife, and manifest a more healthful environment for all forms of life on the planet.

Additionally, with fewer people consuming meat, land previously used to raise farm animals – and used to grow tremendous amounts of food for those animals – is turned over to the wilds of nature. When a person chooses to follow a sunfood diet, they are also choosing to eliminate their share of the fossil fuels, toxic chemicals, and resources used to maintain the global meat, dairy, and egg industries.

"Health depends largely on the foods we eat, and even the commerce of the world is concerned mainly with food supply. By understanding thoroughly, therefore, the meaning of the diet reform movement, we acquire new ideas of living. To become a genuine diet reformer is to recognize that all true and lasting reform begins with oneself. It means further that man will not only become a new creature with a more radiant health, but that he will be better able to promote the higher life of love and brotherhood."
– Dugald Semple, *The Sunfood Way to Health*

On a sunfood diet your power will awaken from a dormant state induced by unhealthful foods, low-quality life choices, and slothful thinking patterns. Your perceptions will enlighten. What you are capable of accomplishing will become clear to you as you transform into a happier, more healthful and satisfied being in tune with your instinct, intellect, talent, and essence.

A plant-based diet that is free of meat, dairy, eggs, and low-quality foods provides for the restoration of your inner nature, which benefits outer nature.

"According to Sapaté and Wien, 'Epidemiologic studies indicate that vegetarian diets are associated with a lower BMI and a lower prevalence of obesity in adults and children. A meta-analysis of adult vegetarian diet studies estimated a reduced weight difference of 7.6 kg for men and 3.3 kg for women, which resulted in a 2-point lower BMI. Similarly, compared with nonvegetarians, vegetarian children are leaner, and their BMI difference becomes greater during adolescence. Studies exploring the risk of overweight and food groups and dietary patterns indicate that a plant-based diet seems to be a sensible approach for the prevention of obesity in children. Plant-based diets are low in energy density and high in complex carbohydrate, fiber, and water, which may increase satiety and resting energy expenditure.' The authors conclude that plant-based dietary patterns should be endourage for optimal health."
– Dr. Michael Greger, NutritionFacts.org; quoting from study, Vegetarian Diets and Childhood Obesity, *American Journal of Clinical Nutrition*, May 2010

"We are the living graves of murdered beasts, slaughtered to satisfy our appetites. How can we hope in this world to attain the peace we say we are so anxious for?"
– George Bernard Shaw

"I am in favor of animal rights as well as human rights. That is the way of a whole human being."
– Abraham Lincoln

"Everyone has control over what they put in their mouth and these choices make a huge difference for our shared environment – our biosphere, as well as our individual environments – our bodies! Choosing organic, vegan raw foods is not only supporting our individual bodies with optimally nutritious foods, but supporting the growth of the whole organic and vegan industry – basically, our health and the health of our planet."
– Rod Rotundi, Leaf Organics, Culver City, CA; LeafOrganics.com

"The fact that the calves are actually killed so that the milk doesn't go to them but to us cannot really be right, and if you have seen a cow in a state of extreme distress because it cannot understand why its calf isn't by, it can make you think a lot."
– Kate Bush

"Being vegan helped me realize I can say and do what I believe is right. That's powerful. Nothing's changed my life more. I feel better about myself as a person, being conscious and responsible for my actions and I lost weight and my skin cleared up and I got bright eyes and I just became stronger and healthier and happier. Can't think of anything better in the world to be but be vegan."
– Alicia Silverstone

"There are many reasons to buy locally grown food. You'll get exceptional taste and freshness, strengthen your local economy, support endangered family farms, safeguard your family's health, and protect the environment.
Getting to know the farmers who grow your food builds relationships based on understanding and trust.
Fruits and vegetables shipped from distant states and countries can spend as many as seven to fourteen days in transit before they arrive in the supermarket."
– FoodRoutes.Org

"Every time a consumer spends a dollar they are placing a vote on the future."
– Howard Lyman, author of *No More Bull*

"Gardening is the most therapeutic and defiant act you can do, especially in the inner city. Plus, you get strawberries."
– Ron Finley, LAGreenGrounds.org

ADAPTT (Animals Deserve Absolute Protection Today and Tomorrow), ADAPTT.org. Gary Yourofsky gives seminars about the truth of the animal farming industry.
FarmUSA.org
GreenPeople.org/AnimalRights.htm
MercyForAnimals.org
United Poultry Concerns, UPC-Online.org
Shark Savers, SharkSavers.org
WeDontEatAnimals.com

GROW FOOD

"The glory of gardening: hands in the dirt, head in the sun, heart with nature. To nurture a garden is to feed not just on the body, but the soul."
– Alfred Austin

THE absolute number-one cause of greenhouse gas emissions is related to food production, packaging, shipping, marketing, and cooking – and especially to diets that include meat, dairy, and junk food.

"Lead with your fork, not your mouth."
– Bernie Wilke

Eat regionally: It uses at least 50 times less fossil fuel. Eat organic: It uses 50 percent less fossil fuels. Eat a vegan diet that is all or mostly raw: it uses over 15 times less water, over 25 times less land, and over 30 times less petroleum than the typical American diet.

Disconnect from the corporate food train that has guided the majority of people to rely on stores and restaurants for food. Grow food using heirloom and nongenetically modified seeds. Aim for variety in your garden. There are 7,000 species of edible plants.

Educate yourself about *veganic* gardening, which uses no bone meal or blood fertilizers. However, soil isn't vegan, and consumes all types of dead bodies.

Creating an amazing culinary garden doesn't have to cost much. Books and magazines about gardening are available at libraries. There are many places to get free seeds, cuttings, vines, and fruiting bushes and trees. Some of the Websites listed below provide information about this. Many people owning land, including people with empty backyards, will allow people to plant there.

Nurture wild edible plants native to your region. Include wildflowers to support local bee colonies. Plant berry bushes and fruiting trees in nearby wildland. Learn how to identify edible plants in your local environment, including what you may think of as weeds, such as dandelion, purslane, young fiddlehead ferns, watercress, milkweed shoots, lambs quarters, chickweed, and sorrel. Also, learn the difference between edible and nonedible mushrooms.

376

Learn about the Dervaes family of Pasadena, California. They turned their small yard into a garden that produces thousands of pounds of fruits and vegetables every year: PathToFreedom.com.

"We live off of what comes out of the soil, not what's in the bank. If we squander the ecological capital of the soil, the capital on paper won't much matter... For the past 50 or 60 years, we have followed industrialized agricultural policies that have increased the rate of destruction of productive farmland. For those 50 or 60 years, we have let ourselves believe the absurd notion that as long as we have money we will have food. If we continue our offenses against the land and the labor by which we are fed, the food supply will decline, and we will have a problem far more complex than the failure of our paper economy. Remember, if our agriculture is not sustainable then our food supply is not sustainable... Either we pay attention or we pay a huge price, not so far down the road. When we face the fact that civilizations have destroyed themselves by destroying their farmland, it's clear that we don't really have a choice."

– Wes Jackson, co-founder of The Land Institute, LandInstitute.org

"Thoughtful and informed people realize that local is the answer. Local seeds which grow well in a certain area need fewer chemicals, practices like crop rotation, composting, and green manure-ing (using crops, especially nitrogen-fixing plants like beans, to return nutrients to soil). All these techniques create a healthier soil which needs fewer chemicals. That creates healthier people."

– Deborah Koons Garcia, director of the documentaries *The Future of Food* and *In Good Heart: Soil and the Mystery of Fertility*

Get away from giving your food dollars to multinational corporate food companies. Grow some of your own food!

Used and discount gardening supplies can be found at garage sales, secondhand stores, and though Websites such as CraigsList.org.

Local vegan restaurants and juice bars may be more than happy to give you bucketsfull of quality food scraps you can use in composters and to build up healthful soil.

Book of interest:
The Forager's Harvest: A Guide to Identifying, Harvesting, and Preparing Edible Wild Plants, by Samuel Thayer

American Community Gardening Association:
CommunityGarden.org

Australian Community Gardens Network,
  CommunityGarden.org.au.
Bay Area Seed Interchange Library, EcologyCenter.Org/BASIL
Bioneers, Bioneers.org
Bountiful Gardens, BountifulGardens.org
City Food Growers, Australia; cityfoodgrowers.com.au
Community Alliance with Family Farmers: CAFF.org
Community Gardening Association: CommunityGarden.org
DollarSeed.com
Earth Garden Magazine, POB 2, Trentham, VIC 3458, Australia;
  earthgarden.com.au. Magazine for sustainable living
Edible Estates, EdibleEstates.org
FedCo Co-op Garden Supplies, POB 520, Waterville, ME 04903; 207-
  873-7333; fedcoseeds.com
Food Empowerment Project, POB 7071, San Jose, CA 95150-7071;
  530-848-4021; FoodIsPower.org
Food Not Lawns: FoodNotLawns.com
Gardenerd, gardenerd.com
Gardening at the Dragon's Gate, gardeningatthedragonsgate.com
Garden Project, GardenProject.org
Growing Organic, GrowingOrganic.com
Harmony Hikes, HarmonyHikes.com. Sergei Boutenko's wild food
  foraging adventure hikes. Sergei is part of the Boutenko family of
  Ashland, Oregon. They have hiked hundreds of miles in the wild while
  surviving on wild plants. With his sister, Valya, he is also the author of
  the recipe book *Fresh*. Access: RawFamily.com.
Hollygrove Market and Farm, New Orleans, hollygrovemarket.com
Institute for the Study of Edible Wild Plants and Other
  Forageables, WildFoodAdventures.com
Island Seed and Feed, Goleta, CA; IslandSeed.com
Kids Gardening, kidsgardening.com.
KitchenGardeners.org
LAGreenGrounds.org
The Learning Garden, TheLearningGarden.org. Venice, California.
  Often have raw food gatherings on weekends.
Mid-City Community Garden, New Orleans,
  midcitycommunitygarden.com
Montview Neighborhood Farm, 38 Henry St., Northampton, MA
  01060; montviewfarm.org. A CSA (community supported agriculture)
  food forest located on three acres of land near downtown
  Northampton.
National Farmers Union Seed Saver Campaign, 2717 Wentz Ave.,
  Saskatoon, SK S7K 4B6, Canada; NFU.CA/SeedSaver.html

National Gardening Association, garden.org.
National Plant Germplasm Service, ARS-Grin.Gov/NPGS
Native Seeds, NativeSeeds.org
New Orleans Food & Farm Network, noffn.org
Organic Gardening Magazine, organicgardening.com
Oregon Tilth, Tilth.org
Organic Seed Alliance: SeedAlliance.org
Osborn International Seed Co., OsbornSeed.Com
Theodore Payne Foundation, TheodorePayne.Org. Promotes the
  preservation and use of native plants. Sells native fruiting trees and
  bushes.
Peoples' Global Action, AGP.Org
Permaculture, Permaculture.co.uk
Planting Seeds Project, New City Institute, Vancouver, CA;
  NewCity.CA/Pages/Planting_Seeds.html
Primal Seeds, PrimalSeeds.Org
Rare Seeds, RareSeeds.com
Ray Mears, RayMears.com
Real Food Challenge, realfoodchallenge.org
Restoring Our Seed, POB 520, Waterville, ME 04903; GrowSeed.Org
The Rhizome Collective, Austin, TX; rhizomecollective.org
Save Our Seed, SavingOurSeed.org
Scatterseed Project, POB 1167, Farmington, ME 04938;
  GardeningPlaces.Com/ScatterSeed.htm
Seed Alliance, SeedAlliance.org
Seed and Plant Sanctuary for Canada, Salt Spring Island, BC;
  SeedSanctuary.Org
Seed Savers Australia, seedsavers.net
Seed Savers Exchange, SeedSavers.org
Seed Savers Network, SeedSavers.Net
Seeds of Change, SeedsOfChange.com
Seeds of Diversity, POB 36, Stn. Q, Toronto, ON M4T 2L7, Canada;
  Seeds.CA
SeedSave.Org
Seeds Trust, SeedsTrust.com
Snow Seed Organic, 831-758-9869; SnowSeedCo.Com
Sow Organic Seed Co., POB 527, Williams, OR 97544;
  OrganicSeed.Com
Square Foot Gardening, SquareFootGardening.com
Synergy Seeds, synergyseeds.com
Tilth, Tilth.org
Tilth Producers, TilthProducers.org

Underwood Gardens, Maryann Underwood, 1414 Ximmerman Rd., Woodstock, IL 60098; UnderwoodGardens.Com. Maryann Underwood's company sells endangered and heirloom seeds; works to preserve genetic diversity of food plants; teaches people the ancient practice of saving seeds; and publishes books and videos on how to save seeds. The Website features a forum where gardeners can share gardening tips, ask questions, and receive feedback.

United Plant Savers, POB 400, East Barre, VT, 05649; UnitedPlantSavers.Org

Victory Seeds, VictorySeeds.com

Wild Man Steve Brill, WildManSteveBrill.com.

Willing Workers on Organic Fams (WWOOF), WWOOF.org

Yards to Gardens, y2g.org

"Growing food is like printing your own money."
– Ron Finley, LAGreenGrounds.org

FRUIT & VEGGIE SHARING ORGANIZATIONS

"Doing things for free encourages people to share. It encourages people to be community, to be family. It provides people the chance to be generous with each other."
– Tree

"When you reap the harvest of your land, you shall not reap all the way to the edges of your field, or gather the gleamings of your harvest. You shall not pick your vineyard bare, or gather the fallen fruit of your vineyard; you shall leave them for the poor and the stranger."
– Leviticus 19:9-10

Eat the Weeds, eattheweeds.com
Fallen Fruit, fallenfruit.org. Fruit share site.
Food Not Bombs, foodnotbombs.net.
Food Not Lawns, foodnotlawns.com.
KitchenGardeners.org
Neighborhood Fruit, neighborhoodfruit.com. Fruit- and vegetable-sharing site.
Veggie Trader, veggietrader.com. People sharing homegrown and wild harvested produce.
Yards To Gardens, Y2G.org

"The other animals who share this planet with humankind have as much right to live here as we do. They are, like us, the sorts of beings who have experiences in their own lives, who value those experiences, and who demonstrate by their actions that they want to continue having those experiences. The least we can do is let them."
– Tim Gier

FARMERS' MARKET LOCATORS

FARMERS' street markets provide direct access to produce grown on family farms in your region.

By shopping with a biodegradable cloth bag and purchasing whole, locally grown foods, you are eliminating packaging and the use of global food transportation, which uses enormous amounts of fossil fuels and other resources.

Australian Farmers' Markets Association, farmersmarkets.org.au. Lists farmers' markets throughout Australia.

CSA California, csacalifornia.org. Community Supported Agriculture is one way of supporting local farmers. Some may provide boxes or bags of locally grown produce that you pick up once a week at your farmers' market, at another location, or is delivered to you.

Farm Direct Co-op, FarmDirectCoop.org. A Massachusetts cooperative of 350 members who receive locally grown produce. Their example of how to run a farm co-op can be duplicated in other regions.

Farmers' Market, FarmersMarket.com

Farmers' Market Finder, search.ams.usda.gov/farmersmarkets

Food Routes, FoodRoutes.org

Local Foods, localfoods.org.uk/local-food-directory. For finding farmers' markets in the UK.

Local Harvest, LocalHarvest.org

London Farmers' Markets, lfm.org.uk

Pick Your Own, PickYourOwn.org. Lists farms in a growing number of countries where you can harvest your own produce.

"One of the problems is that the government supports unhealthy food and does very little to support healthy food. I mean, we subsidize high fructose corn syrup. We subsidize hydrogenated corn oil. We do not subsidize organic food. We subsidize four crops that are the building blocks of fast food. And you also have to work on access. We have food deserts in our cities. We know that the distance you live from a supplier of fresh produce is one of the best predictors of your health. And in the inner city, people don't have grocery stores. So we have to figure out a way of getting supermarkets and farmers markets into the inner cities."
– Michael Pollan

NATURAL FOODS STORE LOCATORS

Australian Farmers' Markets Association, farmersmarkets.org.au. Lists farmers' markets throughout Australia.

CoOpDirectory.org

FoodRoutes.org

Organic Consumers Association, OrganicConsumers.org. For a list of natural foods stores, including co-ops and buying clubs, click on "find organics."

Veg Project, 4547 E. 16yth Ave., Denver, CO 80220; 303-399-6479; kindle (at) vegproject.org; VegProject.org. Veg restaurant collective. The site contains listings of vegetarian restaurants. It was started by Kindle Fahlenkamp-Morell. Also runs veggietrip.com, which contains information about vegetarian restaurants around the world.

"Once I learned how to be a healthy vegan by eating the right foods, my performance improved dramatically."
– Brendan Brazier

"As vegans, we have much to be proud of. We stand firmly against the overwhelming pressures to conform to the dominant culture, we refuse to accept the fictions of ubiquitous carnistic propaganda, and we withstand the incessant seductions to fall back asleep and follow the path of least resistance."
– Dr. Melanie Joy

"Waking up to the animal holocaust is deeply painful. Not only are you confronted by the sheer size of it all, 10 billion land animals in the U.S., 58 billion globally each year, but when you share what you have learned with your friends and family members, who you deeply respect and love, they show indifference at best. You feel like you have come upon genocide that everyone is trying to hide and ignore. And you can no longer participate. And you can no longer keep quiet. And then you are painted as militant, extreme, judgmental, et al. It is deeply painful on so many levels."
– Gary Smith

"It's bizarre that the produce manager is more important to my children's health than the pediatrician."
– Meryl Streep

VEGETARIAN RESTAURANT LOCATORS

IN addition to the restaurants and cafes listed in my book *Sunfood Traveler*, which are serving raw cuisine, the following Websites provide information about vegetarian restaurants around the planet:

Happy Cow, HappyCow.net
Mercy for Animals' vegetarian restaurant guide, VegGuide.org
Raw Food Planet, RawFoodPlanet.com
Soy Stache, SoyStache.com
Vegan Steven, VeganSteven.com
Vegetarian Resource Group, VRG.Org
Vegetarian Restaurants, Vegetarian-Restaurants.Net
Veggie Trip, veggietrip.com

If you are interested in raw vegan restaurants, and other businesses and media related to raw veganism, feel free to join my Facebook group page: Raw Vegan Restaurants, Chefs, Retreats, and Produce. All posts must be on topics relating to raw veganism, including posts about raw vegan restaurants, cafes, chefs, food trucks, caterers, authors, books, blogs, Websites, retreats, seminars, events, videos, and information specifically related to raw veganism.

> "All creatures are deserving of a life free from pain."
> – Maura Commings

> "I know of no other animals who are more consistently curious, more willing to explore new experiences, more ready to meet the world with open mouthed enthusiasm. Pigs, I have discovered, are incurable optimists and get a big kick out of just being."
> – Lyall Watson

> "With complimentary self-description, humans exonerate themselves of wrongdoing. Food-industry enslavement and slaughter cause suffering and death of colossal magnitude. Yet, consumers of flesh, eggs, and nonhuman milk count themselves among 'animal lovers.'"
> – Joan Dunayer

SPROUTING

"Scientists have studied sprouts for centuries to better understand their high levels of disease-preventing phytochemicals, and how they contribute to better health, from prevention to treatment of life-threatening diseases. Major organizations including the National Institutes of Health, American Cancer Society and Johns Hopkins University have reinforced the benefits of sprouts with ongoing studies that explore various sprout varieties for their nutritional properties and to validate health claims.

According to Paul Talalay, M.D., in the American Cancer Society *NEWS*, 'broccoli sprouts are better for you than full-grown broccoli, and contain more of the enzyme sulforaphane which helps protect cells and prevents their genes from turning into cancer.' His findings are consistent with several epidemiologic studies that have shown that sprouts contain significant amounts of vitamins A, C and D. Sprouts are widely recognized by nutrition-conscious consumers and health care professionals as a 'wonder food.'"

– *Good Sprout News* of the International Sprout Growers' Association; ISGA-Sprouts.Org

EATING fresh sprouts is an excellent way to get phytonutrients (plant nutrients), such as enzymes (vital to all life), amino acids (for building protein), chlorophyll (abundant in greens, especially baby greens), biophotons (vital nutrients that are tiny specks of light in living cells, and often referred to by sunfoodists as "vital life-force energy"), antioxidants, high-quality oils (including omega-3 fatty acids, which we need for brain and nerve health), fiber, and other nutrients.

Sprouting is also one of the least expensive ways, besides growing your own garden, to get raw greens and all of their beneficial components into your diet, which is important for anyone wanting to experience vibrant health.

The magic of a seed is that it is a plant-making kit. Seeds are amazing in that they can be eaten by an animal, pass through the digestive tract, and start to grow only after they have left the animal's digestive tract. Magically, what seeds need to grow is provided in the nutrient-rich feces. That is how many plants are spread through nature, by being eaten by animals, who then unknowingly provide themselves as a vehicle to transfer the seed to a new location, where it grows.

Exposing seeds to moisture takes the seed out of its dormant state, shutting off the enzyme inhibitors, which mostly exist in the skin or shell, and igniting the nutrient factories that build the structure from a seed into a plant. The first few days of a plant's life is a time of exuberant energy and a microscopic storm of nutrient-making activity. By consuming the sprouts, you are transferring the concentrated vibrant nutrients of the young plant into your body.

> "What is the great secret that has been eluding the investigations of scientists and lives of laypersons for centuries? Enzymes. You are only alive because thousands of enzymes make it possible. Every breath you take, thought you think, or sentence you read, is a result of thousands of complex enzyme systems and their functions operating simultaneously."
> – Ann Wigmore, author of *The Hippocrates Diet*

Some of the beneficial components of sprouts include antioxidants. These are natural plant chemicals that work in the plant to protect it from various stressors, such as the invasion of bacteria and fungi. When we consume the sprouts, the substances that work to protect the sprouts then work inside us to protect our health.

Because some of the chemicals that form in sprouts specifically fight the invasion of harsh bacteria, sprouts can also help to improve digestion and rid the digestive tract of certain types of bacteria that can cause illness.

As long as you have an area that is between about 50 to 100 degrees Fahrenheit and has indirect sunlight, you can grow sprouts anywhere on the planet (although some seeds are more likely to grow when in the temperature range of between 60 and 90 degrees Fahrenheit). You don't need anything special to grow sprouts. All it takes is something like a big glass jar and a screen to cover the top. You can also use a bowl covered with a screen, or a sheer cloth. Of course, you also need clean water to first soak the seeds, then to rinse them. We often germinate seeds in a bowl covered by a plate, which also makes it easy to rinse as we put water in the bowl, then hold the plate on with our thumbs as we tip the bowl over the sink or outside in the garden, and let the water seep out.

Probably the most common method of growing sprouts is to use a big jar covered by a screen, keeping the jar tilting almost upside down at an approximate 45° angle in a big bowl to drain excess water.

Some people use mesh bags to sprout seeds. This also makes it easy to rinse the seeds.

There are a variety of sprouting trays and machines on the market that can make it easier to sprout seeds. Some sprouters automatically spray and rinse the sprouts so that you don't have to. I've never owned one of those fancy gizmos. Some people like them. We do fine with bowls and jars.

There are a variety of seeds that are good for sprouting. Seek those that are from organic sources.

Make sure your soaking and sprouting bowls, jars, screens, and/or mesh bags are clean, or else you may find that you will also be growing some unwanted bacteria – turning your germinates rancid.

During the soaking time remember that seeds can die if they remain in water too long. If it is cold, you may want to soak a longer period; if it is warm you want to sprout a shorter period. In warmer weather the seeds will also need to be rinsed more often. As you get more familiar with sprouting, you will learn what works best for the types of seeds you are using, and the environment of the room.

Unless you have an automatic sprouting machine that regularly mists the sprouting seeds, you will need to rinse them one to three times per day with clean water to keep them clean, fresh, and hydrated (moist). It is good to have a screened strainer for rinsing the smaller seeds, and a colander with smallish holes for rinsing the larger seeds/beans.

Sprouting takes place faster in warm weather.

Also, people often use the word _sprout_ when they really mean _germinate_. But that is a technicality. For instance, you may hear people say _sprouted garbanzo hummus_, which is really germinated garbanzo hummus. The difference between a _germinate_ and a _sprout_ is that a germinate is only when the root has appeared, such as _germinated_ garbanzo beans used to make raw hummus, and a _sprout_ is when the leaf has started to appear, or is in full form, such as alfalfa sprouts, sunflower sprouts, bean sprouts, and sprouted wheatgrass. But people seem to have a thing against the word _germinate_, and maybe because it reminds them too much of the word _germ_, so they will continue to use the word _sprout_ for both sprouted and germinated seeds. Commonly some of the seeds that are only germinated rather than sprouted include buckwheat, garbanzo, chia, and quinoa.

There are also a lot of raw recipes that call for _soaked_ seeds or nuts, such as _soaked_ almonds or _soaked_ sunflower seeds. Soaking seeds and nuts for a time (usually less than a few hours) turns off the enzyme inhibitors, ignites the factory of the seed in making enzymes, amino acids, essential fatty acids, biophotons, and other nutrients, including vitamins and antioxidants. Soaking makes nuts and seeds more nutrient-rich and easier to digest. Commonly, some of the seeds that are soaked rather than sprouted include nuts, such as almonds, macadamias, cashews, Brazil nuts, and other nuts (yes, nuts are seeds).

People who are into the *Living Foods* diet commonly will soak their seeds and nuts before eating them, to make them truly living foods rather than dormant seeds and nuts.

Most types of grain germinates are sweetest when the tail on the seed has just started to grow. The longer the tail grows, the less sweet it will become.

Once seeds have passed the germination stage and start to develop leaves, they are then sprouts.

Sprouts benefit from exposure to light, such as indirect sunlight, as this will trigger the development of chlorophyll in the sprouts.

Within a plant, chlorophyll transforms sunlight and CO_2 into sugar and oxygen. Chlorophyll is molecularly very similar to human blood plasma. There are strong nutritional qualities in chlorophyll as it helps strengthen the immune system in fighting off infections, and helps rid the body of toxins, especially those that gather in the liver. Because chlorophyll helps generate new cell growth, it also is important in healing wounds and illnesses.

Some sprouts are more chlorophyll-rich than others. With a content of about 70 percent chlorophyll, wheatgrass is perhaps the richest sprout of all.

If you are not going to use the sprouts right away, you can slow their growth by putting them in the refrigerator, or in a cold room (not freezing). Rinse and drain once a day with clean water and you should be able to keep them in a cold, slowed growing state for two to four days, or more.

You can also slow soaked seeds from sprouting fully by keeping them in the refrigerator. Then, when you are ready to sprout them, remove them from the refrigerator, rinse, and let them grow in room temperature.

Sprouts are living, breathing plants. They need air. Don't put them into a sealed container. A screened jar or a casserole dish with a glass top left slightly open work well because they both allow for air to enter the container. A jar with a screen fastened around the top and turned almost upside down at an angle in a jar works best for many seeds because it prevents them from sitting in water while also letting in air. As they sprout at room temperature, remember to rinse them two or three times a day to keep them from rotting.

One way of keeping sprouts fresh in the refrigerator is to store them in a bamboo bowl covered by a second bamboo bowl that has a dozen or more small holes drilled into it. This also provides an easy way to rinse them once a day by pouring water into the bowl, covering with the top bowl, and tilting upside down over the sink or outside to eliminate excess water before putting them back into the refrigerator.

Some people will drink the soak water as it contains enzymes that are released by the seeds.

Just as long as the soaked seeds are kept moist and you don't let them dry out, you break down the enzyme inhibitors, and nurture the seed to become a plant.

Again: Sprouts must be rinsed, and most are best if they are rinsed two times per day, although some may need rinsing only once per day. The more you get used to sprouting, the more you will learn which seeds require more attention, and which require less.

When the sprouts have reached the size you want them, put them in direct sun for an hour or more. By doing this you will ignite the chlorophyll and nutrient-making factory within the sprouts, greatly increasing their nutritional value. Make sure not to allow sun to bake them or let them dry out. Keep them covered with a screen or sheer cloth to keep little buggy friends away.

Eat Sprouts, EatSprouts.Com
International Sprout Grower's Association, ISGA-Sprouts.Org
Mumm's Sprouting Seeds, Sprouting.Com
Sprout Man, SproutMan.Com
Sprout People, SproutPeople.Com
Tim Tyler's Sprout Farm, Sprouting.Org

FRUITING TREES AND BUSHES

FRUITS and berries are some of the most nutritious foods you can eat. One way to guarantee that you have access to fresh fruits and berries is to plant some of your own fruiting trees and bushes. If you don't have your own land, consider planting them on a cooperative neighbor's property, or on nearby wildland. I know people who hike into a canyon near their home where they have been planting fruit trees and berry bushes. Little by little they are creating an amazing fruit forest. They are also saving money, getting exercise, improving their nutrition, and disconnecting from the corporate food chain.

California Rare Fruit Growers, CRFG.org. Paul Thomson and John Riley founded this association in 1968. There are now chapters with thousands of members in many countries

California Rare Fruit Growers, San Diego chapter, CRFGSanDiego.org

California Rare Fruit Growers, CRFG.org/nurlist.html. Site listing nurseries selling both rare and common fruiting trees and bushes.

California Tropical Fruit Trees, TropicalFruitTrees.com. Vista, CA. California Tropical Fruit Trees sells a variety of both rare and common fruiting trees and berry bushes.

Common Vision, CommonVision.org. California-based organization plants fruiting trees at schools and other community facilities, and also helps reforest areas that were formerly forested.

Northern Nut Growers Association, NutGrowing.org

"Globalized industrialized food is not cheap: It is too costly for the Earth, for the farmers, for our health."
– Vandana Shiva, author of *Making Peace with the Earth*

"What we need to do is to grow veganism by embracing it as a valid, acceptable, and logical choice in our everyday lives. We need to put forth positive examples of veganism, and to live as proud vegans. We should not run from our choices, or mask them in cutesy terms. Instead, we should live what we are proudly, and build a genuine movement of people who demand an end to the human exploitation of animals."
– Bob Torres

COMMON FOODS

The following are what most Americans limit themselves to in their diet. These foods appear over and over again in different forms, and are most often grown or raised using synthetic farming chemicals.

Wheat: In the form of bread, bagels, crackers, cakes, cookies, pastas, donuts, scones, and cereals. Baked items may contain a variety of unhealthful ingredients. L-cysteine or cystine derived from human hair or bird feathers may be used as a dough conditioner. Some baked goods, such as commercial pastries, cakes, and cookies, may contain beef fat (lard), butter, processed salts, and a variety of chemical dyes, preservatives, scents, and flavorings. Commercial bread may contain ammonium sulfate, which is used as a fertilizer on farms, but is used in some bread to provide nitrogen for the yeast to grow. Wheat of all types, including spelt, and also rye and barley contain gluten, which can play a role in mood swings, anxiety, depression, lack of energy, and a variety of other health problems.

Meat: Mostly beef, but also pork, lamb, chicken, turkey, fish, crustaceans, amphibians, reptiles, and wild animals. Please read Howard Lyman's book *No More Bull*.

Corn: Cooked corn, corn chips, corn syrup [aka corn sugar], tortillas, corn flakes, soda and candy (most soda and candy made these days are sweetened with corn syrup). Additionally, many farm animals today are chiefly fed corn, which means meat and dairy are a type of corn product.

If you haven't seen the documentary, "King Corn," you are in for a learning experience about industrial food. Please watch it.

Milk: Milk, yogurt, butter, cheese, cottage cheese, creamer, ice cream, cream, kefir, whey, and casein. Also may be listed on ingredient labels as "milk fat," and "butter fat."

Eggs: Including mayonnaise, meringue, and glaze.

Potatoes: Including baked and fried, and potato chips.

Vegetable oil that has been exposed to high temperatures in processing and/or cooking: corn oil, palm oil, canola oil, soy oil, olive oil, sunflower oil, etc.

Sugar: Including corn syrup (aka corn sugar), cane and beet sugar (white sugar, brown sugar, powdered sugar, raw sugar), agave, etc.

Iceberg lettuce: While iceberg lettuce isn't as empty in nutrition as some people would have you believe (it does contain amino acids, antioxidants, vitamins, minerals, and biophotons), it is good to choose a variety of lettuces and other greens, and not limit yourself to iceberg lettuce as your main green-leafed vegetable. Grow lettuce.

Bananas: Please eat organic bananas. Banana plantation workers have suffered severe health problems caused by the pesticides used on nonorganic banana plantations. If you live in a large city, you can likely purchase organic bananas by the case at a fruit wholesaler.

Apples: Usually one or two types, rather than variety. Often the apples have been cooked into baked or fried items, such as pies or turnovers, or are in cooked applesauce or pasteurized (heated) apple juice. Like other fruit, apples are most nutritious when eaten raw.

Oranges: Usually as pasteurized orange juice, and more and more often in the form of a juice that only consists partially of orange juice with the rest being artificially flavored, dyed, sweetened, and scented water.

Celery: Conventionally grown celery has been found to contain so many farming chemicals that it has been listed at the top of the so-called "dirty dozen" foods grown using chemicals. Eat organic celery. It is easy to grow using the stem butt; simply cut the bottom off the stalk of celery, put it in soil, and keep it moist. It will grow.

Carrots: Peeled and processed carrots may have been treated with bleach. Prepared foods may contain carrots dyed with chemicals.

Broccoli

Tomatoes: Including ketchup, salsa, and pasta and pizza sauces.

Onions: Often as powder containing salt, preservatives, and/or MSG.

Processed salt: Table salt has been heated and processed to the point that it is not a good thing to eat, is harsh on the tissues, and is a contributing factor in cardiovascular, kidney, liver, and blood system diseases. It may contain various chemical or metal additives to prevent caking. A better quality is unprocessed sea salt, or pink salt.

Mustard: Most often in the form of bottled mustard containing processed salt and artificial dyes, sweeteners, scents, and flavors. Mustard is easy and less expensive to make at home, using raw ingredients. (True Dijon mustard contains red wine, and not vinegar.)

Low-quality dried herbs and spices: Including those that contain processed salts; low-quality oils; MSG; and synthetic chemical dyes, flavors, scents, preservatives, and drying agents.

Cola and soda: In 2011, the average American drank nearly 50 gallons of sodas and colas, amounting to more than 400 calories per day. "Soft drinks" aren't so soft on human health. They contain loads of health damaging ingredients. They are sold in petroleum plastic bottles, or cans lined with petroleum derivatives that are known to cause cancer, learning disabilities, birth defects, and hormonal changes. Some brands of soft drinks contain brominated vegetable oil, which is also used as a fire retardant. In the drink, the brominated vegetable oil helps keep an even flavor. In humans, it can lead to memory loss, nerve disorders, and skin lesions. Cola contains extract of the kola nut that interferes with the ability to absorb minerals. Corn syrup plays a role in obesity, diabetes, heart disease, and related health problems; interferes with the ability of the intestines to absorb nutrients, and shortens cell life. Regular drinkers of soda have higher cholesterol, are likely to have fatty livers and increased skeletal fat. The caffeine in cola helps lead to adrenal fatigue, and causes mineral drain. All of these substances in cola play a part in weak bones and osteoporosis. Sodas, candy, icing, cakes, cookies, and other sweets may be dyed with coal tar extracts, which are not healthful.

Coffee: Often from companies that damage the environment and generally don't support human rights. More forests are being cleared to grow a variety of coffee that doesn't need to be grown in shade. This is killing massive numbers of wildlife, damaging soil, reducing diversity, bringing species closer to extinction, raising temperatures, and reducing the absorption of carbon. If you choose to drink coffee, make sure it is organic, shade grown, and from nonslave labor.

Food additives: Including MSG, emulsifiers, and synthetic preservatives, dyes, flavors, scents, etc. Many of the thousands of synthetic food chemicals have been proven to cause cancer, learning disorders, mood swings, hyperactivity, headaches, and allergies. For more information, access SweetPoison.com, and the Website of The Center for Science in the Public Interest at CSPI.org.

Instead of following a diet limited to just a few ingredients, consider the wide variety of edible plants, including those that are native to your region of the planet.

When you follow a diet that is rich in raw plant matter and free of low-quality foods and animal protein, you will have more energy, your brain will function at a higher level, and you will desire a more active lifestyle. Your zest for life will be present, and will become obvious through your actions.

How much food are you eating when you eat something? Are you eating fruits, vegetables, nuts, and seeds, or some combination of them, that you see in front of you when you follow a plant-based diet? Or are you eating a whole lot of grain and fishmeal used to feed farmed animals, which is a practice that produces a small piece of meat? Why are we depleting the oceans to feed fish to farmed animals that are naturally vegetarian and would never ever eat fish from the ocean? Why are we clearing land of ancient forests, sending species into extinction and raising global temperatures, to feed farmed animals when we would be healthier eating fruits, vegetables, nuts, and seeds, and allowing the forests to remain as homes to diverse species?

Please join me in following a plant-based diet. Please, localize your diet by eating all or largely locally produced foods as much as possible. Wherever possible, grow some of your own foods, and support local organic farmers. Compost your food scraps into soil. Cook less, or not at all. By doing so, you will be healthier, and so will our home, Earth.

"The reaons I decided to go vegan were both health-related and ethical. I went vegetarian initially for ethical reaons. But as I learned more about the unhealthiness of dairy, I gradually started eliminating it from my diet. But it wasn't until I started to think and read more about the horrible ways many dairy cows are treated that I decided to go all the way."
– Matt Frazier

"Good health is about being able to fully enjoy the time we do have. It is about being as functional as possible throughout our entire lives and avoiding crippling, painful, and lengthy battles with disease. The enjoyment of life is greatly compromised if we cannot see, if we cannot think, if our kidneys do not work, and if our bones are fragile or broken."
– T. Colin Campbell, Ph.D., Cornell University; author of *The China Study* and *Whole: Rethinking the Science of Nutrition*; TColinCampbell.org

"Choosing to consume animal products is a choice to partake in the exploitation and intentional slaughter of sentient beings. Given our wide variety of food choices today, we can easily refuse to partake in such exploitation."
– Dan Cudahy

ADDITIONAL QUOTATIONS

"I know of no more beautiful prayer than that which the Hindus of old used in closing: May all that have life be delivered from suffering."
– Arthur Schopenhauer

"We can become prisoners of our earliest indoctrination, or we can choose to look critically at our assumptions and align our lives with our values. Choosing to live vegan is how we are able to do that best."
– Jenny Brown

"To become vegetarian is to step into the stream which leads to nirvana."
– Buddha

"Suffering is suffering, whether experienced by animals or humans. The physiological process is identical."
– Mirko Bagaric, Head of Deakin Law School

"I can't imagine that if you're putting something in your body that is filled with fear or anxiety, or pain, that that isn't somehow going to be inside of you."
– Ellen Degeneres

"Consuming animal products is a choice only insofar as society allows you to choose to do things that are obviously and indisputably morally wrong. Are you free to choose to hold racist views? Yes, you are. It is morally wrong to judge others solely by skin color? Yes, of course it is. So saying that something is a 'choice' says nothing about its morality. We cannot morally justify consuming animal products. Period. Consuming those products may be a matter of 'choice,' but only in a most superficial sense. It is not a matter of choice for anyone who takes morality seriously."
– Gary L. Francione

"I was vegetarian from age 19 until I got pregnant with my first son in 2005. He was allergic to dairy in my breast milk, so I cut it out. After Fred was born, I read *Eating Animals*, by Jonathan Safran Foer, and it convinced me that it was worth it to go 'all the way,'

and so I eliminated eggs and all trace dairy – like in baked goods and my beloved candy bars I indulged in from time to time. My love for animals since childhood feels complete now that I am vegan, and it feels really right for every reason: health, ethical, environmental. It is an amazing lifestyle and I find it easy and inexpensive. Our boys eat a variety of foods that many kids have never heard of, and they also get sweets and fun foods in their lives, too. We make it work because it matters to us to do it, even if it's sometimes challenging."
     – Mayim Bialik

"I think I could always live with animals. The more you're around people, the more you love animals."
     – Walt Whitman

"I expect to pass through this world but once; any good thing therefore that I can do, or any kindness that I can show to any fellow creature, let me do it now; let me not defer or neglect it, for I shall not pass this way again."
     – Ettiene De Grellet

"Compassion for animals is intimately connected with goodness of character; and it may be confidently asserted that he who is cruel to animals cannot be a good man."
     – Arthur Schopenhauer

"I don't think it makes sense to start assigning value to one species over another. Who has the yardstick that measures value?"
     – Mary Lou Randour, Ph.D.

"It is just as wrong to kill an animal as it is to kill a human being, and only human chauvinism, speciesism and the inordinately high opinion the human race has of itself prevents it from accepting this simple fact."
     – Charles B. Edelman

"As an invertebrate zoologist who has studied crustaceans for a number of years, I can tell you the lobster has a rather sophisticated nervous system that, among other things, allows it to sense actions that will cause it harm. ... [Lobsters] can, I am sure, sense pain."
     – Jaren G. Horsley, Ph.D

"If you eat an avocado and you bury the pit in the ground, chances are, if in the right climate, that pit might grow into an avocado tree. If you eat an apple, and you bury the seeds in the ground, chances are you could expect an apple tree to emerge from the ground. This also applies to all fruits and vegetables with

seeds. When you eat these foods, and include the seeds, you nourish your body with that same life-force energy that could have eventually sprouted into a tree, or plant. Now think about this... If you bury a cow, or a pig, or especially the remains of a dead cow or pig, or any other animal, what happens? It decays. When you eat animals, you deplete your body of nutrients, restrict yourself from gaining life-force energy, severely damage your body system, coat your organs with mucoid plaque from the decaying remnants, age prematurely, and if you are lucky, you may die from heart disease rather than cancer. The animals decay in your body just as they would in the ground. What will it be?"
– Jesse Jacoby, author of *The Raw Cure*

"He is a heavy eater of beef. Methinks it doth harm to his wit."
– William Shakespeare

"Instead of using their food, water, topsoil, and massive amounts of land, and energy to raise livestock, Ethiopia could for instance grow teff, an ancient and quite nutritious grain. Seventy percent of all their cattle are raised pastorally in the highlands of that country where less than 100 pounds of meat and a few gallons of milk are produced per acre of land used. If this land were used for the growing of teff, Ethiopians could produce over 2,000 pounds of food per one acre with no water irrigation. The end product could provide a much greater amount of much needed nutrients and even stimulate improved economics with business opportunities to sell teff (as well as many other types of produce) to other countries. Therefore, conversion to plant-based food systems for local regions in developing countries would feed more people more nutritiously with more efficient use of their resources, improve long term soil fertility, create economic opportunities, all of which would provide a path toward breaking the poverty and hunger cycle."
– Dr. Richard A. Oppenlander, ComfortablyUnaware.com

"Since I became vegan, I have noticed that I'm happier! (Which is something that everyone wants, but very few can achieve.) I may worry and get upset when seeing and empathizing with the suffering of animals, but at the end of the day having compassion for animals has made me a better person and has enabled me to enjoy a richer life."
– Andres Grijalva

"Many years ago, as I traveled around the world, I noticed the vast number of animal species that other people ate. And it dawned

on me that there were literally thousands of animals I didn't eat. Dogs or cats. Bears or bats. Tigers or turtles. Horses or hamsters. Rosellas or rats. Nor did I drink the milk of goats, yaks, or donkeys, giraffes, or cats. I decided to go only 5 animals more. I simply added cows, sheep, pigs, chickens, and fish to the list. It was a breeze."
   – Philip Wollen

"All the talk today about how undesirable it is to consume horses carries the implication that our immense ingestion of other livestock is perfectly acceptable. We are advised not to eat horses, nor dogs, rabbits, or cats – no matter how close to starvation we might be. But devouring limitless numbers of cattle, pigs, sheep, lambs, chickens, turkeys, and ducks is quite all right.

This causes us to overlook the real problem, which is not horsemeat, but meat consumption in general. The world cannot feed itself if it continues to make meat a common staple. Millions upon millions of livestock require vast amounts of grain and water, ultimately far more than the environment will be able to provide.

Aside from the survival problems raised by the consumption of immense quantities of land, water, and grain in producing meat, there is another menacing aspect: all the poisons and torture that happen along the way from the feedlot to the supermarket. For the health of the planet and for our own health and for the sake of the livestock, we should stop eating animals. Rather than calling for more regulation of meat production, we need to move entirely away from meat meals.

Originating from the top of the food chain, all animal products menace our health. Pesticides and other toxic run-offs work their way into the food and water consumed by livestock. So with wild and farmed fish, and seafood. Finally, perched at the highest rung on the food chain, we humans feast on the accumulated toxins that concentrate further in our bodies."
   – Michael Parenti, author of *The Face of Imperialism*

"I think that people should start eating less meat. In case you haven't noticed, meat is made out of animals. How would you feel if you were a baby pig separated from your mother and about to be turned into bacon? We don't eat dogs and cats because they are cute. Well, pigs can be just as cute if you give them a chance."
   – Isaac Bustos, Age 9

"If you are neutral in situations of injustice, you have chosen the side of the oppressor."
   – Desmond Tutu

"Those who describe animals as not having any thoughts or feelings come closer to that description than the animals they are trying to describe."
– Edward Alberola

"The world is not a factory and animals are not products for our use."
– Arthur Schopenhauer

"It is ironic, don't you think, that the majority of humans who lack the heart to stop participating in the killing and eating of sentient animal beings will inevitably die as a result of heart disease?"
– David Chase Taylor

"Let your life be a counter-friction to stop the machine."
– Henry David Thoreau

"Neutrality helps the oppressor, never the victim. Silence encourages the tormentor, never the tormented."
– Elie Wiesel

"Veganism is about changing the future. It's not about looking to the past and figuring out how to eat and act from there. It's about showing people it's time for our society to evolve."
– Ginny Messina and Jack Norris

"I do feel that spiritual progress does demand at some stage that we should cease to kill our fellow creatures for the satisfaction of our bodily wants."
– Gandhi

"Flesh eating is simply immoral, as it involves the performance of an act, which is contrary to moral feeling: killing. By killing, man suppresses in himself, unnecessarily, the highest spiritual capacity, that of sympathy and pity towards living creatures like himself and by violating his own feelings becomes cruel."
– Leo Tolstoy

"Since visiting the abbatoirs of South France, I have stopped eating meat."
– Vincent Van Gogh

"I have no doubt that it is part of the destiny of the human race in its gradual improvement to leave off eating animals."
– Henry David Thoreau

DOCUMENTARIES TO WATCH

Please watch these documentaries:
- **The Big Fix**, TheBigFixMovie.com
- **The Corporation**, TheCorporation.com
- **Crazy Sexy Cancer**
- **A Delicate Balance**, ADelicateBalance.com.au
- **Dirt: The Movie**, DirtTheMovie.org
- **Earthlings**, Earthlings.com
- **Farmageddon**, FarmageddonMovie.com
- **Fat, Sick, and Nearly Dead**, FatSickAndNearlyDead.com
- **Food Beware**: The French Organic Revolution
- **Food Fight**, FoodFightTheDoc.com
- **Food, Inc.**, TakePart.com/FoodInc
- **Food Stamped**, FoodStamped.com
- **Forks over Knives**, ForksOverKnives.com
- **Fresh**, FreshTheMovie.com
- **The Future of Food**, TheFutureOfFood.com
- **Gasland**, GaslandTheMovie.com
- **Glass Walls**, Meat.org
- **Got the Facts on Milk?**, milkdocumentary.com
- **In Organic We Trust**, InOrganicWeTrust.org
- **Killer At Large**, KillerAtLarge.com
- **King Corn**, KingCorn.net
- **May I Be Frank**, MayIBeFrankMovie.com
- **Meat the Truth**, MeatTheTruth.com
- **Meat's Not Green**, Meat.org
- **Meat Your Meat**, Meat.org
- **Processed People**, ProcessedPeople.com
- **The Real Dirt on Farmer John**
- **A River of Waste: The Hazardous Truth About Factory Farms**, ARiverOfWaste.com
- **Super Size Me**
- **Vegucated**, GetVegucated.com
- **We Feed the World**
- **What's On Your Plate?**, WhatsOnYourPlateProject.org
- **The World According to Monsanto**

"I've been vegan since I was about 3 years old, and involved in animal rights for years. I've seen a number of animal rights films throughout the years. None has affected me as profoundly as *Earthlings*."
– Joaquin Phoenix

WEBSITES OF INTEREST

ACTrees.org
AmazonWatch.org
American Community Gardening Association: CommunityGarden.org
AncientTrees.org
AppleLuscious Organic Orchards, AppleLuscious.com
Michael Arnstein, TheFruitarian.com.
Bautista Dates, Mecca, CA; 7HotDates.com; KissMe (at) 7HotDates.com.
The Bautista family has a mail-order date company so they can sell the dates they grow directly to the public.
Beyond Pesticides, BeyondPesticides.org
Bioneers, Bioneers.org
California Rare Fruit Growers, CRFG.org. Paul Thomson and John Riley founded this association in 1968. There are now chapters with thousands of members in many countries
California Rare Fruit Growers, CRFG.org/nurlist.html. Site listing nurseries selling both rare and common fruiting trees and bushes.
California Tropical Fruit Trees, TropicalFruitTrees.com. Vista, CA. California Tropical Fruit Trees sells a variety of both rare and common fruiting trees and berry bushes.
Chris Kendall, TheRawAdvantage.com; nutritionist, yoga practitioner, professional skateboarder
City Farm Organic Produce Markets, 1 City Farm Pl., East Perth, Australia; cityfarm.org.au. Saturday 9:00-12 noon. Organic produce and nursery
Community Garden, CommunityGarden.org
Co-op Directory, CoopDirectory.org
EarthEcho.org
EarthFirst.org
EarthFirstJournal.org
EarthIsland.org
Eat Fruit Feel Good, eatfruitfeelgood.com
Eat the Weeds, eattheweeds.com
Edible Forest Gardens, edibleforestgardens.com
Edible Schoolyard, EdibleSchoolyard.org
811 Directory, el-camacho.com/811friendly. Information about the LFRV lifestyle, includes listings of stores, places to travel, roommates, farms, etc.
EndangeredSpeciesInternational.org
Fallen Fruit, fallenfruit.org. Fruit share site. This began in Los Angeles with property owners who had fruit trees and were willing to allow other people to harvest the fruit and share it with others.

Farmers' Market Finder: AMS.USDA.Gov/FarmersMarket

FoodNotBombs.net

Food Not Lawns: FoodNotLawns.com. Promotes the growing of organic food gardens instead of manicured lawns.

The Food Revolution, FoodRevolution.org

Food Routes, FoodRoutes.org

ForestsForever.org

TheFruitarian.com. This is Michael Arnstein's Website.

Fruitarian Nirvana, fruitariannirvana.ning.com. A social networking site for those interested in LFRV.

Fruit Co-op, califruit.webs.com. Good source for dates and raw almonds.

Fruit for Our Children, New Zealand, fruitforourchildren.com.

The Fruit Shack, 55 Dunn Bay Rd., Dunsborough, Australia; fruitandvegshack.com.au.

Gardenerd, Gardenerd.com

Green Guerillas, New York, NY; GreenGuerillas.org.

Guerilla Gardening, guerrillagardening.org.

Home Orchard Society, HomeOrchardSociety.org

How to Go Organic, HowToGoOrganic.com

ILoveMountains.org

InternationalRivers.org

Jourdan's Beautiful Food, Florida; jourdansbeautifulfood.com. Tropical fruit.

Kitchen Gardeners, KitchenGardeners.org

Label GMOs, LabelGMOs.org

Local Harvest, LocalHarvest.org/store/local-csa.jsp

Local Harvest, Santa Cruz; CALocalHarvest.org. Searchable database of farmers' markets, small farms, and related groups and businesses.

Mad Cowboy, MadCowboy.com

Monsanto Watch, MonsantoWatch.org

MonsantoSucks.com

MountainJustice.org

NativeForest.org

Natural Resources Defense Council, NRDC.org

Neighborhood Fruit, neighborhoodfruit.com. Fruit- and vegetable-sharing site.

NoImpactProject.org

Non GMO Shopping Guide, NonGMOShoppingGuide.com

North American Fruit Explorers, NAFEX.org

OceanProtection.org

OccupyMonsanto360.org

OilSandsTruth.org

Organic Consumers Association, OrganicConsumers.org

Organic Food & Farmers' Markets, Australia; organicfoodmarkets.com.au. Site lists organic farmers' markets in Sydney area.

Organic Foodee, OrganicFoodee.com

Organic It's Worth It, OrganicItsWorthIt.org

Organic Seed Alliance, SeedAlliance.org

Pesticide Action Network, PANNA.org
Percy Schmeiser, PercySchmeiser.com
Permaculture, Permaculture.net
Pesticide Action Network, San Francisco, CA; PANNA.org
Pick Your Own, PickYourOwn.org. Lists farms where you can harvest your own produce. Blake2007 (at) PickYourOwn.org
PlasticFreeTimes.com
PlasticPollutionCoalition.org
RAN.org
Rare Fruit Society of South Australia, rarefruit-sa.org.au.
RawfullyOrganic.com. An organic food co-op in Texas founded by Kristina Carrillo-Bucaram, KristinaBucaram.com; Kristina (at) RawFullyOrganic.com; FullyRaw.com.
RawNaturalLiving.com. Matthew Warner is the author of *Fruitarians Are the Future.*
ReefResiliance.org
Real Food Challenge, RealFoodChallenge.org
Responsible Technology, ResponsibleTechnology.org
Rodale Institute, RodaleInstitute.org
SanctuaryForest.org
SaveTheRedwoods.org
SeaShepherd.org
SeaTurtle.org
Take Part, TakePart.com
30 Bananas A Day, 30BananasADay.com
Tropical Fruit World, TropicalFruitWorld.com.au. Gold Coast, store with variety of fruit.
269Life.com
Union of Concerned Scientists, UCSUSA.org
Urban Organic Gardener, UrbanOrganicGardener.com
Vegetarian USA, VegetarianUSA.com
VeggieFul.com
Veggie Trader, veggietrader.com. People sharing homegrown and wild produce.
VoteHemp.com
The War on Bugs, TheWarOnBugsBook.com
WildEarthGuardians.org
Willing Workers on Organic Farms, OrganicVolunteers.org
Worldwide Opportunities on Organic Farms, WWOOF.org
WorldWaterCouncil.org
Urban Organic Gardener, UrbanOrganicGardener.com
Yards to Gardens, y2g.org

"Some people talk to animals. Not many listen though. That's the problem."
– A.A. Milne, *Winnie-the-Pooh*

"Let me clarify: I am not a vegan because I 'love animals.' Rather, veganism is about justice. It is not a 'lifestyle choice.' It is not a 'personal preference.' Veganism is not about you or me at all. It is about the fundamental right of nonhumans not to be used, owned, labeled, branded, enslaved, exploited, and generally commoditized to serve our interests and convenience."
– Kerry Wyler

"Baby steps are for babies. Let's treat people like adults. Let's speak to their highest potential. Let's generously provide them the information and guidance they need to go vegan. Let's be honest about our moral obligations to nonhuman animals. And let's be unequivocal in advocating veganism as the moral baseline for respecting the rights of nonhuman animals. We can – and should – present veganism as the first step toward respecting nonhuman animals."
– Timothy E. Putnam

"I understand that advocates are frustrated and, in many cases, probably afraid to even hope that the vegan world we long for might ever come to be, but the answer is not to promote a message of half-way measures simply so the public can stomach it. Those of us who know the truth about animal exploitation and have been fortunate enough to have the realization that veganism is the only answer have a duty to share that truth with others, regardless of how many times we are rebuffed and feel belittled or isolated as a result. No matter how many people close their eyes and ears, every now and then someone will understand, and to that person, your message will be absolutely life-changing."
– Angel Flinn

"We need to begin showing people that specieism is as abhorrent and inconsistent as any other prejudice, and that any rational person already holds the principles which should lead them to accept veganism in the first place."
– Rob Johnson

"Of all the wrongs I have committed in life, I consider being violent to nonhumans by consuming and using them in all forms the most regrettable one."
– Vera Cristofani

"The awful wrongs forced upon the innocent, helpless, faithful animal race form the blackest chapter in the whole world's history."
– Edward Freeman

See: 269Life.com

GLOSSARY OF NAMES

A • Glossary of names

Abele, Ridgely, 50, 294; **Abrams,**
Donald, MD, 87; **Adams,** Carol J., xv;
Affleck, Casey, 143; **Alberola,**
Edward, 399; **Aleksandra,** 343;
Alzheimer, Rudolph, 117; **Anand,**
Sonia, 93; **Anderson,** Mike, 49;
Anderson, Pamela, 189, 298;
Anderson, Ray, 171; **Anderson,**
Tracey, 288; **Andre** 3000, 143; **Angell,**
George T., opening pages; **Angelou,**
Maya, 115; Anhang, Jeff, 231; **Annin,**
Peter, 274; **Aoki,** Devon, 189; **Aren,**
Rai, xii; **Armstrong,** Lance, 50, 294;
Arnstein, Michael, 35, 68, 293;
Arnstein, Victoria, 68, 293; **Asch,**
Sholem, 176; **Assange,** Julian, 171;
Attwood, Charles, Dr., 181; **Aurelius,**
Marcus, 42; **Austin,** Alfred, 376

B • Glossary of names

Barnard, Neal, Dr., 19, 34, 53, 55, 76,
89, 118, 120, 135, 137, 147, 148, 218,
310, 313, 322, 327, x; **Basinger,** Kim,
221; **Baston,** Harry, xvii; **Bekoff,**
Marc, 221, 302, xi; **Bell,** Raja, 144;
Bello, Walden, Dr., 229; **Bentham,**
Jeremy, 40, 213; **Berger,** John, 173;
Berkoff, Nancy D., 33; **Berry,** Rynn,
35, 39, 93, 186, 194, 327, 335; **Best,**
Steve, Dr., 11, 271; **Beston,** Henry,
237; **Bialik,** Mayim, 396; **Biggle,**
Lloyd, 161; **Bigwood,** Rob, 50;
Blades, Reuben, 129; **Blake,** Sienna,
210, 226; **Blaustein,** Andrew, 158;
Bock, Alan, 153; **Boik,** John, 73;
Bonaly, Surya, 294; **Boutenko,** Sergei,
94, 378; **Boutenko,** Victoria, 318, 327;
Bowlby, Rex, 221, 291; **Bradley,**
Timothy, 50, 143; **Brand,** Russel, 28,
143; **Brazier,** Brendan, 50, 186, 294,
383, xiii; **Brophy,** Brigid, 265; **Brower,**
David, 166; **Brown,** Harold, opening
pages, xiii; **Brown,** Jerry, 395;

Brownell, Kelly, 125; **Bruce,** Amanda,
Dr., 125; **Brunton,** Paul, Dr., 174;
Buddha, openging pages, 263, 395;
Burke, Edmund, 171; **Bush,** George
W., 162; **Bush,** Kate, 375; **Bustos,**
Isaac, 398; **Butler,** Virgil, 27; **Byron,**
Lord George, 287

C • Glossary of names

Calton, Jayson, Ph.D., 81, 82;
Cameron, James, 260; **Campbell,**
Chris, 294; **Campbell,** Colin, Dr., 21,
46, 53, 60, 58, 68, 90, 94, 110, 122,
123, 136, 146, 191, 192, 197, 292, 308,
310, 325, 337, 394, x; **Campbell,**
Tomas M., Dr., 202; **Capaldo,**
Theodora, 266; **Carillo-Bucaram,** 37,
298; **Carr,** Kris, 187; **Carrington,**
Hereward, 95; **Carson,** Rachel, 164,
165, 171, 213, 260; **Caruso,** Pino, 115;
Cassini, Oleg, 271; **Castelli,** William,
2; **Cehun,** M., 107; **Ceronetti,** Guico,
131; **Chanakya,** Arya, xii; Chapela,
Ignacio, 368; **Charles,** Prince, 134,
368; **Chavez,** Cesar, 72, 135; **Chin-
Dusting,** J., 107; **Clifton,** Mary, Dr.,
94; **Clinton,** Bill, 143; **Clinton,**
Chelsea, 189; **Coats,** C. David, 288;
Coburn, Heather, 344; **Coffin,** Ed, xv;
Cohen, Jamie, 72; **Cohen,** Robert,
Dr., 202; **Coleman,** Vernon, 66;
Conniff, Richard, 105; **Cook,**
Christopher, 226; **Cousens,** Gabriel,
112; **Cousteau,** Jacques Yves, 273; vii;
Cowles-Hamar, David, 26, 27;
Cristofani, Vera, 404; **Cromwell,**
James, 26; **Cudahy,** Dan, 394; viii;
Cummings, Maura, 384

D • Glossary of names

d'Lamartine, Alphanse Marie-Louis,
226; **D'Amdamo,** Peter, 15; **da Vinci,**
Leonardo, 147, 150, 192, 208, 261,
277, 303; **Damiano,** Anthony, 226,
328; **Danzig,** Mac, 50, 294, 295;
Darwin, Charles, 6, 11, 215, 242, 271;
Davis, Brenda, 19, 35, 39, 93, 175,
186, 327, 335; **Davis,** Daisie Adelle,
124; **Davis,** Karen, 27, 41, 260, 228;

E • Glossary of names

F • Glossary of names

G • Glossary of names

H • Glossary of names

I • Glossary of names

T • Glossary of names

U • Glossary of names

V • Glossary of names

W • Glossary of names

Y • Glossary of names

Z • Glossary of names

INDEX

C • Index

D • Index

E • Index

F • Index

G • Index

I

H • Index

I • Index

J • Index

O • Index

P • Index

Q • Index

R • Index

S • Index

T • Index

U • Index

V • Index

W • Index

Y • Index

Z • Index

ABOUT THE AUTHOR

"If a cluttered desk is a sign of a cluttered mind, of what, then,
is an empty desk a sign?"
– Albert Einstein

TURNING to a vegan diet to regain his health after several near-death
experiences, and learning the hard way that standard medical care
can be anything but health-infusing, John McCabe began writing books
exposing the corruption of the medical industry.

McCabe's first book was *Surgery Electives: What to Know Before the
Doctor Operates*. First published in 1994, and now out of print, it was an
exposé of the financial ties of the medical school, hospital,
pharmaceutical, and health insurance industries whose unethical business
practices result in the deaths of tens of thousands of ill-advised people in
the U.S. every year. The book was endorsed by some congresspersons
and by all of the patients' rights groups in North America.

McCabe also wrote a similar book specific for those considering
cosmetic surgery. *Plastic Surgery Hopscotch* was published in 1995 and
detailed many of the risks involved with the various surgeries, and in
dealing with the medical industry in general.

Realizing that medical care in Western culture is largely the end
result of horrible dietary choices, McCabe then turned to writing about
how a plant-based diet can prevent and reverse a wide variety of diseases
while also protecting the environment.

Becoming an advocate for plant-based nutrition free of disease-
inducing animal protein, synthetic chemicals, and heat-generated toxins,
McCabe coined the term *raw vegan*, and began using it in his writings on
the topic. *Raw vegan* quickly became an internationally recognized term
defining what is becoming an increasingly popular dietary choice of
unprocessed, unheated, fresh, organic, plant-based foods free of the
components that trigger disease, but rich in the nutrients on which
humans thrive in health.

After more than a decade of helping others to write some of the
most popular raw vegan books, in 2007 McCabe's *Sunfood Living: Resource
Guide to Global Health* was published by Random House and North
Atlantic Books.

McCabe is also the author of the reference book *Sunfood Traveler: Global Guide to Raw Food Culture*. In addition to chapters covering various topics of interest relating to the raw vegan lifestyle, the book contains the most comprehensive list of raw vegan restaurants, cafes, retreats, catering companies, and businesses ever published.

Using a wide variety of scientific studies concluding the benefits of a diet rich in raw fruits and vegetables and free of animal protein, McCabe wrote the 2011 book, *Sunfood Diet Infusion: Transforming Health and Preventing Disease through Raw Veganism*. Overhauled and republished in 2012, the book quickly became one of the most well-read raw vegan books on the global market.

To reach other markets outside of the raw vegan community, McCabe's book *Vegan Myth Vegan Truth* was published in 2013. In it, McCabe repurposed some of his previous writings while adding additional chapters and a vast quantity of quotations from a variety of people voicing their concerns for animals and advocating for the health, cultural, and environmental benefits of a vegan diet.

As a way to expose the dire situation of the damaged environment, including from ocean acidification, mountaintop removal, fracking, tar sands mining, clearcutting, animal agriculture, monocropping, plastic trash, and the spread of industrial pollutants, and to help educate people on the need for a more sustainable society, including the need to shut down the animal farming cartels and stop the GMO companies, McCabe wrote a little book titled *Extinction: The Death of Waterlife on Planet Earth*. In it, McCabe continues his advocacy for a plant-based diet free of synthetic chemicals, and argues for humans to stop mass breeding and killing billions of animals, to stop killing billions of wild animals, and to turn to Nature-friendly sources for energy, packaging, building, and food. In the summer of 2012, the book became a best seller, reaching the top of the book-selling charts in the UK.

McCabe is also the author of *Marijuana & Hemp: History, Uses, Laws, and Controversy*, which details the world's most useful plant, and how corrupt politicians have worked with corporate leaders to outlaw industrial hemp farming in the U.S. and many other countries. While the book covers many issues relating to marijuana and hemp, it presents information on the need to utilize hemp as a sustainable resource for materials used in construction, fabric, fuel, cleaning, plastic, and food.

In the plain, unfancy, low-cost *Raw Vegan Easy Healthy Recipes: Simple, Low-fat, Health-Infusiong Cuisine*, which was published in 2013, McCabe provides a variety of recipes that are no-nonsense, low-fat, rich in nutrients, and diverse enough to satisfy a wide variety of preferences. It is a little recipe book that will be a nice addition to the kitchen of any person interested in healthy dietary choices.

As an author of numerous books and a ghost co-author of many books by other writers, McCabe has had his hand in more raw vegan books than any other writer.

Through his books, and those he has helped to write, McCabe has had an international influence, playing a role in creating a raw vegan culture that is flourishing in some regions while beginning to blossom in countries the world over. While California is considered the epicenter of raw vegan cuisine, interest has gone global. From South Africa to Northern Europe, New Zealand and Australia to Asia, and throughout the Americas and many island nations, raw vegan culture continues to evolve into a force that has become an industry and lifestyle influencing everything from what is being grown on farms and in home gardens, to what is being served in restaurants and sold in stores and at farmers' markets.

Combined with his other books, McCabe's philosophical, theoretical, and inspirational book *Igniting Your Life* helps people to implement healthful teachings into their daily life and awaken their senses through pure, unadulterated, plant-base nutrition. *Igniting Your Life* book contains thousands of quotations from influential people throughout history. Adapting its teachings can spur a life previously undiscovered, and perhaps one far beyond what the reader had previously considered possible.

McCabe encourages people to plant and protect trees and forests; to protect animals and wildlife habitat; to protect the environment; to practice yoga; to walk or to ride a bike instead of driving a car; to use cloth shopping bags instead of "paper or plastic"; to use biodegradable cleaning and otherwise environmentally safe household products; to work against the genetic engineering of food (such as by Monsanto); to work for GMO labeling laws; to stop the spread of nuclear energy and creation of nuclear weaponry; to work to legalize industrial hemp farming so it can be made into paper, clothing, food, building materials, energy, and other materials while supporting family farmers; to disconnect from the corporate food chain by planting organic food gardens and supporting local organic farmers; and to live close to Nature by following a plant-based diet consisting of organically grown, non-GMO foods free of synthetic food additives, MSG (monosodium glutamate), corn syrup and other processed sugars and salt.

To contact the author:
John McCabe
C/O: Carmania Books, POB 1272, Santa Monica, CA 90406-1272, USA

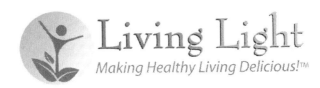

Living Light

Making Healthy Living Delicious!™

LIVING LIGHT CULINARY INSTITUTE is the world's leading gourmet raw vegan chef school. Located on the beautiful Mendocino coast of Northern California, it was founded in 1997 by Cherie Soria, who is known as "The mother of gourmet raw vegan cuisine." Her graduates are a virtual who's who in the world of raw foods.

People from over 50 countries have attended the institute to study raw vegan culinary arts and the science of raw food nutrition to become certified chefs, nutritional consultants, instructors, and recipe book authors. Many of the raw restaurants and raw catering companies around the world are owned by graduates of Living Light.

To subscribe to the Living Light newsletter, access their site, RawFoodChef.com. Scroll down and enter your email address in the "subscribe" box.

Besides Living Light Culinary Institute, Cherie and her husband, Dan Ladermann, own and operate several other eco-friendly, raw vegan businesses. Together, they wrote the book *Raw Food for Dummies*, which was published in 2013.

The Living Light Café, with its full menu, and Living Light Marketplace share the same building as the Institute. The Marketplace also has an online store providing gifts for chefs and products for healthful living. (Access: RawFoodChef.com/store/marketplace.) The historic Living Light Inn is located nearby in a restored mansion.

Cherie and Dan have received numerous awards and accolades for Living Light International, including Best of Raw Chef Training Program, and Innovations in Culinary Arts. Living Light is recognized as one of the leading raw food businesses in the world.

Many of the world's top raw vegan chefs have attended the institute, including Chef Ito of Au Lac restaurant in Orange County, California, and Chad Sarno, who has opened restaurants in England and Europe, and many other recipe book authors, food instructors, and nutritional consultants. Many raw food restaurants employ graduates of Soria's institute. (Sign up for the Living Light eletter by accessing: RawFoodChef.com)

When seeking raw chef training, consider if you are doing it for professional reasons, or simply for fun and to increase your variety of foods and food prep skills.

If you are going for a career in raw food – such as by owning or running a restaurant, café, food truck, or catering service, or if you have desires to become a private chef – you may want to look into any training programs that you are considering, and determine if they are worth the money; how much they charge per hour of training; if the training is hands-on or if you are simply going to watch "teachers" prepare foods while they talk; and if they are legitimate. Find out if they are certified with the state or other government branch that qualifies teaching facilities. For your professional degree to be of value, you need the best training you can get, going through a training program that is legitimate and not breaking any laws regulating educational providers.

Living Light Culinary Institute is a fully licensed teaching facility. Access: RawFoodChef.com

•••

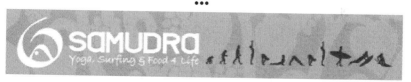

In addition to Living Light as an epicenter of raw food, there is also **Samudra**. Located in Dunsborough, Western Australia, the facility runs yoga and surf retreats. Their raw food café and organic store opened in 2008. Chef training courses began in 2010. They have also been adding culinary gardens and fruit orchards to provide the healthiest food possible to their guests and students. (Access: Samudra.com.au)

Eat
a plant-
based
diet.
Know
that you can
change the world by
changing your diet.
Protect and preserve forests and the habitat of wildlife.
Plant mass quantities of native trees and wildflowers.
Grow organic food. Support organic farmers.
Outlaw the genetic engineering of plants.
Legalize industrial hemp farming.
Compost your kitchen scraps.
Nurture your talents.
Uplift the weary.
Do yoga.
Ride a bike.
Love your way.
Peace your path.
– John McCabe, *SunfoodTraveler.com*

v

WHAT PEOPLE ARE SAYING ABOUT
JOHN McCABE'S BOOK *Igniting Your Life: Pathways to the Zenith of Health and Success*

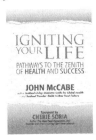

"*Igniting Your Life* will kindle your innermost desires."
– **Cherie Soria**, author *The Raw Food Diet Revolution*. Founder and director Living Light International. RawFoodChef.com

"**An** uplifting and empowering collection of worldly work."
– **Sheridan Hammond**, Australia. Samudra.com.au.

"**We** defy you to not be inspired by this book!"
– **Matt Amsden**, author *RawVolution*, and **Janabai Amsden**, ELR restaurant, Santa Monica, CA. EuphoriaLovesRawvolution.com

"**An** impressive collection of eclectic quotations and thoughtful commentary. Inspiring and motivating."
– **Victoria Moran**, author *Living a Charmed Life: Your Guide to Finding Magic in Every Moment of Every Day*. VictoriaMoran.com

"**In** this book McCabe encourages readers to recognise their true potential and work towards a better way of living."
– **Sienna Blake**, Australia's *Vegan Voice* magazine: Veganic.net

"**A** great compilation that shouts inspiration from every page. The more I read it, the more I can relate to it. Gold stuff!"
– **Harley Durianrider Johnstone**, Australian Division One biking athlete and co-founder of 30BananasADay.com

"**After** only a few hours of reading, I was already writing life plans and lists of things I needed to change in my life."
– **Rob Hull**, publisher, London's *Funky Raw* magazine: FunkyRaw.com

"**Open** any page, anytime, and become inspired to live the life of your dreams."
– **Rhio**, author *Hooked on Raw*, New York; RawFoodInfo.com

"**A** fantastic book."
– **Penni Shelton**, RawFoodRehab.ning.com

PLEASE, PLANT SOME TREES!

TREES and forests are major keys to life on this planet. Without them, we would all die.

The average human living in North America uses paper and wood products that amount to hundreds of trees during their lifetime. To replenish the trees we use is a noble venture.

Please be involved with planting and protecting trees and forests. Support organizations that work to do the same.

Learn the types of trees that are native to where you live. There are over 970 species of trees that are classified as endangered. It is likely that some of them are native to your area. Find out which ones they may be, and then plant some of them.

"Trees shade our ground, create topsoil, clean the air and help the land attract, hold, and filter water. The trees and their roots purify the water as the rains fall. Clean streams keep millions of aquatic and other species alive."
– Tim Hermach, President Native Forest Voice; *Forest Voice*, Spring 2006; ForestCouncil.org

"Destruction of forests is a leading cause of global environmental breakdown, including global warming."
– AncientTrees.org, 2006

"We have nothing to fear and a great deal to learn from trees, that vigorous and pacific tribe which without stint produces strengthening essences for us, soothing balms, and in whose gracious company we spend so many cool, silent and intimate hours."
– Marcel Proust

American Chestnut Foundation, ACF.org
Alliance for Community Trees, ACTrees.org
American Forests, AmericanForests.org
Ancient Trees, AncientTrees.org
Budongo Forest, Budongo.org. African site.
Campaign for Old Growth, AncientTrees.org
California Rare Fruit Growers, CRFG.org
California Tropical Fruit Trees, TropicalFruitTrees.com.
Common Vision, CommonVision.org.

Earth First!, EarthFirst.org
Forest Advocate, ForestAdvocate.org
Forest Council, ForestCouncil.org
Forest Ethics, ForestEthics.org
Forests Forever, ForestsForever.org
Forest Protection Portal, Forests.org
Friends of the Trees, FriendsOfTheTrees.net
Friends of the Urban Forest, FUF.net
Global ReLeaf, GlobalReLeaf.org
Gifford Pinchot Task Force, GPTaskForce.org
Living Tree Paper Company, LivingTreePaper.com
Australia's Men of the Trees, MenOfTheTrees.com.au
North American Native Plant Society, NANPS.org
Native Forests, NativeForest.org
Natural Resources Defense Council, NRDC.org
Northern Nut Growers Association, NutGrowing.org
Protect Our Woodland, ProtectOurWoodland.co.uk
Rainforest Action Network, RAN.org
World Rainforest Information Portal, RainForestWeb.org
Sanctuary Forest, SanctuaryForest.org
Save the Memorial Oaks Grove, SaveOaks.com
Save the Redwoods League, SaveTheRedwoods.org
Sequoia Forest Keeper, SequoiaForestKeeper.org
TasForests, TasForests.Green.net.au. Tasmania, Australia.
Tree Musketeers, TreeMusketeers.org
Tree People, TreePeople.org
Trees for Life, TreesForLife.org
Trees for the Future, TreesFTF.org
Trees Foundation, TreesFoundation.org
We Save Trees, WeSaveTrees.org
North Coast Earth First, NorthCoastEarthFirst.org

"History will not only judge us by our mistakes, but by what we do to fix them."
– Jacques Yves Cousteau

THE GLOBAL MEAT INDUSTRY and THE GRAIN INDUSTRY THAT SUPPORTS IT

- #1 cause of rainforest and wildlife habitat destruction, sending many species into extinction.
- #1 cause of predator reduction on every continent.
- #1 cause of the dead zones in the oceans.
- #1 cause of global warming gasses.
- #1 cause of displacement and destruction of indigenous cultures in South and Central America.
- #1 cause of slave labor in South America.
- #1 cause of fatal land fights in South America.
- #1 use of GMO crops, toxic farming chemicals, land, water, government subsidies, and urban road building.

Meanwhile:
- #1 user of South American meat and grain: The fast foods, canned meat, and packaged foods industries outside of South America.

"The intentional, unnecessary deaths we inflict on sentient individuals of other species worldwide – mainly for food choices – is greater in five days than the deaths we've inflicted on humans in all wars and all genocides in recorded human history. Even if every nonvegan cut their current animal product consumption by 90 percent, it would take us only about 41 days to kill as many nonhumans as we've killed humans in recorded history.

Our treatment of individual sentient nonhumans as renewable resources – as property, things, commodities – is a moral blind spot. The reason for this moral blind spot – the reason we contribute, individually and collectively, to this extreme and senseless violence – is that we have been heavily indoctrinated into speciesism throughout our lives. Additionally, by nature, we often 'rationalize' this indoctrination and ignore unpleasant facts for various reasons."
– Dan Cudahy

- Human dietary requirement for animal protein: zero.
- Humans flourish on a largely or all raw vegan diet rich in fresh fruits and vegetables.

MeatTheFacts.org/wp/category/deforestation; Meat.org; RAN.org; SaveTheRainforest.org; VRG.org; FarmUSA.org; EarthIsland.org/Journal; PETA.org; SunfoodTraveler.com; DrMcDougall.com; ForksOverKnives.com; PCRM.org

WHAT ARE THE LEADING CAUSES OF ERECTILE DYSFUNCTION AND PROSTATE CANCER

IN men, one of the first signs of cardiovascular disease is erectile dysfunction (ED). **On a vegan diet, many men notice that *it* functions better.** It is no coincidence that the countries with the highest consumption of meat, dairy, and eggs also are where more ED prescriptions are filled.

"Men who consume animal protein are more likely to experience prostate cancer and erectile dysfunction. As T. Colin Campbell states in *The China Study*, 'The totality and breadth of the evidence, operating through highly coordinated networks, supports the conclusions that consuming dairy and meat are serious risk factors for prostate cancer.'"
– SUNFOOD DIET INFUSION: Transforming Health and Preventing Disease Through Raw Veganism; **SunfoodTraveler.com**

"This hardening of the arteries that comes from a lifetime of eating beef and other high-fat foods, it doesn't just cause heart attacks, it can also make you impotent."
– Dr. Neal Barnard; NealBarnard.org

The saturated fat and cholesterol in meat, dairy, and eggs slow the blood flow and clog the veins, arteries, and capillaries. The Neu5Gc molecule in dairy (milk, cheese, butter, cream, yogurt, kifir, ice cream, whey, and casein) and in nonhuman mammal meat makes prostate cancer, and other cancer, more aggressive. Real men don't eat animals, eggs, or baby food (milk). To prevent erectile dysfunction and prostate cancer, follow a low-fat vegan diet rich in raw fruits and vegetables.

IT'S ABOUT RESPECTING NATURE AND EARTH

"Following a vegan diet rich in raw fruits and vegetables is the single most effective way you can reduce your carbon footprint. Even better if you grow your own food.

If you are a meat eater and think that eating meat, dairy, and eggs is your business, and none of mine, think again. Similarly to how _Mad Cowboy_ author Howard Lyman and others have stated it, I repeat the defense to the stance of vegans: If your diet style is relying on the mass breeding of animals, then it is my business, and it is the business of everyone on the planet. It impacts us environmentally, socially, physically, and economically. Your diet style pollutes the air I breathe, the water I drink, and the food I eat. It has led to, and is leading to the extinction of species. The entire animal farming industry, including the resources needed to support it, is the main cause of global warming and ocean acidification, which threatens all life on the planet.

A vegetarian diet uses substantially fewer resources than a wasteful and unhealthful meat-based diet.

A plant-based diet is not only healthier for humans, but also for farm workers, the land, plant life, the water, the air, the animals, and Earth."

– John McCabe, author, _Sunfood Traveler: Global Guide to Raw Food Culture_; SunfoodTraveler.com

"Make ethical choices in what we buy, do, and watch. In a consumer-driven society our individual choices, used collectively for the good of animals and nature, can change the world faster than laws."

– Marc Bekoff

"Earth and sky, woods and fields, lakes and rivers, the mountains and the sea, are excellent schoolmasters, and teach some of us more than we can ever learn from books."

– John Lubbock

"By spreading vegetarian education rather than vegan education, we collaborate in the subjugation (however unintentionally) of nonhuman animals. The baseline is veganism. The fact that it is not immediately appealing for 100 percent of all people everywhere is not the point. Veganism is the goal. It can be incrementally achieved, but it remains a goal. To ask for anything less, anything with wider appeal, anything that appears to be a more popular message, is to sell out the rights of animals. Want to make veganism more popular? Start by talking about it."

– Barbara DeGrande

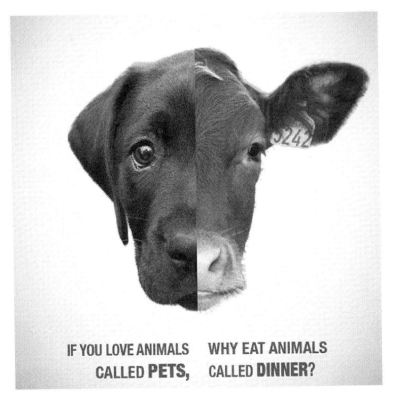

IF YOU LOVE ANIMALS   WHY EAT ANIMALS
CALLED **PETS,**   CALLED **DINNER?**

"Any glimpse into the life of an animal quickens our own and makes it so much the larger and better in every way."
– John Muir

"Know that the same spark of life that is within you is within all of our animal friends. The desire to live is the same within all of us."
– Rai Aren

"The world is in greater peril from those who tolerate or encourage evil than from those who actually commit it."
– Albert Einstein

"The world will not be destroyed by those who do evil, but by those who watch them without doing anything."
– Arya Chanakya

"Those who have the privilege to know have the duty to act."
– Albert Einstein

"Humans – who enslave, castrate, experiment on, and filet other animals – have had an understandable penchant for pretending animals do not feel pain. A sharp distinction between humans and 'animals' is essentioal if we are to bend them to our will, make them work for us, wear them, eat them – without any disquieting tinges of guilt or regret. It is unseemly of us, who often behave so unfeelingly toward other animals, to content that only humans can suffer. The behavior of other animals renders such pretentions specious. They are just too much like us."
– Carl Sagan

"Killing is a denial of love. To kill or to eat what another has killed is to rejoice in cruelty. And cruelty hardens our hearts and blinds our vision, and we are unable to see that they whom we kill are our fellow brothers and sisters in the one family of creation."
– G.L. Rudd

So no, in my experience, there is no such thing as humane animal products, humane farming practices, humane transport, or humane slaughter."
– Harold Brown, former cattle farmer

"Deliberate cruelty to our defenseless and beautiful little cousins is surely one of the meanest and most detestable vices of which a human can be guilty."
– William Ralph Inge

"As long as people will shed the blood of innocent creatures there can be no peace, no liberty, no harmony between people. Slaughter and justice cannot dwell together."
– Isaac Bashevis Singer

"As long as humans continue to eat animal pieces, they will never know what peace is."
– Rich Lysloff

"What is man without the beasts? If all the beasts were gone, man would die from a great loneliness of the spirit. For whatever happens to the beasts, soon happens to man. All things are connected."
– Chief Seattle

"I first became vegan for health reasons, which for me translates to performance gains. Soon after I stopped eating meat I realized that there were many more reasons other than just health to be vegan. Aside from the health, environmental, and animal welfare

concerns, I also began to dislike the way in which society views meat consumption. The slick marketing and complete removal of any thought that the ground-up plastic-wrapped piece of meat bought in a supermarket was recently an animal walking around in a field, not too differently from your dog. Society makes contributing to killing an animal completely acceptable and anonymous, others do all the messy work – breeding, raising, killing – all you as the consumer have to do is walk into a friendly, clean supermarket in the shopping mall and buy a piece of meat wrapped with a cartoon picture of a smiling cow on it."
– Brendan Brazier

"To the beaten pig, I hear your screams; to the scalded chicken, I feel your pain, and to the stunned cow, I see your suffering. It is real to so many of us who value your life on earth as much as our own. We are no more important than you. We are so sorry that humans possess so little mercy for those whom they have the power to abuse. We will do everything we can to end your misery until the day we die. You are not alone'"
– Andrew Kirschner

"I was fighting against animal abuse and one day I simply realized that the mass slaughter of animals for food is one of the worst forms of abuse in our world today. We get upset when we hear about the guy down the street with his dog chained up outside on a short leash in all kinds of weather, but we overlook the abuse in the farming industry."
– Rikki Rockett

"It's troubling when people get upset with vegans for pointing out the suffering, rather than getting upset with themselves for causing it."
– Jo Tyler

"I really don't get the nonvegans that say things like, 'Vegans need to get over themselves,' or, 'Vegans think they are so much better than others.' It is because we got over ourselves and don't believe we are better than anyone else that we are vegan. Thinking you are better than someone is believing that someone should die for you to be able to have a sandwich or a coat. Being stuck on yourself is believing that a baby should die so that you can have the breast milk that was intended for them. Thinking you are better than someone is believing your wants are more important than another being's desire to live. Being stuck on yourself is believing that billions of day-old male chicks being ground up alive is fine as long

as you get your scrambled eggs. Thinking you are better than someone is being totally fine with billions and billions of sentient beings being brutally raped, tortured, kidnapped, and slaughtered every year so that you can fit in with society."
– Erica Tattooedvegan Floyd

"I hate when people dismiss veganism as a 'personal choice.' It's not, it's a moral obligation. Would those same people also assert that murdering someone, or beating a dog, or raping a child is a 'personal choice?' When your actions directly impact the lives of others, it's no longer a simple 'personal choice.'"
– Ed Coffin

"Until a vegan enters the room, people don't see themselves as meat eaters. They are merely eaters, and it is we vegans who have made them aware of what they are doing. Often this is discomforting."
– Carol J. Adams

"At the moment our human world is based on the suffering and destruction of millions of nonhumans. To perceive this and to do something to change it in personal and public ways is to undergo a change of perception akin to a religious conversion. Nothing can ever be seen in quite the same way again because once you have admitted the terror and pain of other species you will, unless you resist conversion, be always aware of the endless permutations of suffering that support our society."
– Sir Arthur Conan Doyle

"A universe is, indeed, to be pitied whose dominating inhabitants are so unconscious and so ethically embryonic that they make life a commodity, mercy a disease, and systematic massacre a pastime and a profession."
– J. Howard Moore

"First it was necessary to civilise man in relation to man. Now it is necessary to civilise man in relation to nature and the animals."
– Victor Hugo

I SAW TRAIN CARS PASSING

I saw train cars passing. Watching them, I realized they were filled with cows being taken to their death as part of the animal holocaust we call "the meat industry."

They were mass bred animals born to mothers who were placed in "rape racks" to be mechanically inseminated with bull sperm.

They were female babies born only to be incarcerated their entire lives by the animal agriculture cartel. During their lives they were raped and turned into milk-making machines.

The vast majority of the male babies born on dairy farms typically are put to death early in life. Bulls are of no use to the dairy industry, because they can't produce milk. Because of that, the male babies are killed. Their flesh is packaged and sold as the meat called "veal." Their stomach lining is sold as a product called "rennet" used in cheese processing. Veal is murdered babies.

Cheese, ice cream, yogurt, butter, kifir, casein, and whey are all derived from the milk of a cow. Milk produced in the breasts of a mother cow and meant to feed a baby cow or baby bull, not a human.

The dairy industry exists because baby animals are murdered and people have been convinced that consuming dairy is good for health.

Humans that consume dairy products are more likely to experience diabetes, arthritis, heart disease, strokes, heart attacks, and cancer.

Cows that are raised for milk and flesh live sad, unnatural lives ended when a ramrod mechanically shoots into their skulls, and/or their necks are slit.

Some of these gentle animals are not dead as their legs are sawed off. They die that way. Hanging. Bleeding. Suffering. Agonizing. Fear rushing through their tissues. Blood splattering.

Their skin is peeled off. Their heads are chopped off. The carcass is cut to pieces.

Bones are removed with much of them used to make things like gelatin, hard candy, soft candy, drug capsules, and "bone meal."

The blood drained from the animals is turned into other products, including fertilizer.

The muscle tissues are packaged and sold as meat for humans to eat.

Their organs may also be used in disease-inducing products like fast food, hot dogs, cold cuts, jerky, and canned foods.

Humans who eat animals often say they love animals. Would they take a saw and slice off the legs of an animal, its body still warm from the blood recently flowing through its veins and arteries and organs, including skin that felt pleasure and pain, tounges that tasted, lunges that breathed, eyes that saw, and brains that thought? Most would not. So they, through their dietary choices, employ the hit men called slaughterhouse workers who work in the most dangerous profession, often suffering deep cuts, some losing fingers and hands.

Many of those slaughterhouse workers are living in the US as undocumented workers, unable to collect workers' comp when injured, afraid to take legal action against an employer for injuries suffered in unsafe work conditions. Living third-world lives in a first-world country.

The meat industry is chains, rape, cages, incarceration, horror, pain, agony, suffering, disease, baby killing, modern slavery, injured workers, monocropping, GMOs, toxic farming chemicals, drugs, pollution, global warming, drained aquifers, deforestation, desertification, ocean acidification, dead zones, spilled blood, burned fossil fuels, and extinction.

The meat industry fuels the heart attack, stroke, colon cancer, Alzheimer's, MS, macular degeneration, breast cancer, arthritis, varicose vein, and erectile dysfunction industries, and the accompanying pharmaceutical and hospital industries.

In the U.S., in recent years about four thousand cows are murdered every hour.

The human nutritional need for animal protein is zero. Humans flourish in health on a low-fat diet rich in raw fruits and vegetables.

Humans would be better off never eating flesh and never breeding another animal for slaughter.

"We need another and a wiser and perhaps a more mystical concept of animals. Remote and universal nature and living by complicated artifice, man in civilization surveys the creature through the glass of his knowledge and sees thereby a feather magnified and the whole image in distortion. We patronize them for their incompleteness, for their tragic fate for having taken form so far below ourselves. And therein do we err. For the animal shall not be measured by man. In a world older and more complete than ours, they move finished and complete, gifted with the extension of the senses we have lost or never attained, living by voices we shall never hear. They are not brethren, they are not underlings: they are other nations, caught with ourselves in the net of life and time, fellow prisoners of the splendour and travail of the earth."
– Henry Baston

HAVE YOU FOUND THIS BOOK USEFUL?
Tell others about it!
Mention it on your Facebook page.
Mention it on Facebook group pages.
Tweet about it on Twitter.
Write a reader review on Amazon.com.
Text your people with a photo of the cover
and encourage them to read it.
Give a copy to a friend, relative, co-worker, neighbor, or lover.
Send a copy to your local newspapers, newsweeklies, animal rights
groups, pet rescue organization, and farm sancutary.
Ask your local natural foods store to sell it.

Keep speaking up for the non-human animals.
Help stop this animal holocaust we call
"the meat, dairy, and egg industries"
that is being run by the animal agriculture cartels.

Spay or neuter your pet.
Don't support pet breeders.

Follow a vegan diet.

Grow a garden.
FoodNotLawns.com
Y2G.org
KGI.org

21973961R00261

Made in the USA
Charleston, SC
07 September 2013